LIGHT YEARS AHEAD

The Illustrated Guide to Full Spectrum and Colored Light in Mindbody Healing

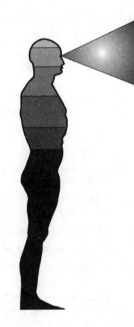

LIGHT YEARS AHEAD PRODUCTIONS™

CELESTIAL ARTS
Berkeley, California

Co-Producers/Directors: *Light Years Ahead,* the Conference, upon which this book is based:
Lee Hartley, Ed.D., and Brian J. Breiling, Psy.D.

Publisher/Co-Editor: *Light Years Ahead,* the Book: Brian J. Breiling, Psy.D.

Project Director/Co-Editor, contributing poet and artist: Bethany ArgIsle, ArgIsle Enterprises.

Cover Design, Art, Illustrations and Logos: Barbara Thomason, M.F.A., Barbara C. Thomason & Associates.

Production support on Cover: Ralph Kehiler, Ralph Kehiler Illustrations.

Book Design/Layout: Albert Howell, Meta4 Productions.

Editorial Staff: Transcription: Evelyn Brown
                   Copy Editors: Lee Hartley, Ed.D.
                                    Nola Lewis, M.S.
                                    Joan Lamb
                                    Melinda McKown
                                    Victoria Randall
                   Medical Editor: Elson Haas, M.D.

First Printing, January 1996.

Library of Congress Cataloging in Publication Data

Brian, Breiling J., 1954 —
Light Years Ahead: The Illustrated Guide to Full Spectrum and Colored Light in Mindbody Healing.
ISBN 089087-762-9
1. Health & Healing.   2. Light Therapy.

---

1   2   3   4   5   6   7   8   9   10   /   99   98   97   96

Quote Releases and Permissions:

Too Much Light, Spectrums, Home of Light, Language of Light, and Dream from *Near Life* (a collection of self-published poems), ©1996 by Bethany ArgIsle. Reprinted with permission of the author.

Excerpt from *Creating Your Own Personal Vision: A Mind-body Guide for Better Eyesight* ©1994 by Samuel Berne, O.D. Reprinted by permission of Colorstone Press, Santa Fe, N.M.

Excerpt from *Drawing From The Light Within* ©1994 by Judith Cornell. Reprinted by permission of the author.

Excerpt from *Once a Month* ©1990 by Dr. Katherina Dalton. Reprinted by permission of Hunter House, Alameda, CA.

Excerpts from the *Preventive Medical Center of Marin Newsletter,* Volume 2, (1) Winter 1993. Reprinted by permission of Elson M. Haas, M.D., San Rafael, CA.

Excerpts from *The Practical Compendium of Colorpuncture* by Peter Mandel, ©1986 by Energetik Verlag, Bruchsal, Germany; and *Esogetics: The Sense and Nonsense of Sickness and Pain* by Peter Mandel, ©1993 by Energetik Verlag. Reprinted by Permission of the author.

Excerpt from *Introducing Spirituality Into Counseling and Psychotherapy* ©1982 and *Call of the Dervish* ©1993 by Pir Vilayat Inayat Khan. Reprinted by permission of Omega Publishing, New Lebanon, N.Y.

Excerpt from *A Return to Love: Reflections on the Principles of a Course in Miracles,* ©1993 by Marianne Williamson. Reprinted by permission of the author.

Excerpts from the mystical poetry of Paramahansa Yogananda from the following sources: *Inner Reflections Engagement Calendar,* ©1994; *Where There is Light* ©1988; and *Whispers From Eternity* ©1988. Self-Realization Fellowship, Los Angeles, CA. Reprinted by permission of the Publisher.

Excerpts from *Catching The Light; The Entwined History of Light and Mind* ©1993 by Dr. Arthur Zajonc. Reprinted by permission of Bantam Books, a division of Bantam Doubleday Dell Publishing Group, Inc., New York, N.Y.

Excerpt from *Seat of the Soul* ©1989 by Gary Zukov. Reprinted by permission of Simon and Schuster, New York, N.Y.

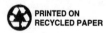
PRINTED ON
RECYCLED PAPER

PRINTED WITH
SOY INK

Photo Credits

ArgIsle, Bethany: Dream Agents, p. 92; Eyes, p. 163; Fear, Can You Hold It Near?, p. 168; collage art photographs courtesy ArgIsle Enterprises, Larkspur, CA.

Baker, Ernest: Lumatron™ Ocular Light Stimulator, p. 150, photograph courtesy Lumatron™ Corporation, Atlanta, GA.

Bolles, Mary, B.A.: Photographs: Bio, p. 298; Audiograms, Pre-Post, p. 311; Visual Field Tests, p. 305, 307, courtesy Sensory Learning, Boulder, CO.

Breiling, Brian, Psy.D.: Photographs: Campimeter, p. 31; Roscalene Filters, p. 204; Dr. Ward Lamb's Experimental Light Therapy Apparatus, p. 204; Dr. Lamb Assessing and Utilizing Light Through the Eyes, p. 206, courtesy Light Years Ahead Productions, Tiburon, CA.

Cedar, Ken: Photographs: Dr. John Ott, p. 52; Ott-Lite Box, p. 102, courtesy Ott-Lite Systems, Santa Barbara, CA

Gabriel, Cousens, M.D.: Photographs: Bio, p. xxvi; logo Tree of Life Rejuvenation Center, p. xxix, courtesy Tree of Life Rejuvenation Center, Patagonia, AZ.

Croke, Manohar, B.A.: Photographs: Kirlian Photograph of Fingertips and Feet Before and After a Single Colorpuncture Session, p. 246, courtesy Colorpuncture and Kirlian Photography, Boulder, CO.

Dinshah, Darius: Photograph: Dinshah Ghadiali from *Let There Be Light*, courtesy Dinshah Health Federation, Malaga, N.J.

Downing, John, O.D.: Photographs: Bio, p. 132; Cameron-Spitler Syntonizer, p. 52; Brain Maps, p. 143, 144, 147, 148, courtesy John Downing, Santa Rosa, CA.

Dubin, Robert, D.C.: Photographs: Bio, p. 118; Space Period, p. 124; Still Life, p. 124, courtesy Robert Dubin, Petaluma, CA.

Green, Jerry, J.D.: Photograph: Bio, p. xxxvi, courtesy Medical Decisionmaking Institute, Mill Valley, CA.

Haas, Elson, M.D.: Photograph: Bio, p. xxx, courtesy Elson Haas, M.D., San Rafael, CA.

Hancock, Betsy, O.D.: Photographs: Edwin Babbitt, M.D., p. 43; Kate Baldwin, M.D., p. 46; Harry Riley Spitler, M.D., O.D., p. 49, courtesy Library of College of Syntonic Optometry, Bloomburg, PA.

Hartley, Lee, Ed.D.: Photographs: Bio, p. 100; Bio, Ward Lamb, p. 200, courtesy Light Years Ahead Productions, Tiburon, CA.

Health Harvest Unlimited, Inc.: Illustration: Chakra design, p. xxxiv, courtesy of the company.

Liberman, Jacob, O.D., Ph.D.: Photographs: Bio, p. 26; Color Receptivity Trainer, p. 39, courtesy Universal Light Technology, Carbondale, CO.

Mandel, Peter, Professor: Photographs: Bid, p. 233; Circles of Transmitter Relay, p. 254; Five Function Circles, p. 251, courtesy Mantel Institute, Bruchsal, Germany.

Olszewski, David, E.E., I.E.: Photographs: Bio, p. 258; Full Spectrum Fluorescent Products by Ott-Lite, p. 270; Ott-Lite Light Box, p. 274; Full Spectrum Desk Task Lamp, p. 275; Ott-Lite shielded tubes, p. 276; Light-Shaker and Tri-Light LED devices, p. 292, courtesy Light Energy Company, Seattle, WA.

Owens, Neil, President: Photograph: Sun-Box, and Sun-Ray, p. 101; Bio-Brite Light Visor, p. 276, courtesy Sun-Box Company, Gaithersburg, MD.

Patton, Terry: Photograph: Sun Up Dawn Simulator, p. 276, courtesy Tools for Exploration, San Rafael, CA.

Pesner, Samuel, O.D.: Photograph: Bio, p. 40, courtesy Samuel Pesner, Los Altos, CA.

Rosenthal, Norman E., M.D.: Photograph: Bio, p. 111, courtesy Norman Rosenthal, Rockville, MD.

Shealy, Norman, M.D.: Photographs: Bio, p. 164; Brain Maps, p. 181; Shealy Relax-Mate, p. 176; Liss Cranial Electric Stimulator, p. 177, courtesy Shealy Institute, Springfield, MO.

Thomason, Barbara C., M.F.A.: Photographs: Light, Sound and Motion Table, p. 294, 308; Audio Tone Enhancer, Trainer, p. 318, courtesy Barbara C. Thomason & Associates, Mill Valley, CA.

Vazquez, Steven, Ph.D.: Photograph: Bio, p. 56, courtesy Health Institute of North Texas, Hurst, TX.

Vente, Robert, Photographer: Photographs: Bio, Akhila Dass and Manohar Croke, p. 232; Brian Breiling, p. 2; Dr. Dass Demonstrating Use of Perlux Colorpuncture Instrument, p. 245; Photron Light Stimulator, p. 151; Kamla Perlux Pen, p. 256, courtesy Robert Vente, San Anselmo, CA.

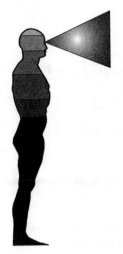

LIGHT YEARS AHEAD

THE ILLUSTRATED GUIDE TO FULL SPECTRUM AND COLORED LIGHT IN MINDBODY HEALING

TABLE OF CONTENTS

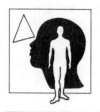

SECTION I
Light In Optometry and Mindbody Healing: Historical and Future Perspectives

Dr. Liberman presents the basis for light's neurophysiological effects on the human body. He describes current and historical literature that confirms the therapeutic value of light and color in the treatment of a variety of physical and emotional disorders.

"What I noticed early on is that light, administered by way of the eyes, seemed to create miraculous enhancement . . . it would open up the field of vision; children would have personality changes, physical changes, academic changes, and performance changes."

"I utilized light as a way of bringing to the surface old, unresolved, unexpressed emotional traumas, which I feel are the roots of the weed we call disease."

Dr. Pesner's presentation addresses the therapeutic application of light from ancient to modern times. His talk highlights the profound physiological and biochemical effects of the major colors of light, as well as providing an overview of theorists' contributions to this growing field. A stirring example of one school-age patient's dramatic response to a magenta and yellow-green light tonation illustrates the power of Syntonic Optometric Principles.

"I guarantee working with light is a life-altering experience; you'll never approach your practice in the same way again!"

SECTION II
Light In Psychotherapy

Dr. Vazquez presents findings from the use of Lumatron™ color and rhythmic light stimulation combined with unique psychological interventions. A powerful live demonstration and other case studies show this synthesis to potentiate emotional and physical transformation far beyond the results of light stimulation alone. Utilizing this approach he has pioneered new dimensions of dream work and rapid trauma relief to elicit deep physiological changes and experiences of spiritual wholeness.

"Brief Strobic Phototherapy is used because it has been found to work faster, and easier, and has a broad range of applications as compared to conventional treatments. In addition, there are some conditions that respond to phototherapy when nothing else seems to work. The result of this accelerated treatment is that it costs less than conventional treatments and yields better outcomes."

Dr. Hartley presents her experience with full spectrum white light and reviews the research for "winter depression," SAD and PMS. Noting that these disorders often go together, she discusses her unique methods of treatment. Case histories demonstrate the power of combining photostimulation from full spectrum and colored light sources and Lumatron™-assisted hypnosis and psychotherapy. She includes a discussion of SAD rating scales.

"I find using the Lumatron™ as a tool speeds up the psychotherapeutic process even more than hypnoanalysis; and by having my clients use a light panel at home, it assists them to put their bodies back into balance. These two light therapy approaches are a wonderful combination!"

Dr. Dubin describes the neurological, physical, and emotional responses of Vietnam veterans' PTSD when they are treated with blue light on the Lumatron Ocular Light Stimulator™. Patients' before and after artwork reveal their transformation. He also discusses his personal involvement with Dr. John Downing's technique of Ocular Light Therapy within a chiropractic setting.

"Light is actually the fundamental physical basis of the universe. All matter is based on light! . . ."

"Sickness or dysfunction is a shortage, lack of, or improper utilization of light . . ."

"Using Dr. John Downing's methods, about 90% of my patients with traumatic stress respond positively to blue light stimulation. It really helps these people integrate their experience and get back to normal."

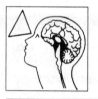

SECTION III
Neurophysiological Effects of
Lumatron™ Light Therapy

Dr. Downing describes the neural pathways through which light enters and affects the visual cortex, limbic system, and brain stem. He presents a wide variety of fascinating case histories in which he outlines the rationale behind colors selected for treatment from either the red or the blue portions of the spectrum. Computerized EEG brain maps, visual fields, and self-report data illustrate the potent effects of Ocular Light Therapy on human functioning.

"Light literally affects every single part of the brain and every cell of the body."

While photostimulation may not replace sex anytime soon, the body's electroencephalographic, neurotransmitter and neurohormonal responses to Lumatron™ red, green, and violet light are similar to that of sexual intercourse. In Part I Dr. Shealy introduces us to his model of disease etiology and treatment methods used at the Shealy Institute. There, light treatment with the Lumatron™ and Shealy Relax Mate™ are an important part of a comprehensive mindbody healing program.

"There is only one major illness, and it's called depression . . . second to depression, the most common problem that we have is magnesium deficiency . . . light stimulation has temporarily changed patients' neurochemistry. We've worked with a series of techniques over the last four years, and we've gotten more than 72% of our 250 chronically depressed patients to stay out of depression. In the last two years we have used Lumatron™ light stimulation as an adjunct."

Dr. Shealy continues his discussion of preliminary clinical findings of the positive effect of Lumatron™ red, green, and violet photostimulation on the levels of 15-20 neurotransmitters and neurohormones, as well as its positive effect on brainwave functioning. The synergistic effects of light therapy coupled with changing mental attitudes, nutrition, and other interventions are highlighted.

"Light is a valuable adjunct and a cost-effective treatment."

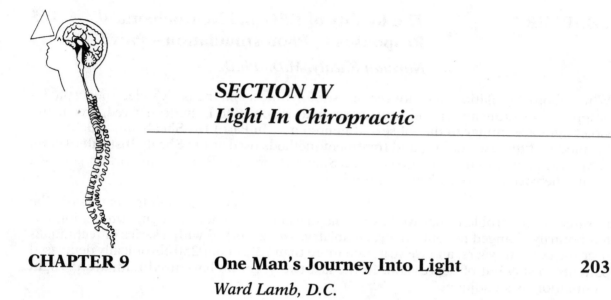

SECTION IV
Light In Chiropractic

Dr. Lamb describes his method of simultaneously applying light directly to the body and through the eyes to effect core energy balance of the chakra system. Two of Dr. Lamb's patients share their journey from chronic unremitting illness to transformation and regaining of health and vitality.

"Color therapy is a very ancient science, so ancient that, we are now rediscovering it as new."

"Today there is all this interest in the brain, and here we have light with direct access via the retina. As a chiropractor, I am interested in affecting the core energy of the body . . . the chakra system. My gut told me when I looked at the light, that here was an ideal modality to approach both the brain and the chakra system simultaneously."

In a continuation of his earlier talk, Dr. Dubin describes his experience blending chiropractic with these two powerful adjunctive therapies.

"The Lumatron Ocular Light Stimulator™ is probably the most powerful tool you'll ever see for opening up the connection between the eyes and the brain! Unless this channel is opened and functioning properly, you will not see a complete healing or a remission."

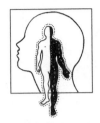

SECTION V
Light In Acupuncture

Dr. Dass and Ms. Croke introduce key concepts of the theory and practice of Colorpuncture and Esogetic medicine based on the life work of German naturopathic physician, Peter Mandel. Similar to traditional Chinese medicine, Colorpuncture balances the flow of life energy in the meridians through the use of colored light placed at various points on the skin. Case histories and Kirlian photographs demonstrate the potency of colored light used in this manner for psychosomatic healing and personal transformation.

"Colorpuncture treatments usually begin with focusing on the body to balance the flow of energy. These foundational treatments help prepare the energy system for higher level treatments that may address the clearing out of old energetic blockages from prenatal, childhood, or past-life traumas and help the patient access information regarding their life's purpose."

Electrical and industrial engineer, David Olszewski and psychotherapist, Dr. Brian Breiling, give an overview of essential concepts regarding the professional and self-care applications of sunlight, full spectrum fluorescents, and monochromatic red light photostimulation with lasers and LEDs. Their discussion offers pragmatic suggestions and warnings for the use of light in acupuncture, pain management, tissue regeneration, PMS, immune disorders, winter depression, and wellness promotion.

"Artificial lighting not only enables us to read and work without the benefit of sunlight, it profoundly affects our bodies' immune and nervous systems."

"The use of light in acupuncture has many potential applications, such as those conditions treated by needles, with similar benefits and fewer side effects."

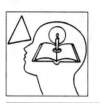

Mary Bolles describes the seven brain centers that process information from the environment and the far-reaching and debilitating effects of learning disabilities. She outlines her regimen which simultaneously uses colored light, sound, and vestibular stimulation. Case examples suggest her protocol's potential to calm, integrate, and organize mental processing. Visual fields, audiograms, and self-report suggest positive effects on children's educational, social, and emotional development.

"Fear may actually be the learning problem . . . and what I see most consistently in clients of all ages is that after the light, sound, and motion treatments, they have less fear. There's an accompanying increase of peace within that person."

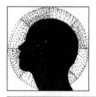

Dr. Liberman elucidates the relationship of light receptivity to consciousness and human evolution. He discusses how unresolved emotional traumas eventually manifest as addictive behaviors and physical illness. He shows how the use of light and color can act "homeopathically" to bring these issues to the surface so they can be resolved, thereby affecting emotional, physical, and spiritual well-being.

"We ourselves are the only healing remedy. Only through the transformation of the self does this remedy become more potent. As we expand our awareness, we need fewer external techniques and technologies. True healing can only be triggered by the core energy that flows between the guide and the seeker. You only need to use the light until you see the light."

SECTION VIII
Light Resources

For ease of access the *Resource Lists* have been divided into sixteen content categories that include:

Light Therapy Authors, Educators, and Practitioners

Products used in Therapy

Educational and Research Organizations

SECTION IX
Bibliography

For ease of access the *Bibliography* has been divided into eleven content categories that include:

Suggested Light Reading

INDEX

SECTION X
Index

Dedications

Brian's Dedication

To my dear friends, Drs. Jacob Liberman, John Downing, Steven Vazquez, and Norman Rosenthal, whose courageous and pioneering spirits have contributed to a renaissance in the therapeutic application of full-spectrum and colored light in both the scientific and lay communities.

To my "heart family" and dream co-creators, Dr. Lee Hartley and Bethany ArgIsle, without whose dedicated help, support, and loving encouragement the *Light Years Ahead Conference* and this book would not have become a reality.

My deepest love, respect, and gratitude to you all.

I honor the light within you.

Bethany's Dedication

To all of you who are at the threshold of finding what it is that will fulfill that "feeling," that motivation, that course of action which will lead to your inner knowing, I dedicate my efforts within these pages to you. Incorporate the best of all you are guided to study and create your own offering – I have had to decipher and discern, unravel and travel to make myself available to common sense and living-loving health care. I have had many challenges and have learned that inside of me is a willingness to Be Well, not just get well.

To the Spirit which makes flowers turn toward the sun and gives us moments of healthy fun; so that we experience a moment of joy on this great Planet, our body. *Light Years Ahead* is a seed of light, and when the time is right, it will take flight through your own unique endeavors. Remain focused, think much, speak less, and keep your devotion and discipline close at all times. For Brian and his first book.

Please, also let it be known that I dedicate each page to trees in the breeze everywhere. The medicine of breathing is the essence of light and life itself.

Acknowledgements

To the following folks, we are most thankful for your perseverant service. There have been a multitude of moments invested by several hearts, and we wish to list them here:

Albert Howell, of Meta4 Productions, a real "Herculean" task master, for your mastery of the line, the page and entire book design. Not only did you decipher a myriad of changes, save us time and money, but your suggestions and ideas "enlightened" and tightened the project at so many turns.

Barbara C. Thomason, M.F.A., Barbara C. Thomason & Associates, gifted artist, photographer, and designer — Job well done for cover and art throughout the book.

Evelyn Brown, thank you for your saintly patience, devotion to details, the late night hours, and typists/transcription powers.

Martha Rigney, of *Light Years Ahead Productions,* for your generous gifts of computer wizardry and radiant encouragement, as well as generating the first official orders for this book.

Nola Lewis, M.S., Research Associate for the Institute of Noetic Sciences, Sausalito, California. Your brilliance shines through your editorial care for the written word.

Joan Lamb, for your eagle eye and angel heart during the final stages of editing.

Melinda "Lyte" McKown, for your early editing.

Ted McClellan of ALTA Indexers, for your pointers.

Victoria Randall, for your "de-lightful" strength of character and skill as a editor, that made you the final word on grammar, content, and style.

We especially wish to thank our "support people" for feeding us and nurturing us with love (which lights up our souls), with food, with encouragement, errands, and healing hands:

Phoenix Deon, singer, chef, driver, true believer, available whenever and wherever we needed your assistance.

Jeanne Hart, of "Cooking From The Heart," for delicious and nutritious gourmet vegetarian and raw foods.

Chris Cooper, Consummate Massage Therapist, who arrived just when we needed a boost, a massage, and some noodle therapy.

For quality visual reproductions we wish to thank:

The Darkroom in San Rafael, California. Special thanks for consistent quality photo reproduction.

Robert Vente, master photographer. Your photos reflect your ability to truly see and be the light.

Terry Patten and Dr. Julian Issacs and all the folks at Tools for Exploration, San Rafael, California, for being so generous with sharing of light technology information and for many products included in our *Resource List*.

*To the following presenters from **The Light Years Ahead Conference**, we thank you for your presentations, as well as special efforts in contributing additional supportive materials.*

Lee Hartley, Ed.D., for your extended labour to birth the first **Light Years Ahead Conference** (which is the basis for this book), as well as your years enlightening others from your wealth of personal and clinical experience.

John Downing, O.D., Ph.D., F.C.S.O., special thanks for pioneering and cultivating the "vision" of the therapeutic use of colored light; a full fifteen years ahead of the mainstream; for inventing the **Lumatron Ocular Light Stimulator**™. It is on the shoulders of your theories and light instrumentation that the majority of these presenters stand.

Jacob Liberman, O.D., Ph.D., F.C.S.O. for your courage to actively speak out on both the physics and metaphysics of light, and for taking the crusade internationally.

Norman Shealy, M.D., Ph.D., for your pioneering research on the neurochemical effects of light and for your generosity to **The Light Years Ahead Conference.**

Steven Vazquez, Ph.D., for your ability to experiment and synthesize a tremendous variety of traditional and non-traditional therapeutics with a deep sense of compassion.

Mary Bolles, B.A., for your enthusiasm and willingness to do whatever it takes to bring out the light in children and adults with learning problems.

Sam Pesner, O.D., F.C.S.O., for your brilliance, humor, and quiet power exuded throughout the conference and this book.

Manohar Croke, B.A., and **Akhila Dass, O.M.D., L.Ac.,** international ambassadors, for the use of light in acupuncture.

Ward Lamb, D.C., pioneer, chiropractor, researcher, and inventor, for your almost sixty years of being a dedicated leader, lighting the way to mindbodyspirit healing.

Robert Dubin, D.C., for your tenacity and sheer power of authentic personhood. Your patients, including the Vietnam veterans, are fortunate for your skill and devotion.

Gabriel Cousens, M.D., for your enthusiastic response and openness to light.

Elson M. Haas, M.D., for your brilliant editing skills and encouraging comments.

David Olszewski, E.E., I.E., for being the practical cornerstone guiding us to the best use of light in our daily lives.

Larry Johnson, J.D., for establishing clarity with regard to business relationships and intellectual property rights.

Jerry Green, J.D., for placing phototherapy practice in the appropriate light of legal insights and for generously supporting this project in both time and guidance.

Concerns and Cautions Regarding Phototherapy

Before reading this book consider the following general and specific concerns:

General Concerns:

1. The purpose of this book is educational, and the information contained herein cannot replace competent medical consultation.

Light Years Ahead only offers *educational information* regarding a range of potential uses of full spectrum and colored light. Keep in mind that the knowledge in this book is not to be interpreted to represent a claim for diagnosis, cure, prescription, treatment, or prevention of any physical, emotional, ophthalmic, or optometric disorder. Although the concepts and techniques of subtle energy healing discussed in this book have been practiced by thousands of people around the world as an alternative and holistic means of viewing the process of healing, this information should not replace competent optometric, medical, psychiatric, psychological, chiropractic, neurological, and/or educational care.

The contents of *Light Years Ahead* represent the views of the individual authors and does not necessarily reflect the opinions and beliefs of *Light Years Ahead Productions*. The authors, editors, publisher, and distributor are in no way liable for any misuse of this material. The information in this book is meant to complement, not replace, the advice of your physician or competent licensed health care professional. If you are under the care of a physician or any of the above health care providers, you should discuss any major changes in your regimen with him or her.

2. Each individual is unique, and this information might not apply to you.

Please realize that the same light therapy approach does not work the same for every individual. Although the experimental case studies in this book are real and are meant to inspire personal exploration and large-group experimental research, you are a unique human being, not a disease. Because this is a book and not a professional health consultation, the information in this book may not apply in your particular case.

We encourage you to pay particular attention to the ways in which both the accepted and experimental light therapies have profoundly affected the practitioners and clients toward a better understanding and realization of personal health. *Light Years Ahead Productions* is neither recommending you use or not use a particular therapy, but that you consider utilizing the best traditional (medical) and alternative (holistic) methodologies, what this book terms integrative mindbody healing, to further your own personal health care.

Specific Concerns:

1. Do not overlook potential pathological conditions that require medical, psychological, or optometric intervention.

A. Severe emotional problems such as (acute or chronic) mood, thought, or dissociative disorders:

For example, of particular concern is the general category of conditions known as mood or affective disorders. Even though full spectrum light therapy is an accepted treatment for seasonal affective disorder (SAD), this and any treatment for all types of mood problems, such as clinical depression, or any of the bipolar disorders (manic depression) should be supervised by either a qualified psychiatrist (M.D.) or psychologist (Ph.D., Psy.D, Ed. D.) or other competent, licensed mental health professional, such as a marriage, family and child counselor (M.F.C.C.) or a clinical social worker (L.C.S.W.) or psychiatric nurse practitioner (R.N.). Self-diagnosing seasonal affective disorder or its subclinical version known as the winter blues can be both difficult and risky, as several other disorders and diseases share symptoms with SAD. Unless you see a physician or psychotherapist to get an expert opinion about your specific situation, you could be overlooking and ignoring a physical or psychological ailment that might worsen with time.

B. Visual pathology.

The content of **Light Years Ahead** is intended to be used as an adjunct to a rational and responsible vision care program prescribed by an eye doctor optometrist (O.D.) or ophthalmologist (M.D.). We cannot rule out the possibility of visual problems following phototherapy in some individuals. People with a history of eye problems may be a special risk.

2. Photoconvulsive Seizures and the use of Light Emitting Devices in Health Care Practice[1]

About one percent of the population has epilepsy (also called seizure disorder). About 3.5% of this 1% (that is .035% or one in 2,850 of the general population) can have a convulsive seizure triggered by flashing lights. The flash rate most prone to causing this reaction is 15-20 flashes per second (Hz). To trigger a seizure like this, the flashing lights must usually be fairly bright, such as a stroboscopic light at a disco. However, some individuals may be triggered by lower intensities, such as those from video games and television. There is a chance that photoconvulsive seizures could occur in the proximity of any instrumentation which incorporates flashing lights. The health care practitioner using such devices should follow these guidelines.

A. For known Photoconvulsive Patients:

Ask the patient if he/she has epilepsy. If so, are they subject to photoconvulsive seizures? If they are subject to photoconvulsive seizures, prohibit them from using flashing light instrumentation.

B. Other Patients:

Other patients may use flashing light instrumentation.

If an unknown photoconvulsive prone patient does have a seizure while using light emitting instrumentation in your office, don't panic. Flashing lights do not damage the brain; they merely trigger a reaction which indicates that this person has a seizure disorder. This early warning sign will be very helpful to his/her medical doctor to properly diagnose and treat the condition. This patient should be referred immediately to a medical doctor, preferably a neurologist.

Seizures which occur in a patient while using light emitting instrumentation may not always be photoconvulsive seizures. They may be non-photo induced epileptic seizures which happen coincidentally. They may also be caused by other medical conditions, such as: encephalitis, meningitis, pregnancy, poisoning, hypoglycemia, head injury, high fever, etc. The patient may resume the use of flashing light instrumentation if his/her medical doctor has ruled out a photoconvulsive seizure and given consent for the patient to resume.

3. Use care in the initial color selection for phototherapy in patients prone towards depression or violence.

Individuals with a history of depression or violence should not begin phototherapy with light from the red end of the spectrum. For example, agitated, depressed or violent patients who are suicidal should not initially be stimulated with yellow light. Similarly, depressed subjects should not be initially treated with green light.[2]

---

1. This segment is excerpted with permission from a treatment guide prepared by John Downing, O.D., Ph.D., F.S.C.O., which was approved by the Epilepsy Information Service, Department of Neurology, of The Bowman Gray School of Medicine, Winston Salem, NC 27103.
2. An additional list of potential negative side effects of phototherapy can be found in *Considerations for Structuring Clinical Practices with Phototherapy, page xlix.*

The Language of Light
Bethany ArgIsle
© 1996

Eyes
are our
windows to life and
our heart's door. Our mirrors
to beauty and one of the ways we
recognize. Eyes have a language they
speak, the language of light. Eyes are
delicate, transparent, ever-changing
with what they reflect
Eyes reach out,
take in.

The eye receives the
image. Light releases
the image, so we see
what we are trained to
see or what the capacity
we have for light
emblazens upon the
screen of life itself.
Too much light dries.
Light can coax.
Light can reveal
what lurks in the
shadows of one's soul.
Landing lights guide
us to launch our lives
and come back again.
Light guides our ride
utilizing our mindbody
as our vehicle.

How To Use This Book

In the winter of 1992, Brian brought me transcribed talks from the first **Light Years Ahead Conference.** At that time, unknown to him, I had just purchased a book entitled *LIGHT: Explore the Amazing World of Light* — From Ancient Sun Myths to the Latest Optic Discoveries that Have Transformed Our Lives. Synchronistic! I had also been working on notes about light for a children's television series. Interestingly, during the production of the book **Light Years Ahead,** while I was watching an educational KQED-TV show, Dr. George (Bud) Brainard, a phototherapy consultant to NASA, stated that, "All astronauts have had light treatments before launch."

As we cross the millennium, more and more there are preparations being made and banks of information committing entire libraries to CD-ROM and other new media activated by light. I believe many of the cruder methods of collecting, storing, and processing information will be refined and, in fact, we will be moving toward light as the "fuel" it has always been.

For the last two decades I have dedicated my time to the production of healing texts and the creation of a preventive health center. I have produced health texts which are easy to access — user friendly — and are at the core of the integration of both ancient and up-to-the-minute healthcare delivery.

We have created **Light Years Ahead** as a primer on light, highlighting only a few of the exciting applications of light in mindbody healing. As you read through each *Section* and *Chapter,* you will note that many of the names of particular treatments, conditions, personalities, healing instruments and institutions have been capitalized, boldfaced, or italicized. Also, we have done this when the information in the text appears on an accompanying chart, so your eye can easily pick things out.

We have designed a book within a book. If you only read the italics, editor notes, bolds, bold italics, you will get an information scan as if you were using your computer. Then if you wish to go deeper into a subject, you can get all the particulars and can easily find your place again, since we have chosen to title the tops of each page not only with chapter titles, but with section icons. The icons are pictographic representations and appear in the *Table of Contents, Sections, Chapters, Bibliography, Resource List* and *Index.* We believe that the *Resource List* (with sixteen categories) and the *Bibliography* (divided into eleven categories) are extensive contributions to the emerging field of light-assisted medicine.

Light Years Ahead is many books in one and can be used in a variety of ways. As a light awareness guide this book can be easily and quickly accessed through the *Table of Contents,* the *Index,* the *Sections* and/or the *Chapters.* For example, if you have a specific interest or condition you wish to look up, such as PMS or SAD, you might initially begin by scanning the *Index* and *Table of Contents,* then later peruse the charts, photographs, drawings and the italic and bold print within a particular chapter.

Light Years Ahead can also be used as an introductory textbook elucidating the past, present and future application of phototherapy. Finally, this book can serve as a resource manual for the exploration of key literature, individuals, products and organizations. For example, the *Bibliography* provides extensive, up-to-date references on the historical and emerging professional and self-care uses of light in medicine, optometry, psychotherapy, education, neurological rehabilitation, acupuncture and chiropractic. Similarly, the *Resource Lists* enable you to contact recognized experts worldwide, including: phototherapy practitioners, researchers, educators, and professional organizations, as well as product manufacturers and retailers.

Beyond our book, you may enjoy "enlightening" your mind by learning more about this "ancient future subject" by attending an upcoming *Light Years Ahead Conference* or workshop. If so please contact us at our *Light Years Ahead* office in Tiburon, California. When you have made one quantum "light leap" in your awareness, we have done our job.

Bethany ArgIsle, Project Director

How To Use This Book

1. For ease of information access **Light Years Ahead** can initially be entered through the *Index, Table of Contents, Sections,* or *Chapters.*

2. Conditions, types of phototherapy, professionals, light instruments, and institutions appear in **bold** or *italic.*

3. Charts in each chapter contain photographs, drawings, and summaries of information.

4. *Chapter* and *Section* locations can be easily found by the use of chapter titles on the top of each page as well as pictographic subject icons.

5. The *Resource Lists* contain sixteen content categories which enable you to contact phototherapy practitioners, researchers, educators, professional organizations, product manufacturers, and retailers.

6. The *Bibliography* contains eleven content categories that provide extensive references on the historical and current uses of full spectrum and colored light in medicine, optometry, psychotherapy, education, homeopathy, and acupuncture, as well as the physics, metaphysics, and business of phototherapy.

Oh, the glory of growth, silent, mighty, persistent, inevitable! To awaken, to open up like a flower to the light of a fuller consciousness!

— Emily Carr

Preface

Lee Hartley, Ed.D.
Director, Light Years Ahead Conference
Co-Founder, Light Years Ahead Productions

It has been said that "We teach what we need to learn." **The Light Years Ahead Conference** was just such a process for me. It was primarily my desire to overcome *dis-ease* in my life and the search for *well-ness* that led me to the books, articles, equipment, and most importantly, the people who were involved in the conference as presenters, exhibitors, and participants. Once I found the path there were many synchronistic moments with one person or piece of information that led from one to another. It has been a fascinating process in which to be involved!

In 1980, while completing my doctorate, I was diagnosed with hypothyroidism. Medication was prescribed to be taken daily. My metabolism had definitely slowed. I became less active and gradually gained weight. In 1987, several new symptoms suddenly appeared: severe digestive problems, many food allergies, psoriasis, and extreme fatigue. These became so severe that, for awhile, I had to alternate working one day with one day resting in bed. It was years before I was correctly diagnosed with chronic fatigue syndrome. In my search to learn what was wrong and what to do, I went to several physicians who wouldn't listen and wouldn't even attempt to solve the mystery.

This led me to do my own research and read many books. One evening I walked past a bookstore and saw in the window Dr. Jacob Liberman's book, *Light: Medicine of the Future*. I knew I had to have this book, but the store was closed. I came back in the morning, bought the book, read it that day, and called Dr. Liberman that evening. I was so excited by the information in his book that I would have been on an airplane to Aspen, Colorado, the next day had he been available. He said that the College of Syntonic Optometry's annual conference was in three weeks in Aspen, and he suggested that I attend and then stay an additional week to work with him. I did, and the outcome was incredible! I felt dramatically better very quickly. I had a rapid increase in energy, and I was able to appreciably reduce the dosage of the thyroid medication. The psoriasis and the food and skin allergies also diminished a great deal. In addition, my unstable neck and lower back, caused by an auto accident eleven years earlier, stabilized and have not needed treatment since that time. My chiropractor told me that it was a "miracle," and I'm still amazed that I experienced such wonderful benefits from only a week of light treatment.

After I returned from Aspen, I was able to borrow and purchase some light therapy equipment that I've continually used at home and in my practice. Although I'm still dealing with some health issues, I keep seeing improvement and feel much better.

I originally heard about light therapy from Dr. Brian Breiling prior to reading Dr. Liberman's book. Later, Brian and I did some networking with several people knowledgable in the therapeutic use of light. These were exciting dinner gatherings where we shared information and mutually encouraged each other. At one of these gatherings Brian suggested that we present a conference on the subject of light.

In the next ten months we created ***The Light Years Ahead Conference.*** It was an incredible amount of work. It is a real tribute to the various light treatment modalities I used that I had enough energy to easily fulfill my responsibilities as Conference Director, as well as continue to operate my own business and see my psychotherapy clients.

For the day-to-day conference work, I'm sincerely grateful for assistance provided me by my secretary, Diane Ventura; our computer expert, Martha Rigney; and Paul Arenson, who did publicity and exhibit sales coordination.

There was often a magic and synchronicity in the production schedule of this conference that kept reminding us that we were all involved in something powerfully synergistic, something that really felt as if it was meant to happen! The two days of ***The Light Years Ahead Conference*** brought together ten dynamic and inspiring speakers that ignited the audience's enthusiasm about the many potentials of light therapy. We all left the event with a definite glow, musing about the "Light Years Ahead."

The idea of more light, more beauty, and more love possesses an irresistable magic.

— Ernest Dimnet

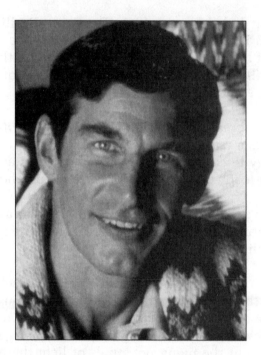

Gabriel Cousens, M.D.

*D*r. Gabriel Cousens is a holistic physician, psychiatrist, homeopath, family therapist, Essene minister, Reiki master, meditation teacher, international peace activist, and co-director of the first Kundalini Clinic in the United States. He is also the author of several bestselling books, including *Spiritual Nutrition and The Rainbow Diet* (Boulder, CO: Cassandra Press, 1986), *Sevenfold Peace* (Tiburon, CA: H.J. Kramer, 1990), and *Conscious Eating* (Santa Rosa, CA: Vision Books, 1993). He has also published articles in the areas of biochemistry, school health, clinical pharmacology, hypoglycemia, and Alzheimer's disease. Dr. Cousens uses nutrition, homeopathy, acupuncture, psychiatry and family therapy, crystal healing, and meditation in his practice. He is happily married and has two children in their early twenties. He is co-director with his wife, Nora, of **Tree of Life Rejuvenation Center** in Patagonia, Arizona, a spa, healing center, and wellness lifestyle community.

Foreword: Shedding Light on the Elements of Health

Gabriel Cousens, M.D.

This is an historically important book that is put together and introduced in a magnificent, thoughtful, and artistic way by Dr. Brian Breiling and Bethany ArgIsle. It is historical in the sense that it brings ancient knowledge about light into the light of our modern awareness, and it is a landmark publication about a budding "new" ancient healing energy.

After reading this book, one can no longer deny, or take "lightly," the importance of light therapy. The comprehensive *Introduction* and the insightful *Chapters* seem to cover almost every reflective angle of light and light therapy. I am thoroughly inspired. For me, it deepens my understanding of one of our most important nutrients and basic elements needed for health and rejuvenation . . . light. It also supports my theoretical work elucidated in *Spiritual Nutrition and The Rainbow Diet:* that nutrition is what we absorb into our overall body-mind-spirit from the many different density levels that have all precipitated from the cosmic force.

This is not a new concept. "In the beginning was the Word, and the Word was with God, and the Word was God" (John 1:1). This familiar concept is given a fuller meaning by ***Light Years Ahead.*** Nutrition all comes from God and is nourished by God or the cosmic force. The cosmic energy, at various levels of density, is the basic nutrient for our bodies. In this context, all levels of energy available to us are considered nutrients–this includes sunlight. Once we understand that various densities of energy are the essential nutrients to all life processes, it allows us to appreciate a paradigm of nutrition which sees material food as just one level of energy density in the context of a larger spectrum of nutrients that aid our healing and spiritual development. Consciousness is the essence of food that we digest.

Historically, there were several examples of people who were able to live on less dense energies than material food: Enoch, Moses, Jesus, Elijah, and Giri Bala. These beings were able to live solely on light and the even less dense cosmic energy. This energetic theory of nutrition allows us to explain how the human system is not completely subject to both the law of conservation of mass and energy and the second law of thermodynamics. **Our ability to both absorb and radiate light directly leads to spiritual development and health.** A decreased ability to absorb light leads to a poorer quality of health and most concretely, a SAD state.

Mastery of the five elements: air (breath), earth (food), water (feelings), fire (light), and ether (mind), are the key elements for health and rejuvenation. ***Light Years Ahead*** supplies the missing understanding of the importance of light in health in a way that is extraordinarily interesting to me. In my work at the Tree of Life Rejuvenation Center in Patagonia, Arizona, I had not become clear on how to bring a deeper understanding of the use of light in the rejuvenation process until I had read this book. I find myself excited and pleased with the doors this book has opened for me.

To help the reader further appreciate the depth of ***Light Years Ahead,*** I would like to share a simple energetic model of healing and health that can serve as a frame of reference. The more we increase the flow of life force in the body, the more healing energy there is and the more health and rejuvenation there will be.

The life force is infinite. We are permeated with it as a spiritual force and its manifestation as a material energetic force in our physical, emotional, and mental bodies. It is our link with the Godhead and the Divine within us. Every cell of our body is oozing with this dynamic energy. Once we understand this Truth, we are confronted with the enigmatic question associated with all disease. If we are permeated with this infinite energy, how do we become "depleted" of the life force and experience a lack of health? We become depleted because of energy-depleting lifestyles and because our emotional, mental, and spiritual blocks create a resistance to the flow of this cosmic energy and to life itself. At the extreme, a blockage of the flow of life force creates death.

Each of the five elements supplies energy and force to help us break through our resistance. These include the therapeutic application of such diverse modalities as breath release work, mental and spiritual disciplines, eating live foods, water therapies and now more clearly, light therapies. Each element when properly used creates enough energy to break up fossilized negative thought forms stored in the mind and body and thus allow more energy to flow freely into the body-mind-spirit complex, creating more healing and rejuvenation. From kundalini, the pure spiritualizing force that becomes released in the subtle body at a certain point in our evolution, to various energy activating diets, our physical, emotional, mental, and spiritual blocks are released when we nurture and activate these vital energies. One of the reasons live foods and fasting are sometimes difficult for people is not the food or lack of it, but the tremendous amounts of physical, emotional, and mental toxins that are released when we go on these diets. People will often stuff themselves with toxic foods to suppress the experience of these cathartic mindbody releases or from what is being released by the kundalini energy.

What is particularly exciting about light therapy is the relative preciseness with which color frequency and intensity enables us to open up the pathways into specific brain structures, such as the limbic system, where so many basic emotional traumas are stored. As pointed out in this book, light energy turns into electrical-neuronal energy. By receiving more light energy through the eyes, the brain uses this energy to optimize itself. Just as when the vital force increases in the body, we have the capacity to release physical and emotional toxins. Thus, the brain and the limbic system and other key structures will be energized enough to release emotional toxins.

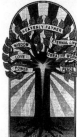

Emotional energy is condensed and stored in these structures when it is suppressed. In this unexpressed form it becomes a biological resistor and creates a dissonant resonance. **Increasing the input of light where this dissonant resonance is stored energizes the stuck dissonance to the point where it must be released by the system.** In this way light therapy energetically stimulates dissonant resonances — *the unfinished business* — to which a person is resistant. Colored Light Therapy used in this way appears to be an irritant, but it is really a wonderful blessing to our health. Light significantly affects every cell and key regulator centers of the body, including: the hypothalamus and pineal gland, the autonomic nervous system, and the more subtle energies of the chakra system.

The different chapters in ***Light Years Ahead*** give the most updated information on exactly how it does this. Reading this book has made me more aware than ever of how important light is in our lives. ***Light Years Ahead*** gives new meaning to Nobel prize laureate Szent-Gyorgyi's description of the essential life process as a little electric current sent to us by the sun.

As we increase our visual fields and get more energy to the brain, all brain functions are specifically enhanced. Sickness is associated with a shortage or poor utilization of light. As Dr. Shealy points out, all is related to all other. "Light — the amount, quality, color, and frequency — influences everything in the brain and everything beneath that." At every level the light is operating, no matter how material. For example, for us human photocells, food is condensed light. That is the basis of my ***Rainbow Diet***. The color of the outer covering of food is a key to what chakra, endocrine, neurological structure, and what organ the food will most affect.

We are human photocells whose ultimate biological nutrient is light. Food, through the process of photosynthesis, brings sunlight energy in the form of resonating electrically active carbon-carbon bonds and electron clouds on double-bonded structures into our physical bodies. This light is then released into our systems as electrical energy. It also stimulates an equal and opposite release of the inner light.

Light Years Ahead is a great book which will stimulate an equal and opposite release of inner light and awareness in all who choose to experience it.

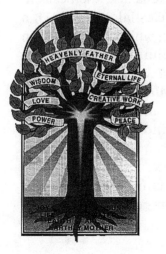

The Tree of Life Rejuvenation Center is dedicated to living, inspiring, and training people to integrate the healing life forces to achieve body, mind and spiritual rejuvenation. The art of physical rejuvenation is combined with psychological and spiritual development in an expansive natural setting that evolves lifestyle into radiant wellness. *See Resource List.*

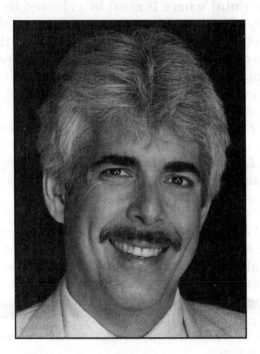

Elson M. Haas, M.D.

Dr. Elson M. Haas is an innovative and active practitioner in the fields of Nutritional and Preventive Medicine, who specializes in what he terms "Integrated Medicine," the incorporation of nutrition, herbology, Chinese medicine, acupuncture, bodywork, and the use of guided imagery into a general medical practice. He is the director of the **Preventive Medical Center of Marin** in San Rafael, California. He is also the bestselling author of *Staying Healthy With The Seasons* (Berkeley, CA: Celestial Arts, 1981), a widely acclaimed book on Eastern and Western preventive medicine, which is currently in its 19th printing. Dr. Hass' second book is a 1200-page compendium entitled *Staying Healthy With Nutrition: The Complete Guide to Diet and Nutritional Medicine*, (Berkeley, CA: Celestial Arts, 1992). Both books were directed by **Light Years Ahead** project director and editor Bethany ArgIsle. His latest book is *A Diet for All Seasons*, with nutritionist Eleanora Manzolini (Berkeley, CA: Celestial Arts, 1995). He and Bethany ArgIsle are also co-founders and partners in Health Harvest Unlimited Inc. and are the originators of Consciousness Fashion products which include Sole-Sox,© Skin Sox, and a line of T-shirts and decals that include the chakras, the acupuncture meridians, and designs incorporating symbols from world religions and other cross- cultural symbology.

Futureword:
Light and Integrated Medicine, The Years Ahead

Elson M. Haas, M.D.

Since sound and light are primary energies, they will play an increasingly important role in the future of medicine. The term I like to use for the current and future medical system is *Integrated Medicine,* because it incorporates and synthesizes all aspects of healing — old and new, technical, physical medicine, and subtle energy medicine. I prefer Integrated Medicine over the reference terms "alternative" or (w)holistic medicine, as it blends together all aspects of medicine and healing that are currently available and useful to us as practitioners and patients. There are several tenets to my approach of Integrated Medicine:

1. The Integration of Basic Family Practice and Preventive Medicine.

Family practice, diagnosis, and treatment can be blended with health supportive and preventive care, such as psychotherapy, phototherapy, counseling, acupuncture, and bodywork. Individual health can be conceptualized and treated within the intimate web of our social relationships to family, work, and self. Health can be conceived as connectedness to being who we truly are and doing what we are really here to do.

2. The Integration of Multidisciplinary Practices.

Combining conventional medicine with more natural methods that include the skillful and judicious use of prescription medicines, nutritional and herbal supplements, osteopathic care, physical therapies, stress management and general lifestyle guidance is an important key to our current and future health-oriented medical system.

3. The Integration of Cross-Cultural Healing Practices.

Although we are now beginning to explore cross-cultural healing practices, in the future we will see more acceptance and use of the ancient and present wisdom of all cultures. The Traditional Five Elements are a central core of Chinese medicine and their balance is the basis for good health. Traditional Oriental diagnosis evaluates the balance of the Five Elements — fire, earth, metal, water, and wood, as well as the internal organs and their energy systems. This particular balance also relates to specific colors, foods and flavors, emotions, climates, and mental attitudes. This whole system and its practical understanding is clarified in my first book, *Staying Healthy With The Seasons* (Berkeley, CA: Celestial Arts, 1981), known as a philosophical and practical, preventive medical text.

In Chinese medicine the *philosopher-physician* is considered the most evolved form of healer. Similarly, I believe the *philosopher-patient* is the way to both create and maintain health as well as to correct and prevent problems. This requires that both doctors and patients pay closer attention to the more subtle levels of life and care for themselves with wise mindbody nourishment, such as creating a balance of diet and exercise, work and play, and attunement to outer and inner life.

4. The Evaluation and Treatment of the Whole Person.

(W)holistic medicine addresses the different levels of human existence — the physical, mental, emotional, and spiritual. Integrated Medicine examines what the individual's whole life is about instead of focusing on just the physical symptoms; it integrates these aspects into the evaluation, treatment, and education of each patient. Sensitive people can utilize energy systems, such as Lumatron™ light therapy or acupuncture, which affect the internal energetic and elemental balance.

5. Preventive Health Care.

The future practice of medicine will be more integrated. We will incorporate the use of modern, physical medicine with more preventive self-care and subtle energetic approaches. The four cornerstones of Preventive Medicine include:

1. Nutrition
2. Stress management
3. Exercise
4. Attitude

These go hand-in-hand to create healthy, functioning and nourished cells and tissues, and a strong foundation for good health and longevity — thus leading to greater energy, vitality and youthfulness. **Phototherapy easily fits into all four of the above dimensions of preventive health care.**

6. Self-Care: Health or Dis-ease is a By-product or Outcome of Lifestyle.

Here we move away from the "fix it" model of Western medicine to the integrated practice of examining wellness as a reflection of how we live, think, feel, and act. These include an examination of our abuses and limitations; nutrition and assimilation (what we eat); stress management (what eats us); and our attitude toward life; genetics and early family experience; past problems and how we dealt with them — all of these, and more, contribute to the person we are today. Realizing and changing the factors that contribute to symptoms and disease is the true path to health.

7. MindBodySpirit Wellness.

In most healing processes we need to become more aware and sensitive to more subtle aspects of both our outer and inner lives, particularly the emotional and psychological issues surrounding our current state and the problems with which we are dealing. Working with more subtle levels of energy, such as acupuncture or light therapy, can shift us or stimulate deeper issues to rise to awareness, enabling us to deal with them more completely and clear them from our bodymind. Thus, they no longer influene the imbalances that may manifest as symptoms or "dis-ease."

One way to accomplish deeper healing is to find a personal process such as light assisted psychotherapy that can generate insight and inner transformation. The real shift comes from how we approach our ill health, both in attitude and in practice. Looking at illness as a positive force for change is useful. Moving away from the questions of, "How can I get rid of this?" or, "What should I take to make this go away?" to more important questions, such as, "Why is this problem or symptom happening now?" or, "Bodymind, what are you trying to tell me?" and, "What do I need to do differently to really heal?" Questions such as these can begin the new healing process in re-integrating the separation that occurs at the different levels of our being which contribute to our illness in the first place. We can each choose consciously to release "life-threatening" thoughts, feelings and actions, so that our own unique vital force, our soul, and spirit can become available to us as we more fully become the self we were designed to be and align with our true purpose for being.

Light, Color, and Subtle Energy Healing

Light and sound are the primordial energies from which life evolved — the essence of nothingness into somethingness. We, too, are an expression of this energy — light, color and sound. Color and sound are vibration and affect all other vibrations. The human body is energy/vibration. We are both space and form, or more accurately, form filled with space . . . lots of space. **Although we live on air, water, and food as nourishment, we are energy and light, and we are affected and nourished by light. The more open, aware, and sensitive to light vibrations we are, the more we can be influenced and healed by the basic light of nature.**

The light of nature manifests itself in the rainbow of colors that we see with our eyes — the sunlight sparkling on the morning dew; the rays of light streaming through the green trees in a forest; the multicolored wildflowers sprinkled over vibrant, yellow-green rolling meadows; the subtle shades of brown and gray at our feet on an oceanside stroll, along with the mixtures of blue and turquoise of the sky and sea; the ecstatic experience of brilliant hues of sunlight or moonlight reflecting on water— these are a few of the infinite examples of how the energy of light affects our being on a daily basis.

Light is energy. Each color is a vibration, a frequency of vibrating energy that intermingles with other life energies. Whether the color is a food, a lightbulb, a painted wall, or our clothes, all have an effect upon us and others. The color wheel generates energies that span the complete spectrum of life experience and, in turn, affect our level of activity and receptivity and the various functions within our body. Light, color, and sound are vibrations of energy that are based on wavelengths and cycles per second of electromagnetic vibration. In those of us sensitive to energy (and any of us can be if we tune into it and take the time to practice) light and color can be felt and sound can be seen. We are vibration; all forms of energy affect us. There are those energies that have a positive influence, such as light and color. Also, there are energies that have adverse effects upon our body and its harmonious and continuous flow of life force. Just as with the color spectrum, the *chakra system* of seven energy vortices represents both the individual qualities of human life and the experience of life in total.

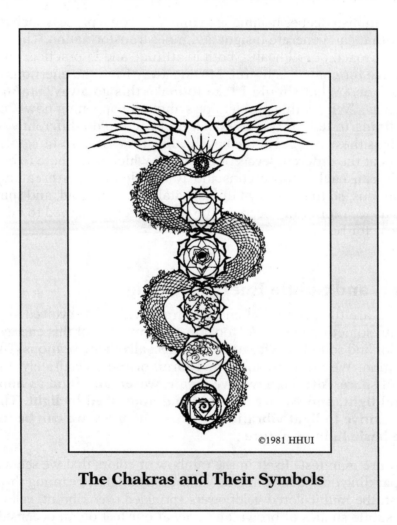

©1981 HHUI

The Chakras and Their Symbols

Bethany ArgIsle and I created the Chakra T-shirt, decal design and poster for our health education company, Health Harvest Unlimited Inc. (see *Resource List* for ordering information) over fifteen years ago when we were extensively studying the metaphysical aspects of life. We also wrote an educational information tag for the shirt which included a chart of the colors and qualities of each chakra. For example, red represents the root chakra of survival (located at the base of the spine) and the body/earth generation point of sexual and healing energy; it is stimulating and warming, with an excess leading to inflammatory conditions and a deficiency causing potential weakness and coldness in the body. On the opposite side of the color spectrum, violet is calming/sedating, helping us to relax and aiding the ability to meditate; it counteracts and balances the color red. This ancient and cross-cultural model for energetic healing is several thousand years old and is a key in the practice of Hindu and Buddhist yoga techniques and ayurveda, traditional Indian medicine. Interestingly, the traditional seven colors associated with each of the seven chakras are also included in the phototherapeutic approaches of Drs. Jacob Liberman, Steven Vazquez, and Norman Shealy. The chakras can be conceptualized as a subtle energy nervous system and correspond to major nerve plexi from the pelvis to the top of the head.

Lumatron™ Light Therapy in the Practice of Integrated Medicine

Utilizing a modality that affects our energy and healing while minimizing negative side effects is the first step toward appropriate health care and a personal healing system. I've been personally inspired by phototherapy from my experiences with the Lumatron™. I did twenty half-hour sessions of red and red-orange between January and February. When I completed the sessions, I felt more energetic, optimistic, and motivated to do things than I usually feel during the winter months. My sessions using the Downing Technique of Ocular Light Therapy® were subtle, yet very powerful. This led me to realize that I had unknowingly suffered a sub-clinical form of winter depression, which many of us suffer to some degree.

I was professionally inspired by the Lumatron™ in my Integrated Medical practice. Approximately a hundred people in my office completed twenty or more sessions of Ocular Light Therapy. **The patients who received the most benefit were those diagnosed with chronic fatigue syndrome, irregular menstrual problems, thyroid difficulties, insomnia and depression.** The majority of these patients noticed similar positive effects. **As a medical doctor, I believe phototherapy affects the human energetic system at the level of core energy, similar to acupuncture, and osteopathic or chiropractic treatment.**

I believe that many people need personal interaction and guidance to move out of their painful experiences of fear, frustration, anger, and helplessness that often contribute to their health concerns in the first place. My experience is that colored light phototherapy would best be combined with the caring interaction of a psychotherapeutic relationship. Reflecting back on all the patients who received colored light phototherapy in my practice, **the best results happened when light therapy and psychotherapy were combined.** The integration of both the constitutional, energetic approach, similar to Dr. Downing's methods, with the psychotherapeutic approach, similar to those of Drs. Liberman and Vazquez, is the ideal combination of "high-tech" and "high-touch" in a phototherapeutic practice.

Phototherapy, with the Lumatron™, is a powerful mindbody healing tool in the armamentarium of Integrated Medicine and one that I believe will play an increasingly important role in the ***Light Years Ahead.***

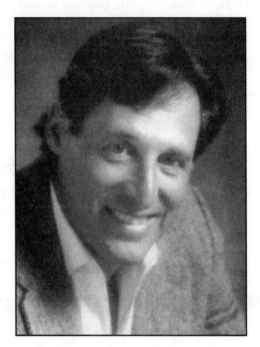

Jerry A. Green, J.D.

*J*erry A. Green, Attorney at Law, received his B.A. from University of California, Berkeley, in 1964, and his J.D. from Boalt Law School in 1967. He has specialized in medical malpractice and health care licensing for over twenty years. He serves as a special consultant to other attorneys on medical issues in malpractice and personal injury cases. As a pioneer of the health care contract, he has authored articles, contributed to professional conferences, and conducted workshops for health practitioners of diverse training and licensure. He lectures and consults for managed care organizations on risk management, informed consent, and medical decisionmaking. He is **President of Medical Decisionmaking Institute** in Mill Valley, California, and author of its professional education program, *Collaborative Planning for Physicians,* which teaches role clarification and shared decision making.

Considerations For Structuring Clinical Practices with Phototherapy

Jerry A. Green, J.D. and Brian Breiling, Psy.D.

Integrative Health Care: The Professional Context of the Practice of Phototherapy

Medical practice attorney, Jerry A. Green,[1] describes the legal differences between two distinct groups of health practitioners — between what he terms the traditional *medical practitioner* and the *holistic* (nonmedical) practitioner. The origin and nature of the differences between these two approaches to understanding health and intervention are based upon more than 2,000 years of divergent methods of theoretical understanding and scientific inquiry. These important scientific distinctions are described by **medical historian, Harris Coulter,** in his three-volume book entitled *Divided Legacy: A History of the Schism in Medical Thought* (Washington, D.C.: Wehawken Books, 1975).

Coulter defines "science" as a methodology for accessing and processing information. Since the time of Aristotle, medical thought has been divided between the individuals who followed *rational methodology* and those whose allegiance was with *empirical methodologies*. This schism continues today with the current allopathic medical model being an outgrowth of the rational school and the empiricists being the forerunners for today's vital energy model used by holistic practitioners. Briefly stated, the rational approach evolved a reductionistic focus on the description, diagnosis, and treatment of pathological conditions. The scientific methodology of the rationalistic school was largely a logical-analytical approach that focused on material matter and the study of the causes of disease. This led to the development of such modern medical treatments as antibiotics and surgery. In contrast, the subjective-observational approach of the empirical scientists developed a holistic model that studied ways to stimulate and balance the individual's unique vital energy (the workings of which were assumed to be unknowable). Today,

---

1. Health contracts, the intricacies of doctor-patient decision making, and the legal distinctions between the medical and the holistic models of health care are complex subjects beyond the introductory scope of this chapter. For more in-depth information, contact Jerry Green, whose address is in the *Resource List: Section One, Light Years Ahead Authors.*

empirical methodologies can be seen in a variety of popular approaches, such as homeopathy and traditional Chinese medicine.

Green states that clinical practice needs to clearly differentiate between medical and holistic practice to clarify the roles of patient and practitioner in order to decrease the risk of professional censure and civil malpractice liability. Clarification of these two distinct forms of health practice also supports the independent professional recognition of holistic practice, lays the foundation for understanding the appropriate allocation of responsibility between the two professional roles, and promotes a meaningful exchange of clinical information with appropriate referrals. **A clearer understanding of these distinctions also clarifies for patients the expectations appropriate to different health practitioners and facilitates informed and responsible health care decision making.**

The *traditional allopathic medical model* has been the dominant approach to medicine for the last hundred years. It has evidenced great success in the treatment of infectious disease and traumatic injury, yet it has done less well addressing the prevention and treatment of chronic and degenerative conditions. The medical approach focuses on the diagnosis and treatment of the symptoms of disease, injury, or other pathological conditions by the use of medication, surgery, and the modification of behavior. **The professional responsibility of the licensed physician is to establish the presence or absence of pathology, which may include the diagnosis and treatment of a pathological condition, observation for the development of a latent or potential pathological condition, and advise regarding the likely outcome or prognosis.** Medical treatment attempts to remove the symptoms of the recognized pathological condition.

In contrast, practitioners of the *holistic approach* focus on the promotion of health and well-being beyond pathology and illness prevention by a variety of practices designed to stimulate, balance and nourish the vital energy. Wellness is distinct from the absence of pathology; rather, it is a state that includes the individual's physical, emotional, cognitive, spiritual, and social response-ability. In this state the individual feels a joy and zest for life, has a sense of peace, happiness and fulfillment, and an awareness and harmony with the natural world.

Holistic practitioners stress the importance of the client assuming a more responsible role in the healing process. Holistic approaches focus on increasing self-awareness and taking active steps towards making health care decisions and lifestyle changes. **Because holistic practices do not offer treatment for pathology, they should not be seen by either doctors or patients as part of medicine.** Methods of energy analysis might include such things as observation of patterns of muscular tension, structural imbalances, quality of movement, levels of physical fitness, self-esteem, mental clarity, emotional insight, and vitality. Sources or potential causes of subtle energy imbalances stem from both external and internal factors. External factors include: toxicity of the air, water, soil, and food; nonnutritive additives in processed foods; noise pollution; radiation; and crowded living conditions. Internal sources of energy depletion entail a lifestyle that includes: chronic, unmitigated stress responses; a lack of optimal nutrition; insufficient, inappropriate, or irregular exercise; poor genetic constitution; birth trauma; a history of family abuse; and/or chemical dependency.

The primary objective of holistic healing is to gain insight and control over patterns of thoughts and actions which affect vital energy patterns. The ultimate goal is to transcend negative energy states and adopt positive lifestyle habits which enhance vital energy. Within the holistic model, chronic energetic depletion or imbalance increases the susceptibility to pathological conditions. While raising or balancing vital energy may have the effect of reducing an illness or facilitating recovery, the existence of depressed vital energy is not pathologic. Self-healing can be facilitated by balancing vital energy, which can be initiated with or without medical diagnosis or treatment.

Today there is a growing public recognition and interest in a host of such holistic "energy medicine" techniques as: ayurveda, chiropractic, acupuncture, homeopathy, yoga, chi kung, fitness training, massage, reiki, shiatsu, applied or behavioral kinesiology, nutritional counseling, and the utilization of such nutrients as live foods, herbs, vitamins and minerals, fasting, increasing awareness and expression of cognitive, behavioral and emotional patterns, meditation, prayer, hypnosis, positive suggestion, visualization, biofeedback, sensory development, the use of colors, sounds and music, breathing exercises, dance, and spending time in nature.

The educational background, skills, and insights of the holistic practitioner will influence which expressions of vital energy to work with and which methods are used to stimulate and balance the life energy. **Nonetheless, it is the holistic practitioner's role to work within their independent scope of professional responsibility and to identify whether clients have concerns regarding pathology, and, if so, refer them to the appropriate medical practitioner.**

While a host of leading-edge physicians have explored energetic premises for years, attesting to their value (see *Bibliography* for texts by Drs. Haas, Cousens, Shealy, Dossey, Siegel and Chopra), the medical model has been the dominant paradigm in health care during the last century. Western society is unaccustomed to thinking about nourishing the life force, and has not yet taken seriously those pioneers who challenge the prevailing scientific model (for example, the **International Society for the Study of Subtle Energies and Energy Medicine**[1] and **The Center for Frontier Sciences**[2] at Temple University).

The traditional medical model does not recognize holistic practices as existing within the accepted standards of the practice of allopathic medicine. Unrecognized methods of medical treatment may be the basis of professional censure (peer review) and may lead to disciplinary action by regulatory agencies resulting in probation, suspension, or revocation of one's license to practice medicine, civil liability (malpractice), or even criminal liability. Since holistic health practitioners are not licensed physicians, energetic perspectives in healing lie outside the scientific paradigm of medical education and training. Unless the physician has undergone additional training in a nonmedical,

---

1. The International Society for the Study of Subtle Energies and Energy Medicine (ISSSEEM) is an interdisciplinary organization for the study of energetic and informational interactions with the human psyche and physiology (either enhancing or perturbing healthy homeostasis). They publish a newsletter known as *Bridges* and an interdisciplinary scientific journal called *Subtle Energies*. Their address can be found on page *381* of this book, under *Referrals and Educational Information.*

2. The Center for Frontier Sciences publishes a quarterly journal entitled *Frontier Perspectives*. Their address is Temple University, Ritter Hall 003-00, Philadelphia, PA 19122. Telephone (215) 787-8487, Fax (215) 782-5553.

holistic practice, competency may be sacrificed by seeking to receive both kinds of services (medical and holistic) from the same individual.

If holistic practices are viewed in terms of nourishing and balancing vital energy, they do not conflict with the scope of medical practice, which reserves medical functions to licensed physicians. The "Unlawful Practice of Medicine" is defined in the California Medical Practices Act, Section 2052 of the *California Business and Professions Code,* as:

> Any person who practices or attempts to practice, or who advertises or holds himself out as practicing, any system, or mode of treating the sick or afflicted in this state, or who diagnoses or treats, operates on, or prescribes for any ailment, blemish, deformity, disease, disfigurement, disorder, injury, or other mental or physical condition of any person, without having at the time of so doing a valid, unrevoked, certificate as provided for in this chapter, or without being authorized to perform such act pursuant to a certificate obtained in accordance with other provision of law, is guilty of a misdemeanor.

Similarly, Section 2903 of the *California Business and Professions Code,* known as the Psychology Licensing Law, defines the "Practice of Psychology":

> No person may engage in the practice of psychology, or represent himself to be a psychologist, without a license granted under this chapter, except as otherwise provided in this chapter. The practice of psychology is defined as rendering or offering to render for a fee to individuals, groups, organizations, or the public any psychological service involving the application of psychological principles, methods, and procedures of understanding, predicting, and influencing behavior, such as the principles pertaining to learning, perception, motivation, emotions, and interpersonal relationships; and the methods and procedures of interviewing, counseling, psychotherapy, behavior modification, and hypnosis; and of constructing, administering, and interpreting tests of mental abilities, aptitudes, interests, attitudes, personality characteristics, emotions, and motivations.

> The application of such principles and methods includes, but is not restricted to: diagnosis, prevention, treatment, and amelioration of psychological problems and emotional and mental disorders of individuals and groups.

> Psychotherapy within the meaning of this chapter means the use of psychological methods in a professional relationship to assist a person or persons to acquire greater human effectiveness or to modify feelings, conditions, attitudes and behavior which are emotionally, intellectually, or socially ineffectual or maladjustive.

Thus the law does not prohibit people from choosing any health practice; it only defines what services must be provided by licensed practitioners. Keep in mind that holistic practices are best considered as adjunctive to medical care, not a part of the medical treatment regimen, and ancillary to licensed services.

The precise context for the practice of phototherapy will await future research and legal decisions regarding professional and paraprofessional role definitions. This may take years to define, judging from the example of full spectrum light research on SAD, which took nearly a decade of quality medical research for physicians to begin to achieve professional acceptance. Although years of controlled research still needs to be conducted (particularly for colored light phototherapy), at this early point it appears that both full spectrum white light and colored light phototherapy may have broad potential applications (yet to be determined) within both frameworks, medical and holistic, of health practice.

For colored light phototherapy to become a recognized part of medical practice may require a decade or more of outcome research. However, at this point in time colored light phototherapy with the Lumatron™ (Photron™) fits within the **Food and Drug Administration** category (Class II) of experimental nonmedical interventions, limited for sale to licensed health care practitioners.

Optometrist Dr. Samuel Berne, in his recent book *Creating a Personal Vision: A Mind/ Body Guide to Better Eyesight* (Santa Fe, NM: Color Stone Press, 1994), states his belief that colored light phototherapy affects the organs indirectly by working on an energetic level. It is possible that colored light phototherapy may be more readily contemplated, both professionally and legally, as within the scope of holistic practice.

Precise categorization may be difficult, as several phototherapy applications may fit in either the medical or holistic category, depending on the licensing of the practitioner and the purpose and context in which phototherapy is used. For example, **Dr. John Downing's** concept of *visual photocurrent* (as measured by the visual field test) may eventually be found appropriate to the medical (optometric, psychological) or the holistic paradigm. An example of a medical use might be for researching the diagnosis and treatment of pathological conditions, whereas a holistic practitioner might use it to balance vital energy. A similar argument could be made for **Dr. Steven Vazquez's** *Brief Strobic Phototherapy.* Future scientific explorations, political discussions, and legal decisions may be needed to clarify the variety of light interventions available in the future.

Light, like food, is ubiquitous. Thus, light therapy, much like nutritional interventions, should not be the sole or monopolistic province of either type of practitioner. Nonetheless, **even if doing phototherapy from the standpoint of a holistic model, it may be important to work in collaboration with a medical doctor, because vital energies may be restored to the point where a regular prescription dosage for a medication may become ineffective, or even harmfully toxic.** An example of this occurred immediately after *Light Years Ahead* author, **Dr. Lee Hartley,** returned from her first series of colored light phototherapy sessions with **Dr. Jacob Liberman.** At that point she visited her internist and needed to have the dosage of her thyroid medicine significantly reduced. Interestingly, the effects of light often bridge both models. For example, Lee's self-reported (holistic) "positive side-effects" of her phototherapy sessions were experienced as a profound positive shift in her energy level and a decrease in muscular tension and pain, both of which were also directly observable as changes in pathology by her (medical) team of physician and chiropractor.

The Integrated Health Contract: Placing Phototherapy in the Appropriate Light

Jerry Green (1982) maintains that quality health care can be obtained through the process of bargaining, rather than through regulatory and professional mandates. Clients need to have a purpose in mind when choosing a health practitioner. By interviewing them before engaging their services, clients can learn about the practitioner's willingness and unique skills which can satisfy their purposes and what is necessary to work with that practitioner. The initial interview of a health professional should be approached as if an adviser were being hired to help implement a plan. Clients may want to shop around and see at least two practitioners to develop clarity regarding a basic plan. The objective of this interview is to reach an agreement regarding basic elements of a plan that defines complementary responsibilities and assists in fulfilling the client's purposes. For example, if the client's primary purpose is to seek diagnosis and treatment of pathology for a severe back problem, they should seek the services of a physician regarding the diagnosis of tissue or structural damage and to receive advice about medical treatments. The client may also want to learn how to reverse the patterns of accumulating tension from a holistic practitioner, such as with colored light phototherapy.

The health care contract is a verbal agreement. Its terms may be implied or expressed written agreements. Express terms need not be in writing to be recognized legally. They may be evidenced in clinical notes, such as in the following *Health Provider's Record of a Preliminary Plan For Medical and Holistic Services.*

The purpose of an integrated, two-part health care contract (plan) is to take into consideration the needs of both practitioner and patient (client) to deal with any concern about pathology separately from any desired plan to nourish, stimulate, and balance the vital energy through a holistic modality. The health plan provides a framework for allocating responsibility between doctors, patients, holistic practitioners, and clients; and it considers the potential need for both medical and holistic services. In this format both parties must clarify their purpose for working together and define their complementary — individual and mutual — responsibilities. This type of decision making gives overt expression to the desires, values, and preferences of consumers while respecting the skills, abilities, and preferences of physicians for assuming responsibility.

The first and most important task for either type of practitioner in the formulation of the health plan is to determine, during the initial intake interview, the client's need for medical services. This includes any questions and concerns regarding the diagnosis or treatment of pathological conditions. The second part of a health contract is to determine what health care interests might be approached from a holistic perspective (e.g., health promotion and the balancing and stimulation of vital energy). There is a time and place for both types of interventions. Understanding the scope of this spectrum of services and the nature of skills required can be negotiated so as to meet both parties' needs and desires at any particular point in time. Consider the following questions found in the **Application For Holistic Services** and the **Health Provider's Record of a Preliminary Plan for Medical and Holistic Services**.[1,2]

The biography of light is like a rainbow; a complex harmony of many features that weaves together the rigorous figures of natural law and the changing human soul to create a transient appearance of colors. The sun low at one's back can write into the mist before us the text of two majestic bows — one the Lord's and the second, Satan's — separated by a chasm of darkness. Graceful pink arcs work their way into the light-filled space beneath the brighter primary bow. The unpretentious intricacy of the rainbow easily becomes a metaphor for human life. The mythic and scientific mingle still within us.

— *Dr. Arthur Zajonc*
CATCHING THE LIGHT: THE ENTWINED HISTORY OF LIGHT AND MIND

---

1. Both forms are based on content from Jerry A. Green's *Holistic Practice Forum*, a two-part independent study program in health decision making and role clarification for physicians and holistic health practitioners that includes sample clinical forms and professional telephone consultation).
2. For a list of professional articles by Jerry A. Green, *see Bibliography: Section 11, The Business of Light.*

Intake Application For Holistic Services:

In order to prepare for an informed choice of health care services of a non-medical nature, you must first evaluate your need for the diagnosis and treatment of any medical condition such as a disease, injury, or other pathological mental or physical condition. I can help you learn the differences between medical conditions and the dynamics of balancing vital energy through colored light phototherapy, which works with health factors which are within your control and are therefore not really amenable to medical treatment. You may elect to consult a physician prior to engaging in this work, work with a doctor concurrently, or you may decide that your concern is insufficient to warrant seeing a physician at this time.

Clients often ask about medical conditions. You are more vulnerable to developing pathological conditions (i.e., illness, injury, disease) when energy imbalances persist for extended periods. However, an energy imbalance does not necessarily suggest the existence of a medical condition. Also, healing or recovery from an illness or injury is facilitated by balancing vital energy, which can be initiated with or without medical diagnosis or treatment.

Because I am neither trained nor licensed to diagnose or treat medical conditions, I ask that you answer the following questions so that we can discuss your need for medical services and clarify the scope of professional services which I can offer you.

1. Does the diagnosis or treatment of any medical condition (i.e., illness, injury, disease, or other mental or physical condition) concern you? Please explain here:

    _____

    _____

    _____

2. Describe any concern about your health in terms of patterns of behavior or imbalances you experience on physical, emotional, mental, or energetic levels:

    _____

    _____

    _____

_____   _____
Date   Applicant

Health Provider's Record of a
Preliminary Plan for Medical and Holistic Services

Client's Name:_____ Date:_____

1. Plan Regarding Pathology

- ☐ Client to receive advice regarding diagnosis, prognosis, and treatment alternatives.
- ☐ Client to obtain services for monitoring a recognized pathological condition during a period of changing lifestyle patterns.
- ☐ Client to receive optometric or psychological diagnosis and treatment.
- ☐ Client to receive medical diagnosis and treatment.
- ☐ Client to receive above services as follows:

The above services will be obtained on (date)_____by

Doctor: _____ (M.D., D.O., O.D., Ph.D., etc.)

Address:_____

Phone:_____

- ☐ Client's concern is insufficient to warrant referral to a medical doctor (optometrist, psychologist, etc.) at this time. Client has agreed to communicate any increase in concern. Practitioner is satisfied that client's choice is not unreasonable.
- ☐ Client has made the above choice(s) after discussing each of the alternatives and its implications.

2. Plan Regarding Vital Energy

   A. Nature of imbalances (adaptations made for experimental phototherapy use):

- ☐ Visual Field Test Results_____
- ☐ Photosensitivity Assessment (see Vazquez *Chapter Three*):_____
- ☐ Stress Management: _____
- ☐ Cognitive/Emotional Patterns: _____
- ☐ Physical Tension Patterns: _____
- ☐ Other: (e.g., dietary and nutritional, etc.): _____

   B. Client's Responsibility

- ☐ Home Phototherapy:_____
- ☐ Vision Exercises:_____
- ☐ Stress Reduction Diary:_____
- ☐ Diet, Nutritional, Exercise Changes: _____
- ☐ Awareness Journal:_____
- ☐ Behavioral Changes:_____

   C. Time Frame and Frequency

      _____Weeks(s)/Month(s): _____Estimated Visits: _____

3. Financial Arrangement:_____

Additional Considerations For Health Plans With Colored Light Phototherapy:

1. Inform clients of the potential risk of colored light to elicit a "healing crisis."

Holistic approaches, such as colored light phototherapy, may promote an aggravation of experiences which are seen as symptoms of pathology by medical model practitioners. These experiences can sometimes be expressions of healing known in the holistic model as a *healing crisis,* or feeling worse before feeling better. Several authors in this book describe the potential for colored light through the eyes to precipitate an exacerbation of previous mindbody symptoms on the way to healing. Dr. Jacob Liberman notes that patients' unfavorable reactions to certain colors of light through the eyes are tantamount to an "allergy to these particular colors," a reaction he believes is associated with unresolved emotional experiences. For example, during a course of this type of phototherapy certain memories and strong emotions may surface and create a state of temporary discomfort which typically diminishes as the material is brought to conscious awareness, verbalized, abreacted, and worked through.

In the process of seeing old unconscious patterns, we may re-awaken memories, emotions, or experiences that were too painful for us to look at at the time . . . In terms of our awareness, there is an outer vision — how we see the world — and an inner vision — how we see ourselves. The clearer we can see inside ourselves, without denial, the clearer our outer vision will become. Light seems to be able to cut through the roadblocks and resistances we have set up; such as, ego, personality, and the rational mind — and helps us discover unconscious patterns about ourselves. It is as though light fills up all the dark places of the inner vision. When we look at light, what we see is a clear mirror of ourselves.

— Dr. Samuel Berne

The following *Client Information on Healing Crisis* is based on a client information sheet from Holistic Practice Forum (Medical Decisionmaking Institute), adapted for healing crisis in homeopathy, and a written agreement to participate in experimental colored light phototherapy by Dr. Steven Vazquez.

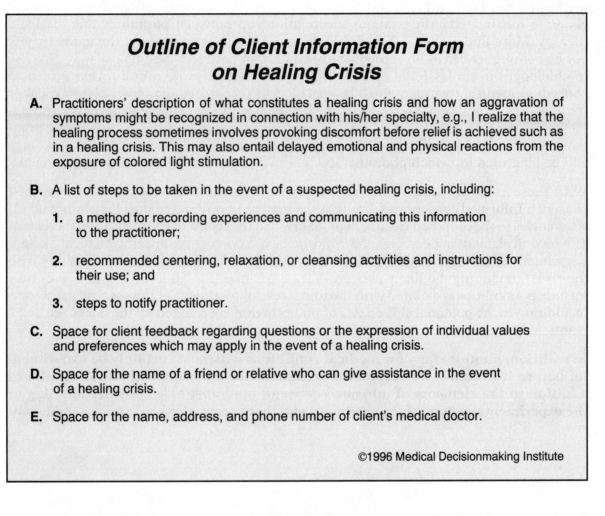

Outline of Client Information Form on Healing Crisis

A. Practitioners' description of what constitutes a healing crisis and how an aggravation of symptoms might be recognized in connection with his/her specialty, e.g., I realize that the healing process sometimes involves provoking discomfort before relief is achieved such as in a healing crisis. This may also entail delayed emotional and physical reactions from the exposure of colored light stimulation.

B. A list of steps to be taken in the event of a suspected healing crisis, including:

   1. a method for recording experiences and communicating this information to the practitioner;

   2. recommended centering, relaxation, or cleansing activities and instructions for their use; and

   3. steps to notify practitioner.

C. Space for client feedback regarding questions or the expression of individual values and preferences which may apply in the event of a healing crisis.

D. Space for the name of a friend or relative who can give assistance in the event of a healing crisis.

E. Space for the name, address, and phone number of client's medical doctor.

©1996 Medical Decisionmaking Institute

2. Practitioner and client both need to acknowledge potential risks of experimental procedures and potential negative reactions from phototherapy.

Keep in mind that colored light therapy is an *experimental* procedure not yet proven by large scale controlled research. Although light stimulation devices are generally safe, potential hazards may exist. In more than sixty years of using colored light and over ten years of using full spectrum light phototherapy, there have been no documented severe side effects following light therapy. Although the editors and authors strongly believe that light is "the medicine of the future," and perhaps one of the most powerful tools for mind-body transformation, we offer the following words to the wise: Light is a very potent intervention and must be used cautiously and with professional guidance. Light, similar to any medicine, requires an optimum "dosage" (light intensity, exposure duration, wavelength, etc.); and you can actually "overexpose" yourself to light. The potential negative effects from phototherapy are listed in a chart on page xlix.

Consent to Treatment with Phototherapy in a Medical Setting

The consent to treatment with phototherapy in a medical setting presents a number of conceptual and methodological questions. To the extent that the efficacy of phototherapy is best understood as a modality for balancing, nourishing, or stimulating vital energy, its use as treatment for medical conditions may represent a misapplication of resources and generate misunderstandings about the relationship between pathology and vitalistic therapy. More importantly for medically licensed health practitioners, the modality will not be comprehended as an "accepted or standard of practice;" and its use may give rise to challenges to professional responsibility. One must also be mindful that informed consent to medical treatment must be specific to a recognized diagnosis of a medical or "pathological" condition, and most medical conditions have existing or recognized treatments. So the first question is whether phototherapy might become seen as a new treatment for an existing medical condition, or whether a new medical concept of pathology will be identified for which phototherapy is seen as a potentially meaningful treatment.

With these considerations in mind, we can outline the basic elements of informed consent[1]. Informed consent requires that the patient be advised of the (1) risks of and (2) alternatives to the proposed treatment modality, and that consent be freely given thereafter. The second element underscores the importance of knowing the specific medical diagnosis, which will tell us the existing medical treatments which must be advised (along with the risks), including the likely prognosis if no treatment is undertaken. The risks may include possibilities associated with the unsuccessful treatment of the specific pathology, in addition to the potential side effects of phototherapy mentioned on the next page, (e.g., emotional instability and aggravation of symptoms healing crisis, etc.).

In addition, phototherapy for medical conditions will most certainly be experimental before it becomes an acceptable treatment for a recognized pathology. So in addition to the elements of informed consent, one must also consider advising of the experimental nature of the treatment and that expectations of cure are unknown.

A new idea is first condemned as ridiculous and then dismissed as trivial, until finally, it becomes what everybody knows.

— William James

---

1. Informed consent is a concept that refers to a verbal dialog between physician and patient that is usually documented in writing.

Potential Negative Reactions from Phototherapy:

1. Full spectrum (bright) fluorescent light
The side effects at this point in time appear to be minimal and infrequent and stop when phototherapy is discontinued: *agitation, insomnia, hypomania.*

2. Red end of the spectrum light and low frequency strobe flicker rates.
The use of low frequency (below 12 Hz) flicker rates of colored light, particularly from the red end of the spectrum (red, orange, and yellow) can lead to the precipitous release of powerful, subconscious, repressed memories, and their emotional sequelae, such as: *grief, rage, anxiety,* and *fear.* Healing crises are typically temporary, yet appropriate clinical supervision is essential for those suffering severe emotional disturbances. If you are not licensed or trained to handle these reactions, seek professional mental health consultation.

3. Blue end of the spectrum light
Light from the blue end of the spectrum is generally much less evocative than light from the red end of the spectrum. Nonetheless, Dr. John Downing warns against unsupervised use of these frequencies in individuals with a history of *depression* or *fatigue,* as it can accentuate these symptoms.

4. Photoconvulsive seizure activity
There is a very remote possibility (approximately one in 2,850 patients) that the use of flashing lights (strobic light) within both ends of the spectrum between 15-20 Hz can induce seizures in those prone to *photoconvulsive epilepsy.* Intake interviews should routinely inquire about history of both epilepsy and photosensitive seizures.[1]

5. UV light
There is a potential for harm with prolonged exposure to certain wavelengths of ultraviolet light, especially doing unsupervised light therapy in tanning salons. Ultraviolet light is an intense form of intervention, and more in-depth research is clearly required to know its beneficial and unfavorable effects. There are documented cases of skin cancer by prolonged, inappropriate exposure to ultraviolet light in tanning salons. However, there are some associated with professionals and photobiologists who maintain we have a "minimum daily requirement" for ultraviolet and sunlight exposure in the appropriate frequency range and dosage. Skin cancer is on the rise as the ozone layer is on the decline. This is reflected by the title of an article in a recent medical journal, "New Sun, New Dermatology."

6. Electromagnetic field (EMF) Radiation from older light devices
There are documented toxic effects of prolonged exposure to high levels (greater than 2.0 milligauss) of electromagnetic fields (EMF) that emanate from electrical appliances, such as: computers, televisions, fax machines, car phones, microwave ovens and yes, even phototherapy instruments such as older full spectrum light boxes (equipped with older ballast versus newer electronic switches.) Preliminary research hints at a possible connection between EMF exposure and deleterious effects on the immune and neuromuscular systems.

Similar to the precautionary recommendation to sit two to three feet from computer screens, the same or greater distance may be necessary for certain older phototherapy devices. As part of consumer protection, manufacturers of these devices should publish this very relevant electromagnetic field data.

---

1. Dr. Downing's discussion on photoconvulsive epilepsy is found on *page xix* of the *Cautions and Concerns Regarding Phototherapy,* and *First Aid Recommendations for Convulsive Seizures* are found in Dr. Downing's chapter, on page *160.*

Outline of Potential Informed Consent to Experimental Treatment with Phototherapy

Although light stimulation devices used here are generally safe, I understand that there may be risks associated with their use. Since light stimulation devices for the treatment of medical conditions are experimental, no claims or guarantees about their effectiveness as treatment for my condition can be made.

I understand the recognized treatment alternatives for my condition, which are:

_____

consist of the following:

_____

Each of these treatments present the following risks and represent the following potential benefits:

_____

_____

_____

The risks of employing phototherapy as an experimental treatment for my condition, given the dimensions of my current health status and my existing sensitivities, are known to include the following:

_____

_____

_____

I have had a reasonable opportunity to review the above and discuss any questions I might have with my doctor, and my consent to treatment with phototherapy is given freely and voluntarily, without inducements.

Dated:_____

(Patient's Signature)

Our deepest fear is not that we are inadequate.
Our deepest fear
is that we are powerful beyond measure.
It is our light, not our darkness,
that most frightens us.
We ask ourselves, who am I to be brilliant, gorgeous,
talented and fabulous?
Actually who are we not to be?
You are a child of God.
Your playing small doesn't serve the world.
There is nothing enlightened about shrinking
so that other people
won't feel insecure around you.
We are all meant to shine as children do.
We were born to make manifest
the glory of God that is within us.
It's not just in some of us; it's in everyone.
And when we let our own light shine,
we unconsciously give other people
permission to do the same.
As we are liberated from our own fear,
our presence automatically liberates others.

—*Marianne Williamson*

A RETURN TO LOVE: REFLECTIONS ON THE
PRINCIPLES OF A COURSE IN MIRACLES

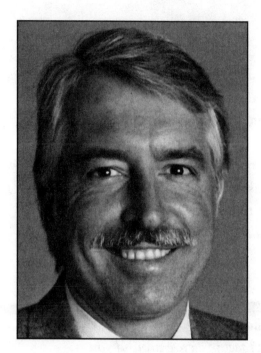

Brian Breiling, Psy.D.

*D*r. Brian Breiling is a body-centered Marriage and Family Therapist who specializes in somatic approaches to the treatment of depression, anxiety, phobias, post traumatic stress disorders, chemical dependency, and adults recovering from physical, emotional and/or sexual abuse. Dr. Breiling is also certified to practice massage therapy, Reiki, hypnosis, biofeedback, and school psychology. His work develops people's mindfulness of physical and subtle energy blockages, using Lumatron™ light-assisted psychotherapy and an eclectic variety of interventions to uncover and release the unconscious "story" behind the mindbody problem. He received his doctorate in Clinical Psychology from the California Institute of Integral Studies in San Francisco. He is in private practice in Tiburon, California. Dr. Breiling, along with Dr. Hartley are the co-founders of *Light Years Ahead Productions* and were co-creators of *The Light Years Ahead Conference,* on which this book is based. He and Bethany ArgIsle are co-editors of this book.

Introduction:
Light Years Ahead

Brian Breiling, Psy.D.

Light From Whom All Blessings Flow . . .

We have not yet assimilated this century's most far-reaching discovery: namely, that energy, or light, is the principle underlying all manifestation. In other words, we have not yet grasped that we, our bodies and our minds, are light.

GEORG FEUERSTEIN,
FROM FOREWORD OF JUDITH CORNELL'S BOOK,
DRAWING THE LIGHT FROM WITHIN

Today we stand on the brink of a new mindbody medicine, where the established materialistic medical paradigm based on the concepts of Newtonian physics is giving way to principles and practices derived from modern quantum theory.[1]

Far from being merely metaphysical "wishful thinking," the very theoretical foundation of quantum physics suggests that at the deepest level of subatomic reality, light is, indeed, the "fabric" of which we are made.

Quantum physics is one hundred years ahead of much of medical science. Its descriptions of reality on the subatomic level and at the level of galaxies are all quite similar; these are views of reality that even have a mystical quality. Interestingly, the reality described by quantum physicists is strikingly similar to the world view and energetic concepts of

---

1. According to quantum theory, matter is comprised of a series of highly complex energy fields. The solidity of physical reality at the macrocosmic level dramatically transforms when one explores the realms of subatomic particle physics. At the deepest levels of microcosmic reality, the atom consists mostly of empty space. At this level all matter is a form of frozen light energy. The word "quantum" is a term in physics meaning "an indivisible unit of energy," such as that found in photons (which is a quantum of electromagnetic energy: i.e., light). Quantum physics is the scientific exploration of models of reality based on the works of Albert Einstein and high particle physics. For more information see Richard Gerber, M.D., *Vibrational Medicine: New Choices for Healing Ourselves*, (Santa Fe, New Mexico: Bear & Company, 1988).

traditional Chinese medicine (i.e., acupuncture and five element theory) and traditional Hindu medicine (known as *ayurveda* — meaning the science of health), concepts which are thousands of years old.

I believe light and phototherapy are the fulcrum of this interface between mind-body medicine and subtle energy healing. Perhaps we are expanding our notions of who and what human beings are from that of *Homo sapiens* to **Photo sapiens** — literally, **"the wise, intelligent knowers of the light."**

Sunlight is one of the most pleasurable, joyful, energizing, and omnipresent blessings in our lives. The radiant energy of the sun is the major source of vitality and power for every organism on the planet. Our species has evolved and thrived under the entire color spectrum of natural sunlight, thus, we are genetically programmed to respond to these specific frequencies of light. Yet, since the Industrial Revolution we have moved our activities inside which creates working and living conditions that keep us away from this life-giving source of energy.

Dr. George (Bud) Brainard, an investigator of light's medical applications, believes that the majority of our indoor lighting is grossly inadequate for our biological requirements. Not only is it not bright enough, but it merely gives us the color of light found typically at five in the afternoon. He suggests that our indoor environments are like working and living in the "Twilight Zone." Today the negative effects of our indoor life-styles are being further compounded by wearing tinted eyeglasses and contact lenses, as well as having tinted windshields and windows that filter out important elements of the spectrum (such as certain ultraviolet frequencies), elements that are prerequisites for the healthy functioning of our minds and bodies. Experts have gone as far as suggesting that **many of us, most of the time, and particularly in the dreary low-light seasons, are actually "starving for light."** This is what I describe as *photophilia* or *chromophilia*, a hypothetical deficiency state in which we may be literally driven to get the appropriate quantity (intensity) and quality (color) of light. A lack of light, both natural sunlight and full spectrum artificial light, can lead to a variety of mindbody imbalances, stress symptoms, hyperactivity, illness, depression, fatigue, and mental inefficiency.

Light is one of our most basic forms of nutrition. Because 90% of the population spends the majority of their time indoors, most of us may be suffering from what **light researcher Dr. Michael Terman,** refers to as *malillumination syndrome.* Similar to the need for vitamins and minerals, it is likely that each of us has our own "minimum daily requirement" for particular light frequencies, or colors. **Our requirements for sunlight or for artificial full spectrum or colored light probably vary according to our mood, the season of the year, our constitutional type, and our overall level of health and vitality.**

> *If our senses conveyed the whole truth to us, we would see the Earth as rivers and glaciers of electrons, each speck of dust as a rolling mass of light.*
>
> — *Paramahansa Yogananda*

Are We Light Starved?

THE PROBLEM: a lack of natural sunlight can lead to ill health with a variety of mental, emotional, and physical symptoms.

THE CAUSES OF LIGHT STARVATION: Photophilia and Malillumination

- **Working and living indoors:** Poorly illuminated environments with inappropriate artificial lighting could have serious health implications. For example, most artificial indoor lighting lacks ultraviolet light (UV), which at the proper intensity is essential to the production of vitamin D and the metabolism of calcium.

- **Unhealthy artificial light:** Most indoor lighting lacks the requisite full-range color distribution and the proper intensity to sustain health and certain functions, such as vitamin D and hormone production. Light's effect on human mindbody health has, until recently, been ignored in architecture, design, and engineering. Both fluorescent and incandescent lighting often have uneven color distribution. For example, incandescent lights have lots of Red but are lacking in Green, Blue, and Violet. Furthermore, indoor lighting is generally not bright enough, amounting to only 1/20th the intensity of outdoor light in the shade on a sunny day. The amount of light that we receive from sixteen hours indoors is dramatically less than the amount we receive from a single hour outdoors.

- **Negative lifestyle habits:** Even in sunny California and Florida the average individual receives little sunlight in a 24-hour period. The additional interferences we have, such as tinted sunglasses and contact lenses, tinted car windshields, and tinted windows, don't allow in the health-giving properties of the entire spectrum of light.

- **Seasons/low light conditions:** In winter in the northern hemisphere the onset for winter depression and seasonal affective disorder occurs in late fall and peaks in February. (These symptoms usually wane in early spring as the days get longer.)

THE SYMPTOMS OF LIGHT STARVATION:

- **Symptoms of lack of exposure to sunlight:** Scandinavian winters have been associated with a higher incidence of irritability, fatigue, illness, lowered immune functioning, insomnia, hypersomnia, depression, alcoholism, and suicide.

- **Vitamin D deficiency:** Sunlight is crucial to vitamin D production.

- **Calcium deficiency:** Calcium levels are lowest in the low light conditions of winter. Calcium is necessary for the growth of bones and teeth. A lack of calcium is related to such conditions as osteoporosis and osteomalacia, the softening of the bones.

- **Neurotransmitter and neurohormonal deficiencies:** Create a disturbance of bodily rhythms, leading to symptoms such as those seen in seasonal affective disorder or its subclinical form, winter depression, phase shift disorders, and jet lag (with symptoms such as: disturbances in sleep, appetite, or mood).

Light is a Vital Nutrient

BACKGROUND: Light Therapy pioneer, Dr. John Ott, states: "Light is a nutrient much like food, and, like food; the wrong kind can make us ill, and the right kind can keep us well." Humans need light of specific intensity and color range to regulate their internal biological clock. Without it, our daily, monthly and annual rhythms get disrupted.

- Our knowledge of light's effect on the human body is in its infancy; yet, researchers continue to discover the power of light in preventive and therapeutic medicine.

- Light regulates and stabilizes our physiology and emotions.

- Light through the eyes affects the brain and every cell of the body.

- Humans have a biological requirement for ultraviolet light, and it is currently unclear how much we need of the other colors of the spectrum.

- Evidence points to the fact that we could all benefit from a greater supply of natural light, particularly during the winter months.

WHAT LIGHT NOURISHES: Light enables us to see, and it plays several vital roles as it enters our eyes and our skin. Light enters the pineal gland (the body's light meter) via the retina. Its neurotransmitter, melatonin, influences the hypothalamus, which is responsible for controlling many of the endocrine functions that are disturbed in depressed individuals such as, *sleep* and *wakefulness,* reproductive physiology, mood, and the timing of the body's biological clock.

- Sunlight shining on the skin triggers the production of melanin, a dark pigment that protects the surface of the body.

- As UV rays from the sun penetrate the skin's surface layer of **melanin**, the body's supply of **vitamin D** is replenished. Vitamin D is known as the **"Sunshine Vitamin,"** and although vitamin D can be obtained from milk and fish, this form is not as biologically effective as the vitamin D produced by sunlight. **Vitamin D_3** is a skin hormone called **solitrol,** which works in conjunction with the pineal hormone, **melatonin,** to control the body's response to light and darkness. Solitrol works antagonistically with melatonin to produce changes in mood and our 24-hour bodily rhythms, as well as affecting our immune system.

- Vitamin D enters the blood stream and goes to the kidneys and liver where it plays a key role in the absorption of **calcium** from foods, as well as the utilization of the mineral **phosphorus**. Nutritionally oriented physician Dr. Elson Haas states that since vitamin D is intimately related to the metabolism of calcium and phosphorus, it is important to the growth and development of bones and teeth in children. Dr. Haas adds that D3, because of its effect on calcium levels, is important in the maintenance of the nervous system, heart functioning, and blood clotting.

The Light Choice For You:
Lightstyle Changes to Light Up Your Life

EXPOSE YOURSELF TO MORE NATURAL LIGHT

• Spend more time outdoors.

We only need 30 minutes of exposure to spring or summer sunlight to produce adequate daily vitamin D levels.

Each 30 minutes of outdoor exercise on a dreary winter day gives the equivalent of a daily session of phototherapy (the idea being to supplement and not replace phototherapy).

Fair-skinned people can receive regular dosages of sunlight in spring, winter, and fall, and even in summer if exposure time is in the early morning or early evening.

Walking in the morning or afternoon is the best time, when light is the brightest.

• **Winter vacations to sunny destinations** in low latitudes with longer and brighter daylight exposure.

• **Relocate to sunnier winter climes.**

CHANGE INDOOR LIGHTING TO APPROXIMATE NATURAL DAYLIGHT

• **Use full spectrum fluorescent light** in order to optimize activity level and mood. This is the nearest thing to sunlight in terms of spectral distribution and brightness.

• **Use color-corrected incandescent lamps** such as neodymium full spectrum bulbs or spotlights corrected with blue filters.

• Keep in mind UV in the right dosage may be beneficial for health.

REMODEL TO ENCOURAGE MORE NATURAL LIGHT

• **Add non-tinted skylights or windows** that bring in more sunlight.

• **Use light-colored paints and carpets** inside and out to reflect more light inside.

White or cream colored walls, ceilings, and floors reflect 60-70% of the light shined on them.

• **Use mirrors** to reflect more light and also give a sense of spaciousness.

7

TRY LIGHT THERAPY

- **Full Spectrum White Light Phototherapy** is an effective treatment, especially during winter months and in populations who are less able to go outdoors, such as the elderly and infirmed.

Indications: SAD, winter depression, shift work adjustment problems, jet lag, delayed sleep phase disorder. Also appears to be effective in PMS, fatigue, and immune system problems.

- **Colored Light Phototherapy** is effective with a wide variety of disorders and has many experimental applications. Consult the Resource List for a qualified health care professional, such as the various contributors or professionals in the Syntonic School of Optometry.

Indications: See following chart in this chapter, entitled Encouraging Experimental Cases Results With Colored Light Phototherapy.

Why is Light An Important Therapeutic Tool?

Our eyes are actually living photocells that convert light energy into life energy. Pioneering optometrist, **Dr. John Downing, inventor of the Lumatron Ocular Light Stimulator**™, a state-of-the-art color phototherapy device, calls these neurochemical/neuroelectric impulses, *photocurrent*. Light enters the eyes and is transformed into photocurrent, which travels via the optic nerve to the entire brain. In Dr. Downing's discussion in *Chapter Six* he states, **"Light affects every part of the brain and every cell of the body."**

Since we are literally *light beings,* or *photo sapiens,* light added into our systems profoundly changes our physical body and the emotions and attitudes that are held within the body and the subtle energy field. Like moths, we, too, are attracted to light. We seem to have an inherent need for light, as well as a natural love and affinity for color. To coin yet more words, we all seem to be *Photophiliacs* and *Chromophiles*.

For over forty years the pioneering work of **photobiologist, John Ott**, has examined the effect of light on humans, animals, and plants. Animals and plants are healthier, live longer, and grow and produce more under natural versus artificial lighting. Light profoundly impacts our health. Lack of light and harmful radiation from computer screens can lead to eye strain, headaches, and circulation problems, such as blood cells clumping, a condition known as roulade.

Recent light research is beginning to significantly impact the architecture and interior design of public buildings, such as schools, offices, and factories. Full spectrum artificial lighting appears to increase productivity, cognitive efficiency, and immune system functioning, while it also appears to decrease accident rates and absenteeism.

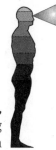

I believe that light is one of the most potent tools for mindbody healing. Light, comprised of both electrical and magnetic energy, may also be the conceptual "missing link" between materialistic medicine and the emerging conceptualizations of quantum healing and subtle energy medicine. The future theory and practice of light medicine could serve to bridge the science of current mindbody medical disciplines such as psycho-neuroimmunology with alternative and traditional medical practices such as homeopathy, acupuncture, and ayurveda.

Within these chapters, you'll see the many uses of light across the spectrum of the healing arts to address a variety of acute and chronic dysfunctions. **Full spectrum white light and colored light have both shown promising therapeutic applications in the fields of optometry, medicine, psychiatry, psychotherapy, chiropractic, acupuncture, and education.**

Dr. Jacob Liberman suggests that light can also be used as a tool for psychospiritual transformation. In effect, "You use the light until you become the light." On this point several of the current authors agree: The combined use of colored light and flash rate "homeopathically," that is, the selection of a color of light that is physically and psycho-logically uncomfortable for the patient, evokes unconscious conflicts and unresolved traumatic memories stored in the body. Psychological and/or physical trauma are often reflected in physical pain and a variety of psychoemotional symptoms.

> *A major key to getting well is becoming comfortable with those aspects of ourselves that were previously uncomfortable.*
> — *Jacob Liberman*

Canadian psychologist, Dr. Warren Hathaway, speaking at the 1992 meeting of the American Psychological Association, stated that **full spectrum lighting in classrooms seems to dramatically affect students' academic achievement, physical development, and overall health and vitality.** His research tracked over 300 ten to twelve-year-olds who were exposed to either energy efficient sodium vapor lamps, traditional cool white fluorescents, or full spectrum lights that were either ultraviolet-enhanced or inhibited. Those students exposed to the full spectrum lights did best overall; they showed greater gains in both height and weight, were absent less often due to illness, and made more rapid academic progress. Also of interest was the observation that those children who were in classrooms that had full spectrum, UV-enhanced lighting also had significantly fewer cavities. A lack of ultraviolet and certain frequencies from the blue end of the spectrum has historically been a hypothesized factor in the onset of SAD. Ultraviolet encourages the skin's production of vitamin D, which may assist the body's calcium absorption, thereby discouraging cavities.[2]

---

2. For more information of the pros and cons of UV light, I refer you to Jacob Liberman's book, *Light: Medicine of the Future,* "UV or Not UV? This is the Question," Santa Fe, New Mexico: Bear & Co.

The authors of **Light Years Ahead** have experienced dramatic successes in treating a wide variety of mindbody conditions with the use of flashing colored light through the eyes. Chiropractor, Dr. Ward Lamb, suggests in *Chapter Nine* that **colored light may also impact the neuromuscular and subtle energy systems when applied directly on the body and simultaneously through the eyes.** A partial list of these authors' clinical experience using colored light phototherapy with a variety of acute and chronic mind-body problems is listed below.

Encouraging Experimental Cases Treated with Colored Light Phototherapy

- Anxiety

- Attention deficit disorder

- Burns

- Depressive disorders (both seasonal and nonseasonal varieties)

- Dissociative disorders

- Dyslexia

- Fatigue and chronic fatigue (CFIDS)

- Food allergies

- Learning problems (attention, concentration, memory, and perceptual processing)

- Hypertension

- Identity disorders

- Immune system problems

- Migraine headaches

- Neuromuscular disorders

- Obsessive thinking

- Pain (both acute and chronic)

- Panic attacks

- Phobias

- Premenstrual symptoms (PMS)

- Post traumatic stress disorder (PTSD) and the abreaction and resolution of traumatic memories

Full spectrum and colored light both appear to have a powerful capacity for regulating and normalizing physiology and emotions. However, light is not a panacea, but a very important part of an integral mindbody healing program, one I believe could benefit everyone. Light researcher Norman Rosenthal, M.D., states, "Light is not a universal mood elevator, but a specific catalytic change agent that is only helpful for certain conditions."

Potential Therapeutic Uses of Colored Light

- To balance the autonomic nervous system

- To regulate neurohormonal and neuroendocrine functioning

- To reveal deeper, underlying musculoskeletal problems in chiropractic

- To balance the subtle energy system

- To enhance depth psychotherapy

- To aid in education and neurological rehabilitation

- To assist in spiritual evolution

What heals us can also harm us if taken improperly in the wrong amounts, wrong types, and at the wrong times. **The theoretical ideal, or *the optimal light treatment*, is a complex issue, one that requires more research and most likely takes into account *the right amount* of light in *the right colors* for *the right person* (considering their particular mindbody problem and constitutional type) at *the right time* of the day and the season of the year.**

Please seek the advice of a competent professional such as those listed in the *Resource Lists, on pages 341-370.*

Too much light can surely burn
Too little light makes me yearn.

—Bethany ArgIsle

Light in Integrative Mindbody Healing: Complementary Medicine

Today, we have the opportunity to design treatment programs for patients and ourselves that sample and combine the very best of health care strategies from around the world. The Europeans have integrated these various health care modalities under the umbrella of **complementary medicine,** believing that each can complement or add to the patient's healing and total well being.

The recent focus of **holistic medicine** is on foods, herbs, and other nutrients as major therapeutic interventions. We are living in a time of a legal and philosophical "turf war" between different approaches to healing, such as the "foodists" versus the "druggists". Gentle self-healing with nutrients, homeopathic remedies, acupuncture, light and more feminine and energetic approaches to healing are in no way incompatible with allopathic medical interventions, such as medication and surgery, and should ideally complement these interventions.

Light is similar to food because it nurtures our mindbody; and light, when used as directed, can be an important adjunctive treatment. Medicine and psychology are also beginning to focus more on health promotion and illness prevention versus disease intervention. Both approaches are necessary within a complementary medicine paradigm.

Integrative mindbody healing is the responsible blending of the rational and scientific with the intuitive. As an informed and responsive health care consumer, it is to your advantage to work in equal partnership with your competent health care professional. Light, both full spectrum and colored, can be an important part of your self-care regimen.

As an informed and "response-able" consumer, please take an "optimistic skeptic's" view of the theory and products offered herein and explore them for yourself. We offer this book to encourage your intelligent exploration beyond the confines of the boundaries of what is currently accepted.

An Historical Perspective of Light Medicine: Back to the Future

Dr. Samuel Pesner gives us a wonderful synopsis of the history and principles of phototherapy in *Chapter Two*. I want to aid your perspective of where we are today in relation to where we have been in the field of phototherapy. Dr. Ward Lamb quips in *Chapter Nine*, "Light Therapy is so old, we're rediscovering it today, thinking its new!" Indeed, color may have been one of the earliest forms of medicine. There is a fascinating history that chronicles the therapeutic use of sunlight and color.

Historically, the Assyrians, Babylonians, and Egyptians all practiced therapeutic sunbathing. Light was purportedly used for thousands of years by the ancient Egyptians and in the healing temples of Greece. Here colors were used therapeutically to heal the sick. Patients were brought into specifically colored rooms. The windows of these healing rooms were covered with special cloths dyed violet, red, blue, green, and so forth. In this way, sunlight entering the room gained important qualities to soothe the mind and heal the body.

For millenia sunlight and color have also played an important role in man's spiritual quest. The ancient Greeks and Romans developed sun and air bathing cults. Highly developed rituals for worshipping the rising sun were integral parts of ancient Nordic and Incan cultures. Our ancestors also associated color with their religions and various spiritual practices, whose purpose was to induce mystical states of awareness. Each god and goddess had a special color which depicted their unique powers and qualities. The architects and clergy of the great cathedrals knew about the effects of colored light on the psyche and spirit, as we see in awe inspiring stained glass windows and the colors used in the celebration of religious rituals during various times of the year and in different seasons.

The association of color and political power continued throughout history. In the Middle Ages in England there were those who were accused and convicted of "color crimes." Only high ranking clergy and the king were allowed to wear purple, and any infringement of this color's use was considered a serious, punishable violation.

Even by today's standards, ancient civilizations were consummate observers of the elements, the seasons, and the colors in nature. They realized how these colors and the seasons of the year affected their well being. Our ancestors spent much more time than we do in nature with the vibrant colors of her elements. They realized the health-giving effects of sunlight and the different healing qualities of different colors of food. The colors of herbs, flowers, and pigments were considered an essential quality for healing. The colors of these plants were believed to correspond to the diseases treated. For example, blood conditions were treated with red flowers and herbs.

Despite light's ubiquitous quality and its long history of use as a healing agent, it was not until the last 120 years that physicians and scientists began to document the effects of light and color. The use of light in modern medicine began in the late 1870s when scientists discovered that sunlight killed bacteria and other microorganisms. The **"Sun Cure,"** the therapeutic exposure to sunlight, was prescribed for diseases as diverse as tuberculosis, cholera, gangrene, diabetes, obesity, chronic gastritis, and hysteria. Some of the earliest medical applications of artificial light occurred in the 1930s in London's Charing Cross Hospital. Here "sunlamps" were used to treat circulatory diseases, such as: anemia, varicose veins, heart disease, and other degenerative disorders.

Some of the first surgical theaters used ultraviolet lights to purify the atmosphere. Physicians found that ultraviolet could reduce air-borne bacteria by 50%. Today dermatologists routinely use small controlled doses of UV to treat herpes and psoriasis, while blue light and full spectrum phototherapy is the treatment of choice for newborns with jaundice.

Dr. Harry Riley Spitler, an optometrist and a physician, is the modern father of the use of colored light phototherapy through the eyes. Interestingly, Spitler's pioneering research on the effects of colored light preceded the rest of the American medical community's investigations on the use of full spectrum light by more than forty years.

13

In 1941 he published his book, *The Syntonic Principle*, outlining his theories on the effects of colored light through the eyes. Since that time Spitler's ideas have influenced a growing international movement of optometrists and other professionals who have successfully treated a wide variety of visual, educational, and mental-emotional problems. Those who follow Spitler's theories and methods of treatment are known as the **College of Syntonic Optometry.**[3]

Not until the early 1980s, with the groundbreaking research of a team of scientists from the **National Institute of Mental Health (N.I.M.H.),** headed by **psychiatrist, Dr. Norman E. Rosenthal,** did modern medicine begin to recognize and examine the effects of full spectrum light on winter depression or seasonal affective disorder (SAD)[4]. Since their early work in the field of light therapy, many other researchers in the U.S., Japan, and Europe have reported that full spectrum light therapy reliably improves the symptoms of SAD and a host of other disorders mentioned above.

Yet it has only been within the last two years that medical researchers have considered colored light therapy as a subject worthy of serious investigation. Before this time all previous phototherapy research conducted by the medical establishment was focused solely upon full spectrum light. Somehow the therapeutic effects of colored light and ultraviolet light were being cast in an "unfavorable light" and not considered within the realm of "respectable science." However, recent medical research by **Dan Oren, M.D., and his colleagues at N.I.M.H.** may be the beginning of a mini-revolution that brings colored light into the "limelight" of more mainstream scientific scrutiny. Dr. Oren's preliminary study found that green light (fluorescent tubes with UV filtered out) is more effective than red light in the treatment of SAD.

Nonetheless, the use of color and colored light has been around for more than one hundred years. **Dinshah Ghadiali is the founder of Spectrochrome, a method of using colored light directly on the body.** In 1948, Dinshah's laboratory was destroyed by FDA agents and his books were ordered to be burned. Unfortunately, it may have taken 45 years for the intellectual prejudice to subside to the point where colored light can, perhaps for the first time, become the subject for adequately controlled clinical investigations.

In all due respect, colored light has somewhat deserved its poor reputation, but it has been "found guilty" mostly by association. Historically there has been a lot of quackery and charlatanism within the field of "Color Therapy" and there is a lot of misinformation in the folklore regarding the supposed effects of different colors.

However, I believe this disrepute is not deserved, insofar as the dedicated optometrists and other clinicians who use colored light following Dr. Spitler's Syntonic Optometric Principles. It is important to note that there is substantial agreement in the works of Dr. Spitler's and Dr. Downing's method, which I very loosely term **"allopathic light treatment**

---

3. See *Resource List: Section Four, The Syntonic School of Optometry Members, page 348.*

4. For an excellent review article on the history and treatment of seasonal affective disorders, the reader is referred to a chapter entitled "Seasonal Affective Disorders" by Norman E. Rosenthal, M.D., and Dan A. Oren, M.D., in *The Handbook of Affective Disorders* (2nd Edition), edited by Eugene Paykel (New York: Churchill-Livingstone, 1992).

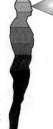

methods" in that they **produce effects opposite from the symptoms treated.** Dr. Liberman's and Dr. Vazquez's contrasting methods, which I term **"homeopathic light treatment methods," tend to temporarily exacerbate or magnify the symptom before it is reduced.** Both methods use colored light phototherapy within a consistent theoretical framework and appear to reliably produce the desired therapeutic results with minimal or no side effects.

In *Chapter Four*, **Dr. Lee Hartley** underscores the idea that **both the homeopathic and the allopathic approaches to colored light therapy can be successfully combined with full spectrum phototherapy to create a positive synergistic effect**. Nonetheless, at this early stage we are still in need of a coherent and unified theory of the therapeutics of light, in all its hues — one that acknowledges and advances the methodologies and mechanisms of action in both the allopathic and the homeopathic approaches to phototherapy.

The ultimate role of colored light in mindbody healing in relation to, and in combination with, full spectrum light will have to await years of carefully controlled research. History and science will be the final judges.

The Light Years Ahead:
The Future of Light Medicine/The Light Age

We are entering a time in history when light is an eminent paradigm. Today, fiberoptics are used as information carriers across the Light Highway. Light is now a way to store information in computers and transfer it almost instantaneously across the globe.

Medicine is burgeoning with new research and applications of light-based technologies. Medical science is discovering more and more ways to use lasers — coherent light — in surgery. Within the field of psychiatry, full spectrum light is earning a much larger role than only the treatment of SAD. It is now being used either alone or with medication to treat a wider range of mental disorders. Oncologists are already using light to augment the effects of chemotherapy in the fight against cancer. Physicians are taking a second look at the promising effects of a fifty-year-old technology, called *photoluminescence*, which uses ultraviolet light to sterilize blood and free it of many different bacteria and viruses.[5]

Light is, indeed, the "medicine of the future." In the conclusion of Dr. Jacob Liberman's bestselling book, *Light: Medicine of the Future,* he contrasts the established materialistic medical paradigm with an emerging model of integral healing and quantum medicine; one in which light technology is united with compassionate and loving professional facilitation, which can lead to the synergistic transformation of body, mind, and spirit.

---

5. For more information on photoluminescence refer to a book by William Campbell Douglass, M.D., entitled: *Into The Light*, which is available from: Second Opinion, P.O. Box 467939, Atlanta, GA 30346-7939.

Addressing this new healing paradigm, Dr. Liberman envisions us entering an **Age of Light,** a future where the use of medications with potent side effects and invasive surgery will be complemented by the noninvasive power of a wide variety of light-based therapeutics. He foresees a time when lasers will increasingly take the place of scalpels; prescription colored light will take the place of prescription medications; chromopuncture, precision fiberoptics, and laser "light needles" will take the place of acupuncture needles; healthy eyes and the ability of *Seeing Beyond 20/20* (to borrow a book title by the **holistic optometrist and vision improvement specialist Dr. Robert-Michael Kaplan),** will take the place of eyeglasses with progressively stronger lens prescriptions; and vibrant "psychosomatic wellness" and healthy longevity will take the place of increasing rates of heart disease, cancer, and chronic degenerative illnesses.

Dr. Liberman also imagines a future where our schools will be transformed from dull, colorless, and poorly illuminated institutions that lack windows and skylights, to inspirational and scintillating learning environments that are colorful and joyful places with ample ambient sunlight and total spectrum lighting. Consequently, our children will be physically healthier, emotionally happier, and intellectually more creative and enthusiastic about learning.

Similarly, he portrays a future where our working environments will be metamorphisized into healing environments, where the business world comes to acknowledge that increased productivity and efficiency can only come from people who are happy, healthy, and enjoy their work. Unhealthy artificial lighting that lacks important spectral characteristics will be replaced by lamps that approximate sunlight. As part of employee wellness promotion, workers will be encouraged to schedule daily sunshine breaks, with adequate skin protection and the appropriate dosage for their constitutional type and the time of year. Doctors will increasingly acknowledge the role that antioxidant rich superfoods, such as spirulina and blue-green algae, play in optimizing our ability to metabolize sunlight.

Further, Dr. Liberman also describes a future in which light-assisted psychotherapy will evolve out of our present-day psychotherapeutic methods, such as traditional analysis, medication, and counseling, which are often aimed at supporting both the suppression and repression of painful memories and the maintenance of the status quo. Instead, traditional ways of emotional healing will be augmented by light therapy methods that are designed to gently bring unresolved emotional issues to the surface in a manner that promotes release and healthy self-expression, as well as the integration and rapid working through of chronically held pain.

I want to briefly mention what I envision as some of the future "megatrends" of light medicine. Holistic physician Dr. Norman Shealy, states in *Chapter Seven* that all illness is essentially related to depression. It is clear that light impacts both mood and immunity in some vaguely understood neurohormonal and neurochemical manner. In addition, almost anything that elevates our mood, including antidepressants or engaging in pleasurable activity, will have an immune-stimulating effect. With the increased interest in psychoneuroimmunology and how the mind can contribute to healing, we are indeed entering a period of "mood medicine." Light therapy in all its colors, in both its

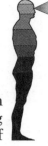

allopathic and homeopathic modes of application, will undoubtedly play a key role in mindbody medicine as we cross into the next millennium. Even as light is currently being used to augment psychiatric and cancer medication, I believe we will discover ways of using light to potentiate and maximize the therapeutic effects of homeopathic remedies, herbs, and other nutritional supplementation.

As the current cost of health care skyrockets, there will be an increasing emphasis on self- healing modalities. Prevention is the only realistic economic choice we have; and phototherapy is not only an effective modality for professional office use, but a powerful self-healing tool that can be used at home.

I also envision a trend towards the increasing synthesis and integration of human knowledge; a blending of the ancient with the modern, the oriental with the occidental, and the scientific with the intuitive. An important part of this synthesis is the integration of the theory and practice of light medicine and quantum physics with traditional psycho-spiritual and subtle energy practices. Every mystical tradition and medical system, with the noteable exception of allopathic medicine, has developed systematic ways to circulate and balance life energy. The nature of light can help bridge the gaps between physics and metaphysics, medicine and spirituality, to give us a practical way to simultaneously accelerate our physical, emotional, and spiritual development.

It is my hope that in the "Light Years Ahead" we take the light and the best of our knowledge of phototherapy into traditional places of "darkness," such as our mental institutions, convalescent hospitals, prisons, homeless shelters, and to people of all ages, races, and social classes whom we have disenfranchised from our hearts.

My Journey Into Light

I am a professional student of the healing arts. In psychology graduate school I had the deserved reputation of being a "workshop junkie" and a recovering "info-maniac." I was always reading the latest books on holistic healing and spending my weekends learning from the latest health guru. I am a "wounded healer," and my passionate search for personal healing has led me on a journey to explore a wide variety of mindbodyspirit approaches that I first used on myself and then later applied in my practice. I feel this search — my real "professional training"— has been mostly guided by forces larger than my personal ego. I feel quite fortunate to have met and studied with Drs. John Downing, Steven Vazquez, Jacob Liberman, and Lee Hartley. My initial encounter with each of these remarkable individuals was "highlighted" by a powerful sense of synchronisity and personal joy — as if I had met an old friend, a true member of my soul family.

My first experience with phototherapy "accidently" came in 1985, when I walked into a local optometrist's office seeking only a replacement for my lost contact lens. This optometrist happened to be phototherapy pioneer Dr. John Downing. After my initial optometric evaluation, John and I talked for over two hours about the work each of us was doing with learning disabled children. I was a school psychologist at that time and was fascinated about using bilateral brainwave biofeedback to assist hyperactive children. John mentioned that colored light therapy could accomplish everything and more than what biofeedback was doing for these children.

I have to admit I was initially ignorant and skeptical about light as a therapeutic modality. As a psychotherapist, I didn't think the eyes had much to do with anything except vision, reading, and movement. This was a prejudice that would take me years of clinical experience to work through, even after I successfully treated many children and adults. **Light is such a simple, yet profound, intervention; one it has taken me nearly a decade of experience to fully appreciate.**

My first experience with phototherapy occurred that same year, as Dr. John Downing's optometric patient. John told me of his 15 years of experience using the Lumatron Ocular Light Stimulator™. People's visual fields increased after a series of two dozen, 20-minute Phototherapy sessions. He suggested I might expect to experience some "positive side effects;" such as: a decreased sensitivity to ambient light; an increase in energy and an increase in such intellectual functions (memory, verbal fluency, and attention concentration), as well as an elevation in my mood. My history was full of difficulties that suggested that I would be a good candidate for **The Downing Technique of Ocular Light Therapy** for such things as chronic winter SAD symptoms that remitted every spring, specific learning disabilities, chronic fatigue, low energy, allergies, and immune system difficulties. By Dr. Downing's criteria I should respond to red light flashed at a rate of 15 cycles per second. I did respond positively and noticed clinically significant improvement in each of these symptoms within a few weeks' time.

Yet, I was a difficult patient. I would miss the requisite five appointments per week for my 20-minute Lumatron™ sessions even though I had noticed benefits after only three or more weekly sessions. **The mindbody effects of light were so incongruous with my previous experience that, at first I denied that light had any real effect — even after I was less fatigued and depressed and had experienced an increase in cognitive functioning (despite my history of learning disabilities)!** I tried to attribute my improvement to other lifestyle changes, such as my diet and exercise program.

Since I wasn't yet sure about light's therapeutic effects, I decided to conduct an experiment. I treated 25 severely learning disabled and multiply handicapped children and several of their parents at a private special education school called The Sky's The Limit in San Rafael, California. **My findings revealed a dramatic increase in the size of all 25 students' color visual fields and a similar reduction in the size of their blindspots, as well as a concomitant increase in scores on standardized tests that measure reading rate, visual-motor coordination, and visual and auditory memory. In addition, there was a decrease in these students' emotionally-inappropriate behaviors as rated by both teachers and parents. I also noticed that these childrens' moods had changed and their overall health, vitality and energy seemed to improve as well.** The inhibited kids had become definitely more expressive and the hyperactive ones had calmed down. Not surprisingly, after the children finished treatments, their parents also wanted light treatments for themselves.

These were pretty impressive results for a small, uncontrolled pilot study. Yet, I still denied that something as simple as light could have such profound effects. It actually took me several more years of exploring a variety of phototherapeutic methods to just begin to comprehend the transformational potential of light in mindbody healing.

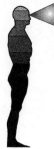

Later I became licensed as a psychotherapist and moved away from my work with the educationally handicapped in the schools. I steered away from phototherapy, even though I experienced it as being a potent tool for children and adults with learning difficulties, because at that time I still did not see light's potential as a psychotherapeutic tool. Then, I re-met Jacob Liberman, and my beliefs about how to work with light really began to shift. As an aside, I initially met Jacob three years earlier through John Downing. The memory of that day is still very clear to me, because what started out as a brief chat turned into an entire day of intense sharing about everything we knew about life, light, and healing. I had had a similar revelation the first time I met another *Light Years Ahead* author, Dr. Ward Lamb. I was profoundly affected by my first and subsequent meetings with each of these individuals.

Three years later I was privileged to attend a workshop put on by Lee Hartley in which Jacob demonstrated a new manner of doing phototherapy (the homeopathic approach) with the Lumatron™. This seemed to accomplish in a few minutes of phototherapy what had taken a few months in more traditional psychotherapy. Both John Downing's and Jacob Liberman's theories and methods of light therapy, as well as their vast wealth of clinical experience, have influenced every single author in this volume. This, in turn, influenced Lee Hartley, Steven Vazquez, and me to begin our experimentation of combining flashing colored light with a wide variety of psychotherapeutic interventions, such as: hypnosis, body oriented psychotherapy, eye movement techniques, and breathwork.

It took me a long time to realize that the eyes are one of the most powerful entry ways into the brain and nervous system and the workings of the psyche. Today I use light-assisted psychotherapy with about 95% of my private practice clients. **My experience using light as a psychotherapist is overwhelmingly positive.** After my long search for personal healing and my exploration of a variety of psychotherapeutic tools, I feel that these methods reliably and consistently work to transform peoples' bodies and minds. **These methods seem to work in a rapid, yet gentle, manner that can increase a client's ability to metabolize emotional experience and move beyond what had previously been troublesome.** I have successfully used these methods as part of ongoing therapy to help people recover and release repressed emotional and physical trauma, such as that encountered with clients who have experienced: incest, physical and emotional abuse, rape, grief, chronic pain, depression, anxiety, panic attacks, and a variety of psychosomatic conditions.

As Dr. Sam Pesner states in *Chapter Two*, "Light will definitely change the way you practice. Light changes lives!" Perhaps you too will contract *photophilia* — an insatiable desire for the light!

Light Years Ahead: The Conference

Light Years Ahead, the book, is based on the first *Light Years Ahead Conference* held in November 1992, in San Jose, California. People from around the world attended this groundbreaking conference that brought together both professionals and lay people interested in the profound healing effects of light through the eyes and on the body. It was a meeting place for the traditional and the nontraditional, an arena where mainstream researchers and a variety of clinicians met and discussed the leading edge in the physics and metaphysics of mindbody healing with light. It felt like history in the making, and there was a definite excitement in the air.

This represented a dream come true for me and my conference Associate Producer, Lee Hartley — a dream conceived ten months earlier while chatting over dinner with our friends and fellow light therapists, Dr. John Downing, an optometrist; Dr. Steven Vazquez, a psychotherapist; and Dr. Ward Lamb, a chiropractor. I casually mentioned my frustration about the lack of networking that prevented the sharing of valuable information and resources in the rapidly expanding field of light therapy. We knew that the medical researchers had their meetings, newsletters, and journals on light research, while the optometrists had theirs. Yet there was no bridge over the chasms of the different philosophical and professional camps. The *Light Years Ahead Conference* built such a bridge; for one weekend we assembled these various light therapy camps under one roof. This was the first time that physicians, optometrists, chiropractors, acupuncturists, psychotherapists, educators, and lay people had an opportunity to dialog, network, and share information related to case histories, clinical approaches, and light technology, as well as speak of their own profound personal experiences with light. *Light Years Ahead* built a community which embraced a variety of professionals and individuals interested in light.[6]

Light Years Ahead: The Book, Its Authors and Subject Matter

Each of the authors in this book brings a unique professional vantage point and a wealth of clinical experience to the field of phototherapy. These individuals are all pioneers in their prospective professions and innovators in both theory and practice. Several of them have invented their own leading edge phototherapy technologies and have enjoyed the "starlight" of international acclaim. We at *Light Years Ahead Productions* believe that these individuals are harbingers of a newly emerging and more enlightened paradigm of mindbody healing.

The professional and legal context for the practice of phototherapy is the subject of the previous chapter written by **Jerry A. Green, J.D.,** and myself. For over 20 years, Jerry has **specialized in medical malpractice and health care licensing. He is the President of Medical Decisionmaking Institute and a pioneer of the health care contract,** which assists medical and non-medical practitioners of alternative or holistic healing modalities to establish themselves within the boundaries of acceptable practice. They discuss the need for practitioners to clearly differentiate between medical (the diagnosis and treatment of pathology) and holistic (stimulating, balancing, and nourishing the vital energies) services, as well as between accepted and experimental modalities in their professional work with phototherapy.

---

6. For more information on light therapy professional training seminars, contact Dr. Lee Hartley of *Light Years Ahead Productions,* listed in the *Resource List: Section One, Light Years Ahead Authors, page 342.*

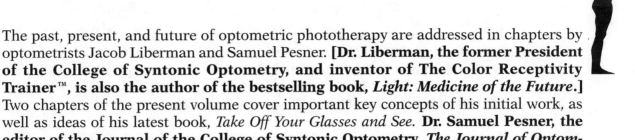

The past, present, and future of optometric phototherapy are addressed in chapters by optometrists Jacob Liberman and Samuel Pesner. **[Dr. Liberman, the former President of the College of Syntonic Optometry, and inventor of The Color Receptivity Trainer™, is also the author of the bestselling book,** *Light: Medicine of the Future.***]** Two chapters of the present volume cover important key concepts of his initial work, as well as ideas of his latest book, *Take Off Your Glasses and See.* **Dr. Samuel Pesner, the editor of the Journal of the College of Syntonic Optometry,** *The Journal of Optometric Phototherapy,* describes the history of light therapy, the early pioneers, and light's theoretical underpinnings from ancient to modern times.

The use of light as a psychotherapeutic tool is addressed by **Steven Vazquez, Ph.D., the originator of Confluent Somatic Psychotherapy and a pioneer in light assisted psychotherapy using the Lumatron™, which he terms Brief Strobic Phototherapy.** His chapter addresses the theory and use of light in depth psychotherapy and dream analysis. A dramatic "live" case demonstration in front of the conference audience highlights the healing potential of Dr. Vazquez's technique. **Lee Hartley, Ed.D., is a psychotherapist who combines both full spectrum, "bright light" photostimulation and colored light-assisted psychotherapy with hypnosis in her clinical practice.** Dr. Hartley's chapter shows how seasonal affective disorder and PMS symptoms often go together and can be successfully treated using these two approaches to phototherapy. Rounding out the section on *Light in Psychotherapy,* **chiropractor and local radio personality Robert Dubin describes his use of the Downing Technique of Ocular Light Stimulation combined with cranial sacral therapy and traditional chiropractic to treat a variety of trauma survivors.** Dr. Dubin presents several fascinating case examples of the successful use of "flashing light therapy" in the treatment of chronic post traumatic stress reactions in Vietnam veterans and auto accident survivors.

The use of phototherapy in chiropractic is discussed by Drs. Ward Lamb and Robert Dubin. **Ward Lamb, D.C., is the innovator of a treatment approach that uses the simultaneous application of light through the eyes and on the body.** Dr. Lamb balances and strengthens his patients' neuromuscular systems by using light to affect the body's core energy or chakra system. Two of Dr. Lamb's patients, whom he refers to as his "courageous recruits," chronicle their journey from the debilitating effects of chronic fatigue syndrome back to vibrant health and well-being with the help of his unique phototherapeutic approach. In a later chapter Dr. Dubin describes the integration, application, and central role of light therapy within the practice of chiropractic and cranial sacral manipulation.

The neurophysiological and neurohormonal effects of Ocular Light Stimulation are the focus of three chapters by Drs. John Downing and Norman Shealy. **Dr. John Downing, founder of The Downing Technique of Ocular Light Stimulation,** has widely disseminated his theories to professionals from around the world. **He is also the inventor of the Lumatron Ocular Light Stimulator™** and the author of a current chapter illustrating with case histories the powerful neurological and clinical effects of Ocular Light Therapy. **Norman Shealy, M.D., Ph.D.,** former neurosurgeon and **founder of the Shealy Institute in Springfield, Missouri, is also the Founding President of the American Holistic Medical Association,** and an internationally recognized expert in the field of mindbody medicine. **The author of numerous professional articles and books,** including *Ninety Days to Self-Health, Occult Medicine Can Save Your Life,* and *The Creation of Health,* Dr. Shealy has recently integrated Ocular Light Therapy into his clinical regimen. He shares with us exciting preliminary research on the neurochemical and neurohormonal effects of Lumatron Ocular Light Stimulation™.

Just before we went to press, it was decided to include two chapters on light in acupuncture. The first chapter is entitled *Colorpuncture and Esogetic Healing.* I believe this new discipline called *Colorpuncture,* **developed in Germany by naturopathic physician Peter Mandel,** is at the forefront of the therapeutic use of light in mindbody healing. The colorpuncture chapter represents the combined efforts of **Dr. Akhila Dass,** a licensed acupuncturist, and her teaching partner, **Manohar Croke,** both of whom studied several years with Dr. Mandel. Dr. Dass and Ms. Croke lead us through several case studies showing the application and potentials of this new technology. The second chapter is entitled *Getting Into Light: The Use of Phototherapy in Everyday Life.* In this chapter **David Olszewski, E.E., I.E.,** with 30 years experience as an electrical and industrial engineer, lecturer and international consultant on the harmful effects of artificial lighting and radiation, presents a scientific and pragmatic understanding of why we should all be concerned with the health effects of the light exposure in our daily environments.

The positive effects of light therapy with educationally handicapped children is the focus of the chapter by **Mary Bolles, the designer of a portable phototherapeutic device known as the Light and Sound Motion Table.** Ms. Bolles' unique approach combines light therapy with simultaneous auditory and vestibular stimulation to dramatically strengthen and organize these childrens' perceptions.

We conclude our book with the section on *Light In Spirituality,* comprised of a presentation by **Jacob Liberman** entitled, *From Light to Enlightenment.* In this inspirational chapter he highlights ideas from his latest book and elucidates the latest paradigms in mindbody healing and the emerging field of quantum medicine.

The Purpose of this Book

Light Years Ahead Productions offers *Light Years Ahead,* the book, as a general primer on the past, present, and future directions in the theory and practice of light therapy. It also contains a *Resource List* for phototherapy practitioners with a wide variety of professional licenses and specializations, light therapy products and their manufacturers, and professional and lay organizations. The *Bibliography* in this volume is a specialized compilation which represents an integral and historical approach which acknowledges the best of physics and medical research, as well as the metaphysics and perennial wisdom related to the application of colored and full spectrum light.

Webster's Dictionary defines science as "knowledge gained through experience." It is in this "light" (of so called "soft science" in contrast to "hard science") that we offer *Light Years Ahead* to inspire and inform the professional and lay communities alike. Even though the "hard" statistical data still needs to be collected, and controlled research still

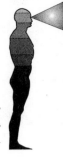

needs to be done, the results of these esteemed clinicians — as well as thousands of other professionals around the world who have used colored light safely and effectively for more than 40 years — cannot be ignored. We hope to encourage the research community to open itself to far wider possibilities for the use of colored light to improve and enhance human health and performance. The types of conditions mentioned in this book represent experimental case studies and are not offered as scientific proof; yet, it is the single case study and the single case "quasi experimental designs" that must predate large scale controlled clinical research.

My purpose in editing this book, as well a co-producing ***The Light Years Ahead Conference,*** is to unite and inspire a "cross pollination" between the various professional and political factions who are currently working with light, including physicians and medical researchers, optometrists, psychotherapists, chiropractors, acupuncturists, and educators. It is my hope that the theories and methods available in these pages will play a key and integral part in the future professional training of these clinicians.

It is also my wish that you use this book and come to know light in all its hues, and better appreciate light's potential for the treatment of a variety of conditions and in the promotion of greater health and well being. I know these chapters will stimulate you to learn more about light's application in integrative mindbody healing and in your area of personal interest or professional expertise.

With great excitement, ***Light Years Ahead Productions*** presents the leading edge work of these luminary clinicians in ***Light Years Ahead.***

> *Knowledge is not but the continually burning up of error to set free the light of truth.*
>
> — *Rabindranath Tagore*

> *Your whole body is light. Light is everywhere and all around you. Every moment God is making you anew, changing your atoms, your cells, and tissues. But your light is covered with darkness by the gross body. So shun your bad habits, be new, pure, perfect and divine.*
>
> — *Paramahansa Hariharananda Giri*

SECTION I

Light In Optometry and Mindbody Healing: Historical and Future Perspectives

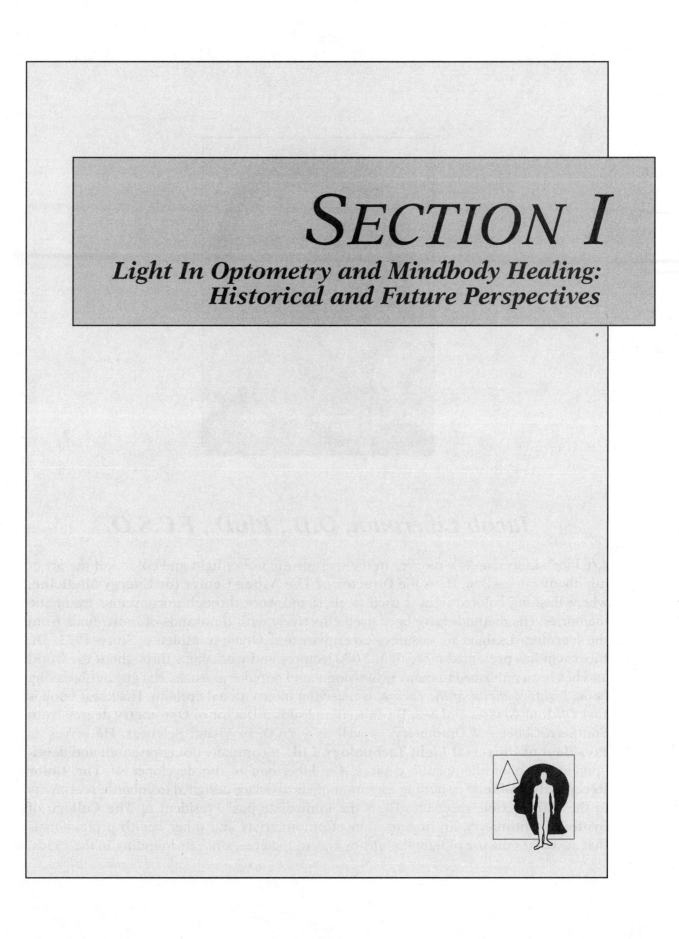

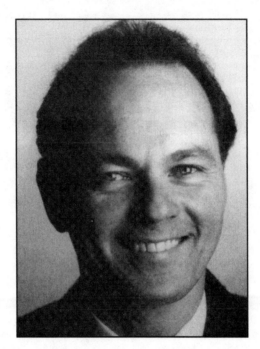

Jacob Liberman, O.D., Ph.D., F.C.S.O.

Dr. Jacob Liberman is a pioneer in the therapeutic use of light and color and the art of mindbody integration. He is the **Director of The Aspen Center for Energy Medicine,** where flashing colored light is used to elicit and work through unconscious traumatic memories. His methods have been used effectively with thousands of individuals from the learning disabled to business executives and Olympic athletes. Since 1973, Dr. Liberman has presented more than 2,000 lectures and workshops throughout the world and has been published in many professional and popular journals. His ground-breaking book, *Light: Medicine of the Future,* is receiving international acclaim. His latest book is *Take Off Your Glasses and See.* Dr. Liberman holds a Doctor of Optometry degree from Southern College of Optometry, as well as a Ph.D. in Vision Sciences. He serves as **President of Universal Light Technology, Ltd.,** a company doing research and development on phototherapeutic devices. Dr. Liberman is the developer of **The Color Receptivity Trainer**™ **,** a cutting edge, non-medical device designed to enhance receptivity to the entire visible spectrum. He is the immediate past President of **The College of Syntonic Optometry,** an organization of optometrists and other health professionals that advocates the use of light therapy by way of the eyes, since its founding in the 1930s.

CHAPTER ONE

Light: Medicine of the Future

Jacob Liberman, O.D., Ph.D., F.C.S.O.

About three weeks ago I was in New Orleans, and one evening I met with Kevin Post, a distributor for the **Ott-Lite®** products. While we were walking and talking about life, Kevin turned to me and said, "So, you use light as therapy, right? You use light for healing?" And I turned to him and said, "Well, Kevin, **you only need to use the light until you see the light.**" And what I found out last night in my conversations with optometrist Dr. Sam Berne[1] is **when you see the light, you have the opportunity to be the light.** And when you "be the light," then there is a whole different aspect of magic that happens.

I would like to share with you some of the things that led me toward the physical utilization of light and some of the revelations that opened up my own inner vision to *see* the light. And then, in *Chapter Twelve*, entitled *From Light To Enlightenment*, we're going to talk about what it means to *see* the light and *be* the light and how that has worked for me personally in the work in which I'm directly involved, in terms of my relationships with individuals in the area of healing.

Goethe, in the middle of his life said, **"Light created the eye as an organ with which to appreciate itself."** And his dying words were, **"Open the second shutter and allow more light to come in."** The second shutter he was speaking of was what some people call the *third eye*, or the *seat of the soul*, the *inner eye*, which is the *pineal organ* as we know it today.

Ken Wilbur talks about **three different eyes**: **1)** *the eye of the flesh, the physical eye;* **2)** *the eye of reason, the mental eye;* and **3)** *the third eye, the contemplative eye,* the eye that Goethe says, "appreciates God."

---

1. A brief description of Dr. Berne's methods of phototherapy and his behavioral optometric methods of vision improvements appear in his latest book, *Creating Your Personal Vision: A Mind-Body Guide for Better Eyesight* (Santa Fe, NM: Color Stone Press, 1994). His address can be found in the *Resource List, Section Two, Lumatron™ Master Practitioners, page 343.*

Having been an optometrist for fourteen years, I knew a lot about the physical eye. I knew a little bit through my own experience about the *eye of reason*. And once in a blue moon I got a chance to experience the *contemplative eye*. **We not only need to integrate our vision to incorporate all of the *three eyes*, as well as opening up the second shutter, but in doing so, we begin to open up our vision in a way that opens up our lives.**

Jonathan Swift said, **"Real vision is the ability to see the invisible."** As we integrate the three eyes, we begin to experience what most people feel is invisible. We now know that most average individuals experience less than one billionth of the stimuli that are present within their environment. My personal experience is that as the *inner eye* opens, as we begin to see what at one time we felt was invisible, we tune into a broader spectrum, not only of the electromagnetic spectrum, but of *subtle energies* that are not even within this electromagnetic spectrum.

It is then that things begin to shift. For me it started in 1973, when I graduated from optometry school. I had been nearsighted and wearing glasses for about ten years; I was on my tenth pair of glasses at the time. Then I went into practice and I was hit with the reality that **the average vision care practice supports people's vision being in constant deterioration, not all practitioners, but the average one**. And it struck me very deeply, because this is what also happened to me. In late 1973, I began doing an experiment on the workings of my mind. At that time I had an idea that the mind was located somewhere within my head. So, if I could find the right button to press in my head, maybe my vision would open up. I began doing things like taking my glasses off, and in the process I realized that a lot of unresolved emotional conflicts kept coming to the surface. At first I thought it was because I took my glasses off that these issues came up. But then I realized that they had been present for a long time, and maybe that was the reason I gave up seeing what I gave up seeing.

My vision began to improve, and I can remember the first time I shared that with a colleague. He said to me, "That's blur interpretation." I had experienced that very same level of invalidation of my feelings and perceptions as a child. I kept doing this experiment and my vision kept opening up. I then began to realize things about our testing methods which are totally absurd.

The eyes are a part of our being. **Shakespeare** said that **"The eyes are the windows of the soul"** — they interrelate with light. The eyes and light are married. So why then, do we do all of our optical testing in the dark?

The eyes have some very interesting aspects. They have an aspect which is the reflection of the part of our mind that analyzes things. We call that *foveal vision, or detail vision.* Then there is an aspect of our vision which reflects the part of our being that feels the environment. This is called our **peripheral vision;** it is the anticipatory, psychic aspect of our sensing system. To me this feeling sense is the most important part of vision.

So, why is it then that when we evaluate someone's vision, we place them in a chair in a darkened room, and we put an instrument in front of their face which totally obliterates the feeling aspect of their vision? Then we give them a pair of glasses where the center of the lens, what we call the *optical center*, is directly in front of the eye. That's the only part of the glass that has the exact prescription, so that any time we look away from the center, we don't see as well.

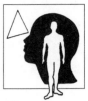

This method is almost a way of "constantly reincarcerating" our vision — to only be the "devil's advocate," to only look for details. However, it eliminates the part of our being that is intuitive and *feels* what is actually going on in the world, the part of us that doesn't have to have it all proven by a double-blind study.

I had some major revelations in the early 1970's about vision. I can remember that my vision kept improving, and when I shared my experience with my senior associate, he said, "Well, let's check your prescription." At that time I was under the illusion that to validate what I was sensing was really so, my prescription had, in fact, to get weaker. I think a real problem was created when we decided we had to prove what we already knew. So for years, I kept checking the prescription and, of course, it only got slightly better. Yet, my vision kept improving. I didn't understand what was really going on with my vision until some time in 1974, when, in the midst of meditating (which I had done since the early 1970s), I had an interesting experience.

The experience I frequently had during meditation was that at times I felt as though I disappeared. I seemed to lose all sense of where I was. And one day I felt this, and I can remember saying, "It feels like I *am* the sky." The reason I described it as becoming the sky is that I felt as though I was seeing from everywhere at the same time. I knew that I was seeing everything, but I couldn't tell you from where. What was important about that revelation is that I realized that **we don't see with our eyes.** The eyes are sensors that take in light; another of these sensors is the skin. But the seeing doesn't happen within the eye, and it doesn't happen within the brain; yet, somehow it seems to happen everywhere at the same time. So the questions in my mind were: "Where are we seeing from? Who is doing the seeing?" I spent years in the process of opening up my vision, and in this process I started seeing things that I never realized existed.

I can remember the first time that I saw the electromagnetic emanation coming off the body, what some people call the *aura*, although back then I didn't know the word. Being a scientist I figured for sure I had a retinal detachment. But I didn't have a retinal detachment, and the experience was very potent for me, because when we see the body giving off light, we begin to understand what our relationship is with the sun and other light-giving bodies. We begin to realize that we are no different than plants, that what we, in fact, call *photosynthesis* in the plant kingdom is probably no different than what we call *metabolism* within our bodies. **We are living photocells.**

The body gives off light, and not only white light, but different colors of light. I didn't understand this until I had a direct experience of it, and presently I've been experiencing this for almost twenty years. I trust my direct experience explicitly. What I realized by noticing that the body gave off light is that the way we interrelate with the sun — the way that we utilize that energy — is the way we either allow it to traverse our being, without in any way controlling it, or the way that we attempt to control it. This then becomes evident in the way that the body re-emanates, re-radiates this light. So, what I'm saying is we think of the sun out there, but we have the opportunity to become the sun.

All of us have seen artists' renderings of great people, be it **Jesus** or **Buddha** or **St. Francis of Assisi,** and many times they're pictured with an *aura,*[2] or with a halo, and I always thought it was something the artist just put in. But after having my own experience of seeing it, I realized that this is what is meant by *to be illumined.* **When I say we**

have the opportunity to become the sun, what I'm saying is that our relationship with light is very crucial to our evolution. This is probably why light is mentioned in regard to evolution, to enlightenment, to being illumined, and so on.

I mentioned before that I had a revelation, a feeling as though I was seeing from everywhere at once, and I came to the conclusion that we don't really see with our eyes. Most people say, "Why, that's impossible! We know that we see with our eyes." Well, if Sam Pesner, who is an optometrist in the front row, took me to his office today and evaluated me, he would find a significantly strong prescription. Yet I haven't worn glasses in sixteen years, and I pass all my driver's tests, and my vision varies between about 20/25 and 20/200 or better. So the question I'm asking is, "Where is it that I'm seeing from?" I only share this experience because **we're in a very important time historically; there are a lot of paradigms that are melting, and crumbling, and the paradigm of how vision works also needs to crumble.** Probably 70% of the individuals in this country wear corrective eyeglasses and, probably more than 90% wear sunglasses, corrective or non-corrective. So all of this led to some very interesting insights in the 1970s when I began utilizing light therapeutically.

I got involved with a group called **The College of Syntonic Optometry.**[3] *Syntonic* comes from the word *syntony* which means "to bring into balance." It was a group of gentlemen who had been involved in this organization that began in the 1920s and was founded by **Dr. Harry Riley Spitler**. Spitler was a man a hundred years ahead of his time. He had four doctorates and he was brilliant! **He came up with an entire system of utilizing light therapeutically, specifically by way of the eyes.** He felt that the light coming in could augment the function of the nervous system and the endocrine system and put the body into balance. I began this work in the 1970s. I used it on my mother and created a miracle within twenty days, which just totally blew me open! I had no idea what to do then. I had discovered something that was magical but I couldn't talk to anybody about it. People already thought that I was somewhat on the fringe, but I had some respectability. But if I was going to start talking about light and seeing auras, I would have been booted out of my profession. So it was a very difficult time for me, coming to these realizations about things that the average person's paradigm didn't yet include. You know, we say that seeing is believing; well, the truth is, if you don't *believe* it, you don't even *see* it. So it's difficult to tell someone about something that is not yet within their concept of reality; there's nowhere to go with it.

I began working in my office, treating a lot of children who had *learning difficulties,* discovering some very interesting things about these children who supposedly had difficulties in school. What I noticed was that they really didn't have that many difficulties, but they were just frightened to be in school.[4] And I remember when I was in school how much I hated it too! Well, not that much has changed; most kids still hate school.

---

2. The aura is an egg-shaped electromagnetic field that surrounds the body. It is composed of frequencies within the electromagnetic (and possibly beyond), color emanations of the subtle energy vortices known as the chakras.

3. See *Resource List: Section Four, College of Syntonic Optometry Members, pages 348-370.*

4. Fear may be the key issue in learning difficulties. For more information see *Chapter Thirteen, page 297:* "Learning Abilities' Dramatic Response to Light, Sound and Motion" by Mary Bolles.

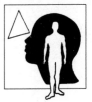

One of the things I know about children is, they know more than we know. You see, they're the next generation and they're a bit more advanced and evolved than we are. They keep trying to tell us things, but we don't listen because we want to be in control. I noticed that when many children are put into — or incarcerated in — what we refer to as learning institutions, which may have very little to do with learning for the most part — a lot of stress develops.

> **These children close down; the way they close down is that the energetic field that surrounds their body collapses, and when it collapses enough, the actual Visual Field — what we measure with a *Campimeter*, or a Visual Field testing device — also collapses**.

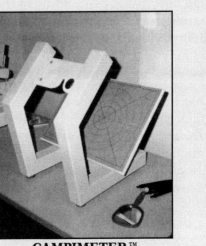

CAMPIMETER ™

So we notice that children who are highly stressed in an academic setting have a visual field which is very tiny. Now, while all of you are looking at me, you're also aware of things happening to the sides. Yet, these children, if they looked at me, may have been able to see only a small part of my face, but they wouldn't have been aware that something was missing, because they had no means of comparison. So, rather than appreciating the world, or their life's experience as a whole, they were experiencing life through a very tiny hole.

The problem is that the field of vision, as I mentioned before, is the feeling aspect of vision or the actual anticipatory part of vision, which allows us to develop relationship. For instance, as I'm looking here, I'm also aware of where I was looking before, and where I will be looking next. You might say that this is the present in relation to the past, in relation to the future. When my visual field collapses so that I'm only in touch with a small piece of the present, I don't know where I am in relation to where I've been, or in relation to where I'm moving. Literally, I'm "lost in space." Many of these children's visual fields collapse even further when this phenomenon occurs.

I noticed early on that light, administered by way of the eyes, seemed to create miraculous enhancement in these situations; it would open up the field of vision. When it did, children would have positive personality changes, physical changes, academic changes, and performance changes. And after awhile, one of the mothers of a child I was treating said, "Well, if you did that with Johnny, how about my migraines?" **I treated her, and three or four weeks later her *migraines*, which she had had for seventeen years, began to dissipate.** When she came back two months

31

later for a progress evaluation, she said, "You know, my migraines are gone, but I forgot to tell you something." I said "What's that?" She said, "Well, before I came to you, I hadn't had my period in a couple of years and within two weeks of the treatment I started getting my *menses* every month, right on time." I said, "Wow, this is very interesting! What's going on here?"

The paradigm kept spreading and I began treating individuals who not only had things such as migraines, but individuals who had been in a *coma*, and even patients who had *multiple strokes*. Some of these patients hadn't spoken for a long time, and then all of a sudden they started speaking. All of these experiences just kept causing me to look deeper. Being a scientist, I needed to understand what I was experiencing. So I began looking at what was really going on.

Now, keep in mind I came from an optometric background and was led to believe that light entered the eye and stimulated the *retina*. It went through the *optic nerve*, to the back of the head, to what we call the *occipital cortex*, the primary visual center or the *striate cortex*. And through some magical means, we saw. However, I wasn't really told much about light. The sun was never mentioned in my education. The only thing we knew about light was that light entered the eye and created something called eyesight or vision. *(See chart on page 134 entitled The Pathways of Photocurrent.)*

The other property I was taught about light was that when it went through a prism, it broke up into its different spectral colors. **Little did I know that humans were physiological prisms, that this invisible energy entered our being and, depending on the way that we used it, either allowed or disallowed the energy to come through. In other words, light was emanated, or re-radiated out energetically through our "other bodies" or** *subtle bodies.*

Now we are beginning to realize that our minds are not confined to our heads, or even to our bodies, but that this physical body is encapsulated by an energetic field which you might call our mind. This energy being received by the body and re-radiated is extremely important. When I began to realize these things, it was over fifteen years ago, and I didn't know much of what I know now.

So I began searching, and I came across a paper written in the late 1800s by a scientist named **Cajal**. In his paper Cajal talks about **his hypothesis that light enters the eye, and aside from going to the centers of the brain having to do with vision, it also touches a part of the brain known as the** *hypothalamus.* Then I looked further; and, in the early 1920s a series of researchers in separate locations seemed to come to the same hypothesis. But it wasn't until the early 1970s that through some very sophisticated scientific techniques we were able to prove conclusively that when light entered the eye, aside from going to the visual centers, it also went to the hypothalamus.

What is the hypothalamus? I came to realize that **the hypothalamus is actually the brain's** *brain.* It's the part of our being that is the major collecting station for all the information from the external environment and from the internal environment, as well as from our psyche. The *stress response* is initiated within the hypothalamus. Many of our *immune functions* are directly sent out, ordered throughout the body from the hypothalamus. The hypothalamus also houses the body's *biological clock*. Just like the watch on

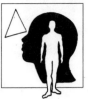

your wrist, the body needs to know when to do what, because all of our life's experiences are cyclic and rhythmic. So a lot of this is handled by the body's biological clock, located within the hypothalamus.

I said, "Wow, this puts light in a much more important position in my life!" I realized that one of the reasons the hypothalamus was so important is that it directly controlled the portion of the nervous system that regulated what was happening within the body, the *autonomic nervous system*. And the hypothalamus also controlled almost all the functions of the body's master gland, the *pituitary*, which affects the functions of the rest of the *endocrine glands*. I said "**Wow, this hypothalamus is 'the CEO' — it's the chairman of the board of the entire body!**"

But then, the scientist inside me said, "Well, who or what is telling the hypothalamus what to do?" And I began looking and I didn't find much. Then I remembered reading in some esoteric texts about the ***pineal,*** which had a whole series of different names. The Greek philosopher **Heroclitus**, in the 4th century, said it was the *sphincter of thought,* or the origin of thought. Indian mystics said it was the *third eye, the eye within* and *the contemplative eye.* **Rene Descartes,** the French philosopher in the 16th century, said that the pineal was the *seat of the soul,* the seat of our consciousness. Science on the other hand, called it the *pineal body,* when we didn't understand what its functions were, if indeed, there were any. Keep in mind that we thought the pineal was a vestigial organ, a mere appendix of the brain. So we called it the pineal body, and then we called it the *pineal gland,* and now within the last ten years, it has graduated; it is now called the *pineal organ.*

What we know about the pineal is that **the pineal is the body's "light meter," it is the body's regulator of regulators**. It regulates everything that's happening in the body, and it's the only part of our being that doesn't receive information from any higher neurological centers. What that means to me is that it's the part of us that's connected to God, — higher energy, energy itself, whoever or whatever that is.

Since the pineal is the body's light meter, it receives information from the environment about light and darkness and spectral characteristics by way of the eyes; it also receives information about the earth's electromagnetic field. I'm sure it receives a lot more information, but that's as much as we can conclusively say right now. All of this is very important, because what we are saying is that it is a part of our being that is receptive to information from the heavens above us (both the qualities of light and darkness), and from the earth beneath our feet. So, it feels as though the pineal gland is the connecting rod between the grounding forces and the heavenly energies. This was my first "glimmer" that the pineal had something to do with this relationship.

As I looked further into how the pineal worked, I was led to believe that light entered the eye, affected the retina, then went to the hypothalamus of the brain, and then the hypothalamus passed this information on to the pineal. **The pineal creates a very interesting hormone called *melatonin,* which is the only hormone in the body that we know of right now that can do anything it wants, anytime it wants, anywhere it wants.** Melatonin is a very powerful hormone that comes into creation from the pineal's relationship with light and darkness, and it is also released because of light and darkness.

So, I came to understand that information was given to the pineal, and the pineal created a messenger hormone which sent that information to every single place in the body without exception. The pineal is basically being told what is happening outside, whether it is light or dark, what time of the year it is, what time of the day it is. The individual cells then use this information to orchestrate their internal function and synchronize themselves with Mother Nature.

In other words, **the pineal is the part of our being that lays the basic foundation for relationship**. This is very important because everything in our life is a function of relationship, the one thing that we know very little about. Recent statistics indicate that less than 50% of all marriages last and, of course, you know we are the only species that has a concept of something called "unemployment," or "exercise," or "vacation." You never see whales on vacation, or trees that are unemployed. Why? My sense is that we are out of appropriate harmonious relationship with our very lives. Maybe this is the reason why our pineals are the size of a pea, whereas, in many animals, the pineal may occupy 50% of their brain at the time they're born. It has something to do with relationship, **and that is a very important thing, because everything in life, everything that happens in terms of health, is a function of relationship.**

My investigation into light, which I just shared with you, seems to be a major foundation for the newly rediscovered field called *phototherapy.* I say "newly rediscovered" because it's not new; it was probably one of the very first healing modalities that we know of. All of the major cultures utilized light. There were people who looked directly into the sun every day and claimed that it would not only heal their physical ailments, but give them the gift of longevity. The Egyptians looked not only into the sun, but at colors as well. They said it would not only heal the body, but it would open up the past memory banks of the observer, almost like a homeopathic remedy. It's as if light would go in and trigger the opening of a part of us that we had kept in the dark. After all, they say we use only 3 to 4% of our intelligence. So what's happening in all those other areas of the brain?

Light has been used for a very long time, expressly for the purpose of healing. I mentioned to you the general usage of light within the field of optometry, called *Syntonics,* where **Spitler's belief was that physical ailments were merely related to an imbalance in the body's autonomic nervous system and endocrine system.** So he said, "If you can put the nervous or endocrine system in balance, you can get the body's health together." Well this was an important step along the way, because prior to that, we looked at the body as a piece of equipment with replaceable parts. People were not looking at the systems underneath that also could have been out of balance. Spitler took the prior work having to do with light a step further.

There's been some tremendous work since the 1970s. **Thomas Dougherty, M.D.,** at **Rosswell Park Memorial Institute**, started working with the idea of utilizing light with certain light-sensitive chemicals in the treatment of *cancer*. In 1972, he started noticing that if he took a certain photosensitive chemical, which he now calls *photofrin,* and injected it into the bloodstream of an individual with cancer, even though the chemical went throughout the body and collected in all the physical tissues, within three days, it began to leave the tissue that was healthy. And it seemed to collect within the tissue that had malignant cells in it. Dougherty found that if he did this with an individual, three days

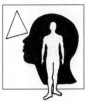

later he could take a **violet** or **ultraviolet light,** shine it on the patient's body and if there was some type of malignant growth somewhere near the skin's surface, that part of the body would fluoresce in response to the light. It would light up and say, "Here I am." **Dougherty then found that if he took red light — now they use laser light *(coherent)*, but at that time he was just using visible, *(noncoherent)* light — and if that light was focused on the spot, within ten minutes the tumor started to self-destruct.** In the last twenty years they've worked on eighteen to twenty different kinds of cancer. It's called *Photodynamic Therapy.*[5] It's done in about seventy to eighty centers within the U.S.A. and Canada right now. The success rate is rather good. I hear that the only side effect is a lot of sensitivity to light for four to six weeks, but they're working on that. Someone also told me that there's some discomfort involved with the treatment, but I have not spoken directly to anyone who's had the treatment, so I don't know yet. **It looks like a very promising possibility for the treatment of cancer.**

I don't particularly like to use light as a drug, and I prefer the use of nonintrusive therapies. **I utilize light as a way of bringing to the surface old unresolved, unexpressed emotional traumas, which I feel are the roots of the weed we call disease.** I'd like to share with you some of the technologies that are presently being utilized in traditional medicine using light.

Dougherty's work has also been utilized by **Lester Matthews** at **Baylor Medical School, Houston, Texas.** He found that if you take a vial of blood, and if that blood has *HIV virus*, or *Hepatitis virus* or *Herpes virus*, and if you inject some of this *photofrin* into the blood, and **run the blood through a clear glass tube and irradiate it with red light, it will knock out 100% of these particular viruses.** Now that doesn't mean that it will eliminate AIDS, because AIDS is not just in the bloodstream; what it does mean, however, is that it is a very nice technology for the sterilization of blood. Therefore, if you have to go into a hospital to get blood, you don't come out with something worse than you went in with. These are just some of the current applications of light.

Another one of the major areas of medicine that has been utilizing light is the area of psychiatry. It has been found within the last dozen years that there is a whole group of individuals that seem to get depressed during the winter time. They call this *seasonal affective disorder (SAD),*[6] when light levels are low and days are shorter. It has been found that if you take light and apply it by way of the eyes, you can trick the brain into thinking the seasons have changed. Initially, the researchers started out with large banks of light, and then they gradually reduced the size of the banks, and increased the wattage of the lights. Now you can actually get light treatment in a pair of glasses that goes on your face,[7] so you can wash your dishes while you're receiving the treatment. If you allow individuals to treat themselves with light every day — originally it was four to six hours, now it could be fifteen to twenty minutes — then, **within three to four days the light can fool the brain into thinking it is no longer winter; it is now spring. Now, the**

---

5. A list of clinical investigators utilizing phototherapy and photofrin in the treatment of cancer is located in the *Resource List: Section Fifteen, Phototherapy for Cancer with Photofrin, page 382.*

6. See *Chapter Four, page 101:* "Make Those Blues Go Away" by Dr. Lee Hartley, for description of light's affect on seasonal affective disorder and PMS.

7. See *Resource List: Section Eight, Full Spectrum Light Products, page 374; Section Nine, Other Phototherapy Instruments, page 376, and Section Eleven, Healing Eyewear, page 378;* for information regarding phototherapy glasses, visors and goggles.

depression and a lot of the symptoms seem to lift, and the person is able to go on with life. This technology is now effective in treating general depression, as well as in dealing with individuals coming off of drug and alcohol dependency. Many of the symptoms of what we call *premenstrual syndrome* **(PMS) can also be alleviated.** In some of the studies patients have been able to reduce the amount of medication they need by up to 90% when it is used in conjunction with light therapy.

There are a lot of interesting technologies having to do with light. I have some different feelings about what's actually going on. **It is not my feeling that** *seasonal affective disorder* **is caused by a lack of light. I think less light is only a catalyst for what is already there emotionally.** I also don't feel that light should be used like a "bandaid on a melanoma." Many of these technologies are effective as tools, but should not be used full time, because then you overlook what is really going on. Unfortunately our medical system has been set up in such a way that the M.D. has become a "Medical Deity." The problem is that they then become responsible for healing us, which means that if they don't, we want to sue them. At the same time, we are disempowered of our ability to take care of our own bodies. We become less and less responsible for taking care of our own health system and our own lives.

We are the remedy. The remedy is not outside of us, and I'm not speaking in just some spiritual, nongrounded sense. **What I am beginning to find is that all disease is the end result of a breakdown in relationship, whether it is relationship within ourselves, between us, with the environment, with the cosmos, or whatever. It is a direct function of the way that we utilize our minds. If the breakdown is within the harmonious, functional relationship, then the cure is to re-create that relationship**.

I'm beginning to understand how the doctor can be the healer, or how the doctor can be the slayer. We think that licensing has to do with what you practice. What I'm beginning to realize is that my license is about giving someone else "the license" to get well. If I can be a living example of what I'm talking about, just by my being very present with another person, I can help facilitate something that happens "magically," and we keep passing on the license to do this. When we do it, they do it; they just seem to get better.

I used to think that it was techniques that would improve one's vision, exercises and so on. Now I get letters and phone calls all the time from people who say, "Gee, you know, I was listening to you sharing your story about your vision, and I noticed that my vision got clear." Now that's called *spontaneous remission*. It doesn't just have to happen with cancer. It happens with everything, as soon as we let go of our old point of view. **If we could just tune in to what we do that creates the** *spontaneous exacerbations* **in our lives, we would have a much greater ability to also notice when that moment of opening occurs and we have spontaneous remission. If we can begin to live that way, then we create a whole field of energy that is supportive of spontaneous remission.** You see, the problem is when I say to someone that my vision has improved, and then the doctor says, "That's impossible," then it is indeed, impossible! So, if I believe him or her (and you know doctors are like gods; that's the way we are brought up), then if I believe them, I take on their concept of reality which eliminates my concept of reality.

Regarding blindness, first of all, there are no blind people. There are people who do not see in the same way as we see, but they are not blind at all. In fact, most of them

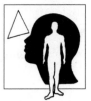

are very "sighted." Spend some time with Ray Charles. What's he seeing that we're not? So, yes, I have worked with individuals who have some limitation in the sight that we think happens in the eye. And sometimes the way I work with these individuals is, I might just go on a walk with them, or I might take them on a guided imagery experience, or what I call an *Open Focus Process,* where I get them to begin to see with their entirety. If you think that you see with your eyes, then it's very, very difficult to shift that paradigm. The way I find that spontaneous remission occurs in the area of vision is by recognizing that we're not totally seeing from our eyes, and we are not only hearing from our ears either. We'll probably find that the areas of mindbody medicine and quantum physics will prove that in the next few years.

What are we actually seeing? We have this illusion that when we look out there, we see something "out there." But what's "out there" is just some dynamically moving little bits of energy that come into existence; they move around, and then they disappear. And my sensors pick up that moving energy, and send that energy to somewhere in "my computer." Then my computer says, "That particular movement of energy means this to me." Next, I take that information and I project it out through this particular projector, onto an invisible screen, and I think that it's "out there." But you're not seeing me, you're seeing you; you're not even hearing me. This information, this vibration coming out of my mouth, is stimulating your eardrum; the information is going into your computer, and somewhere in your computer it's saying, "That particular movement of molecules means this . . . to me." Then I project it out, and I'm fooled, because I think you're saying it, but what you're hearing is yourself, and what you're seeing is yourself. So when you talk about someone who has a limitation in sight, then you have to take a look at who's doing the seeing. **What I find with people who have difficulties in what we call "seeing" is that they have made some aspect of their life's experience "invisible," and if we continue to do that long enough, it will manifest as something on the physical level**.

When we think of malingerers, the truth is we think they're lying. Just like the word *psychosomatic*. I guess it's supposed to mean that the mind or the psyche has something to do with the soma, the body. But what it really means is that we think they're "crazy," they just made it up, and it's all in their imagination. So, we have to switch our language. We don't yet really have a health care system; what we actually have is a sickness care system. It really isn't life insurance; it's death insurance. So, if we don't shift the language, then we have a totally different impression of what's actually going on.

I find that, rather than trying to create a theory and hope that my clinical experience fits my theory, I just notice what happens, and stay away from having to have some theory about what's actually going on. I just notice what's happening and notice how it changes.

QUESTION: What do you feel about eyes that are aging, in relation to your idea?

DR. LIBERMAN: Eyes that are aging, or minds that are aging?

QUESTION: Could be both.

DR. LIBERMAN: Could you be more specific?

QUESTION: Eyesight that fails because the practitioner says, "Well, your muscles are getting weaker, changing, and you don't see . . ."

DR. LIBERMAN: So you're talking about the "my-arms-aren't-long-enough syndrome?" I think that's just part of the same *telepathic agreement field* that we've had about other things. Why do I say that? Well, in 1975, a masseur I went to in Miami, a fellow named Saul, came to me as a patient. Now, I didn't know how old he was; I figured he was in his early 50s, but actually he was 63! He'd been a vegetarian for over twenty years. And he just came in because he liked me and he wanted to show me that he could see better than 20/20 at a distance and better than 20/20 at near without any glasses on at all. So, when I shared that with my colleagues, they said, "Well, you know, it's a mistake; you have to test him again. His pupils were too small." Everybody had a reason to make it an anomaly. **We should study the "healthy anomalies," rather than the pathology.** Then I remember a man I examined in Hawaii once. Interestingly enough, he was another fellow that looked like he was in his 40s. He was also 63 and was on a similar kind of vegetarian diet, a different lifestyle altogether. He didn't seem to step to the beat of the average drum and with him, too, I found this same phenomenon.

Now I'll take you a step further. I have a patient from New York, named Joseph, who came to me last year. He had a lot of *allergies,* sixty or seventy different kinds of *environmental hypersensitivities.* I never had a sense that it was something physical, so I treated him in the way that I usually treat people. He came to me for two weeks. Not only did all of his hypersensitivities disappear, but what was really interesting is that when he came in, he also wanted a vision test. He read perfectly up close and perfectly at a distance, 20/20, no glasses. The question really is, "Where are these people seeing from?" These are the spontaneous remissions. Why should we make them out to be anomalies! We should be studying what's going on here. **I believe it all comes down to being in touch with the self, and in touch with our "belly brain."**

Perhaps I can inspire you to do an experiment on the workings of your own mind. You may then have a similar revelation. As we begin to do that, and as we begin to be brave enough to step out in public and say, "Yes, this is what happened to me; this is my experience . . . when more and more of us begin to do that, then we touch the part of ourselves that has had these experiences all the time. When we begin to shift the paradigm, magic will happen!

Can you imagine how it would be if we had two national registries? One had all of the people on it that were just diagnosed as having some life-threatening illness, and the other one had the names of all

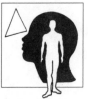

the people on it who were told they had a life-threatening illness and then had a spontaneous remission. Then imagine what would happen if as soon as someone found out that they were supposedly going to die from something, the first thing we did was to couple them with an individual who was told the same thing and was still living. Now, what do you think would happen to the paradigm the moment that happened?

QUESTION: Dr. Liberman, has there been any research on the effect of light with specific diseases such as multiple sclerosis (MS), Parkinson's, or amyotrophic lateral sclerosis (ALS)?

DR. LIBERMAN: **Remember, you're not dealing with diseases; you're dealing with people. You can call it anything you want; it doesn't really make any difference; it's affecting every cell in the body. You can call it any number of different names. When you're right on the money, you'll notice that every single function in the individual will open up simultaneously; everything just opens right up!** So, the way I approach it is, I don't care to have a name for it. It doesn't make any difference anymore. That's more limiting than it is helpful.

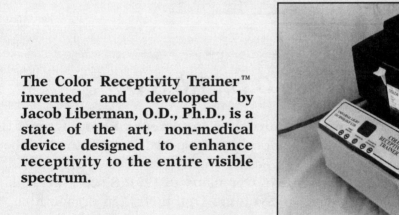
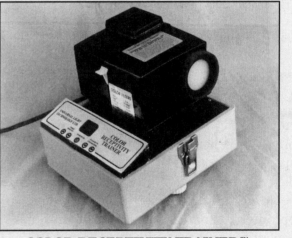

The Color Receptivity Trainer™ invented and developed by Jacob Liberman, O.D., Ph.D., is a state of the art, non-medical device designed to enhance receptivity to the entire visible spectrum.

COLOR RECEPTIVITY TRAINER™

The purest and most thoughtful minds
are those which love color the most.

— John Ruskin

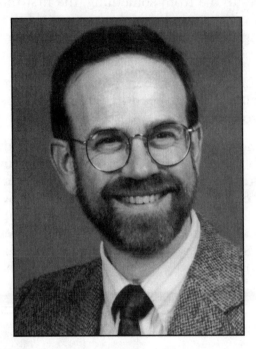

Samuel Pesner, O.D., F.C.S.O.

Dr. Samuel Pesner is the **Editor of The Journal of Optometric Phototherapy.** He practices general optometry in Los Altos, California, with special interests in phototherapy, neuro-optometry and vision therapy. Dr. Pesner received his Doctor of Optometry degree from the Southern California College of Optometry in 1971. Since 1987, he has been an active member of **The College of Syntonic Optometry,** an organization of optometrists and other health professionals that advocates the use of light therapy by way of the eyes, since its founding in 1935. He became a Fellow of the College in 1993.

CHAPTER TWO

Light Therapy: An Historical Overview

Samuel Pesner, O.D., F.C.S.O.

Today I'll be giving you an historical overview of the field of light therapy. Most of what I'm going to tell you is old stuff. You know we've been right on the cutting edge with Dr. Liberman's and Dr. Shealy's[1] presentations about what's new and what's happening in the field of light therapy. What I'm going to tell you about is what has happened over the past hundred years or so, and realize some of what I'm going to tell you is wrong, because we know today that what the original researchers did was based on some faulty information. They certainly didn't know as much as we know now about what goes on in the brain and our psychological process, and so forth.

First, I want to do a quick survey. Would everyone here who is an optometrist please stand. I want to see who's here. Alright, about seven or eight of us. Okay, good. How many M.D.s do we have? One hand came up there. I know there was one other, so we've got at least two. Chiropractors? Nurses? How about people in the area of psychotherapy, psychiatrists, psychologists, counselors? OK, great.

I was in the park the other day walking my dog, and a spiritual healer was walking her dog also, and we got to talking about the tricks that our dogs could do. She said that her dog could do some really neat tricks, and I said, "Well, what can she do?" She said, "Okay, you just sit down here on the bench," and I did, and she patted my lap, and the dog jumped into my lap. Then she said, "Sit." And the dog sat. Next she said, *"Heel!"* and the dog put his paw on my forehead, like this! It was a miracle! And today, too, we are here to talk about *healing* "miracles." I do some pretty miraculous and magical things in my practice with light.

---

1. See *Chapters One, page 27, and Fourteen, page 321,* for Dr. Jacob Liberman's presentations and *Chapters Seven, page 165, and Eight, page 185,* for Dr. Norman Shealy's presentations.

I want to start by sharing with you a case history of one patient I've seen. Three years ago I examined a five-year-old girl who was brought in for her first eye examination. Her mother said that Kara had no problems with her eyes. Kara didn't think she had any problems with her eyes, either, and, in fact, she could see 20/20 and all of her visual skills were normal as well. She looked perfect. And on my diagnosis line I wrote, "Perfect." I always figure we'll laugh about that in a year or two when the patient comes back. Three years later, in May of this year, she came back. She was complaining of *blurred vision*, and she had seen her teacher double that day in school. She was *contemplating suicide at age eight* — not a very happy girl and, yes, she had a bunch of symptoms.

One of the things optometrists do, as Dr. Liberman alluded to earlier, is a test called the **Visual Field Test,** and that's done on an instrument that's called a **Campimeter.** It's a rather small instrument, a foot-and-a-half wide by maybe a foot tall. This is placed about twelve or thirteen inches away from the patient's face, and inside there's a black or gray sheet of paper which looks like a series of concentric circles or a "bull's-eye." We take a small, white, red, green, or blue target which is about the size of your pinky's fingernail, about a quarter of an inch in diameter, and we move it in from the side and say, "Tell me when you can see this. As soon as you are aware of it coming in from the side, say, 'NOW.' When Kara said, 'NOW,' the visual field was the size of a quarter.

One doctor said, "I get these patients who would be called 'malingerers,' all of whom have very small tubular visual fields; this has been written up in textbooks for years and years." And here it was. I have an eight-year old patient with *tubular-shaped visual fields. Her visual acuity, which had been 20/20 at age five, was now about 20/70, and she had all these psychological problems.*

To make a long story short, **I started her on light therapy using a magenta light and a yellow-green light, about ten minutes on each color.** After four sessions I got a phone call from her mother saying, "Kara is fine now; we don't need to come back." I said, "I'd like to see her, just for my records." Her mom said, "Okay." She brought Kara in. All I did was talk to her a little bit and check her visual acuities, which were now 20/25, very close to what we would consider normal, average. I said, "I would like to do this a little bit longer. I really don't feel like we're done." So they agreed and they came back three more times, and then a few days after that. That was **seven sessions, twenty minutes each of total exposure to the light.** They came back after seven sessions, and I did visual fields once again. **This time Kara's visual acuity was 20/20, and her visual fields had expanded almost out to the limits of the page.** I was also able to do some visual fields with color targets, which I didn't attempt before, because there was no reason to do that with her vision constricted as far as it was; it would have been meaningless.

After treatment she was now happy; she was seeing 20/20 and most of her emotional problems had pretty much gone away, except for the fact that in school she was being mistreated by her classmates. There were three girls following her around, hitting her, kicking her, and just basically making her life miserable. At that point I referred her to a clinical psychologist who specializes in children and parents, and I said, "I've got her seeing again and thank heaven we've only got two weeks until school lets out. Hopefully, her next year's classmates will be a little kinder than the ones she has now." But she obviously needed some counseling.

So, I did my part as an optometrist, and now other people will have to do theirs. Ultimately, of course, the child and the mother have to do their work as well, and that's where it touches me as an optometrist. **One of my goals is to interplay with other health professionals — psychologists, chiropractors, and M.D.s; everybody has a role to play.** As we learn more and more, of course, we'll be able to do more and more for our patients, either as individuals or in groups.

On to "Light Therapy: An Historical Overview." So where does this field come from? As Dr. Liberman mentioned earlier, in ancient Egypt light was used in healing rooms, and it was also used to make diagnoses. Treatment was also done in light rooms at Heliopolis, which means the "City of the Sun." We know that light therapy happened in ancient China, Greece, and India, and probably in places that don't exist anymore.

So, where did light therapy start? In the **Bible, God said, "Let there be light. And there was light. And God saw that the light was good, and God divided the light from the darkness . . ."** I don't want to get religious on you here, but light has been around since the beginning of time. One of the things we know now, is that **we are all made of light. Because we are made of light, when we add light into the system, we change the system, the system being ourselves.** Thus, light therapy has been around for a long time, and it's been used successfully for a long time as well.

In more recent history, in the last hundred or so years, we've had a flurry of research activity. One of these researchers was **Augustus Pleasanton who, in 1876, used blue light to stimulate the glands, the nervous system, and the organs,** and he wrote about this. His results were very interesting, and I'm sure these results influenced those who came after him. The next year, **in 1877, Seth Pancoast used red and blue light to stimulate and/or relax the autonomic nervous system.**

In 1878, Edwin Babbitt, M.D., did two things: First, he had an instrument that he called the *Chromodisc* that put light on the body; he also talked about *solar elixirs*, or sun-charged water. Maybe some of you remember grandparents who kept a bottle of *blue water* on the porch. And if somebody got burned or had a *sore throat*, the blue water was used to effect a cure. Those blue bottles were old milk of magnesia bottles. So, it's not the water, per se; it has to be something organic in the water, something that absorbs the sunlight and the energy therein; it's that which effects the cure. But blue water, red water, orange water, all of them have an effect when they've been made the right way, which is pretty simple to do. And that's something that needs to be looked into. It's an old, old science that has been lost, more or less, and it's something that someone should do some research on.

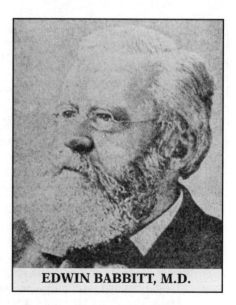

EDWIN BABBITT, M.D.

Babbitt said:

> *Any process, light or heat, that draws blood to the skin, relieves congestion of the liver, spleen, lungs, stomach, intestines, and spinal cord. All vital organs have direct connection with the skin through the blood vessels. Application of light rays in one spot can affect the entire bloodstream through circulation and elimination of toxins.*

That quote was from his book, entitled *The Principles of Light and Color,*[2] published in 1878. It's the basis for about half of what we're talking about here today, as far as light therapy as a curative tool, or as a noninvasive method for effecting change within your body.

In 1926, G.C. Sander said:

> *When the body is in a normal condition, it may be able to filter out from the white light or sunlight, whatever color vibration it needs. However, if a person is not in normal health, the necessary color must be supplied.*

This is the point of using different frequencies or colors for different conditions. I'm talking "old-time knowledge." The things that you're going to be hearing about are based on older work that has now evolved.

In 1920, Dinshah Ghadiali, a man from India, who held numerous doctorate degrees, developed a program called ***Spectro-Chrome,*** based on three principles:

Three Principles of Spectro-Chrome

1. The human body reacts to light.

2. Colors relate to physiological function.

3. Color Tonation (tonation is exposing the body to specific colors) aids bodily function.

---

2. Edwin D. Babbitt's book *The Principles of Light and Color* (published 1878), was enthusiastically received by the people in the field of Color Healing, yet violently opposed by the medical community in his day. He claimed to be able to cure a variety of ailments, by the therapeutic application of sunlight passing through various colors of glass. He was an avid inventor of such tools as **"Chromo Flasks,"** and the **"Thermo-Lume Cabinet,"** as well as a type of stained glass window that could be used in healing. Babbitt associated each color to a particular element and mineral. Although his chromo therapeutic devices are illegal in the United States, in his native Britain there are a number of color therapists who still use and sell these inventions to this day.

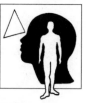

Dinshah Ghadiali's Tonation Areas for Spectro-Chrome

In Dinshah's Spectro-Chrome work he determined specific body areas where the various colors of light should go in order to get certain things done. The part of the body you are going to tonate is called an "Area." The Areas are numbered from 1 to 22 and contain the major organs and structures:

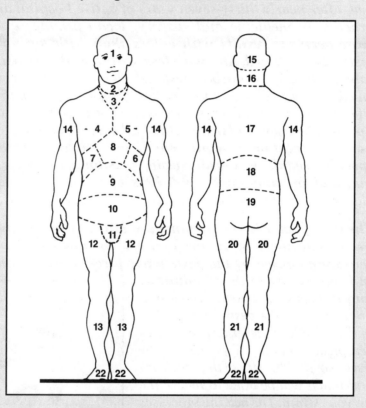

1.	Pituitary, pineal, brain (front)	**11.**	External reproductive
2.	Neck	**12.**	Thighs
3.	Thyroid, parathyroids	**13.**	Shins
4-5.	Lungs, heart, thymus, mammaries (directly below area 3)	**14.**	Arms
		15.	Brain (back)
		15-19.	Spine, spinal cord
6.	Spleen	**16.**	Nape of neck
7.	Liver (also area 8), gallbladder	**17.**	Lungs (back)
8.	Stomach (also area 6), pancreas (front)	**18.**	Kidneys, adrenals, pancreas (back)
9.	Intestines (also area 10)	**19.**	Rectum, buttocks
10.	Bladder, appendix, internal reproductive	**20.**	Back of thighs
		21.	Calves
		22.	Feet

This is just to let you in on the fact that when we talk about *tonating* some part of the body, if we talk about tonating, say, *Areas 4* and *5*, what we're talking about is the person's chest, and so on.

Next, I want to read to you some quotes that **Kate Baldwin, M.D., F.A.C.S.,** wrote and lectured on as a result of her work as a student of Dinshah.

> *For about six years I have given close attention to the action of colors in restoring the body functions and I am perfectly honest in saying that, **after nearly thirty-seven years of active hospital and private practice in medicine and surgery, I can produce quicker and more accurate results with colors than with any or all other methods combined, and with less strain on the patient**. In many cases the functions have been restored after the classical remedies have failed. Of course, surgery is necessary in some cases, but the results will be quicker and better if color is used before and after operations. **Sprains, bruises, and traumata of all sorts respond to color as to no other treatment. Septic conditions yield regardless of the specific organisms. Cardiac lesions, asthma, hay fever, pneumonia, and inflammatory conditions of the eyes, corneal ulcers, glaucoma, and cataracts are relieved by the treatment.***
>
> ***The use of color in the treatment of burns is worth investigating by every member of the professions. In such cases the burning sensation caused by the destructive forces may be counteracted in from twenty to thirty minutes, and it does not return.** True burns are caused by the destructive action of the red side of the spectrum, hydrogen predominating. Apply oxygen by the use of the blue side of the spectrum and much will be done to relieve the nervous strain. The healing processes are rapid, and the resulting tissue is soft and flexible.*

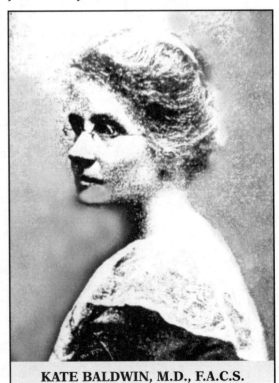

KATE BALDWIN, M.D., F.A.C.S.

Dr. Baldwin's quote was made in 1926! She was the Chief Surgeon at a hospital in Philadelphia, and that was after thirty-seven years of medical practice. She used light a lot in her practice at the hospital and almost exclusively, as I understand, in her private practice.

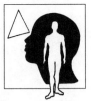

So why aren't we still doing this today? Well, let's talk about the FDA. In the late 1940s and early 1950s, the Food and Drug Administration, in their "infinite wisdom," decided that what Dinshah was doing was "quackery." And they issued injunctions against him, forbidding him to disseminate the information or to ship his instruments across state lines. They only allowed him to have his own personal library and stay in New Jersey. So, this work was squelched by "our government" in the late 1940's and early 1950's. Due to the efforts of Dinshah's sons, this information was kept alive, and it's still possible to get hold of the information and do it for yourself. And there's even some hope as of last May, (I think Jacob Liberman would be able to update us on this) that our government and the FDA might be a little more willing to look at these ideas again in a more "favorable light."

Now, I want each of you in your different professions to think about how the knowledge of light therapy will affect you and your relationship with your clients. Each one of us is coming from a different place, and when we leave here after this two-day conference, we're going back, changed by the information we've shared, to very different work places. This is exactly what happened to me five years ago when I started with *Syntonic Optometry*. **I guarantee you that working with light is a life-altering experience. You'll never approach your practice in the same way ever again!**

Dinshah assigned attributes to colors. If you think about these color responses as a series of patterns as we go through the colors towards the other end of the spectrum, you'll see that each color has its own unique effect, and there's even some logic to it.

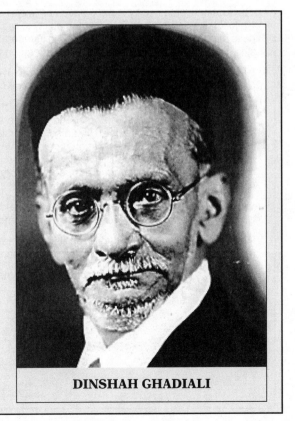

Dr. Dinshah passed away in 1966. He was trained in medicine in India and received numerous honorary doctorates in the United States. His work is being carried on by his son **Darius Dinshah (in Malaga, New Jersey)** at the **Dinshah Health Society,** which is still functioning and is very much worth looking into. They have a newsletter, and their book is called *Let There Be Light.* You should have this book as part of your basic light therapy library, so that you'll have the underpinnings to move forward with your own work. To contact Dinshah Health Society, See *Resource List: Section Fourteen, page 381, Referrals and Educational Information.*

DINSHAH GHADIALI

Summary of Dinshah's Color Attributes

Scarlet is obtained by a combination of ***Red and Blue Light;*** it's a kidney and adrenal stimulant; it also raises blood pressure, increases heart rate and is an emotional stimulant.

Red stimulates the sensory nervous system; it's a liver builder and liver stimulant; it increases the blood count and circulation and causes expulsion of debris through the skin. "Hot stuff." Red is hot; it warms and it speeds things up.

Orange is a lung builder and a respiratory stimulant, a thyroid builder and stimulant, a parathyroid depressant, a bone builder, a tissue stimulant and a decongestant.

Yellow stimulates the motor nervous system and is a nerve builder for both the sensory and motor nervous systems. It stimulates the lymphatic system; it stimulates the intestinal tract.

Lemon is obtained by *a combination of **Yellow and Green Light.*** It's called The ***Chronic Alternative*** by Dinshah. What this means is when you're treating a condition that's been there for awhile, when the restorative and the recuperative powers of the body are depleted, then you need to be giving Lemon, or Yellow and Green together. Thus Lemon will promote healing in persistent disorders. It also dissolves blood clots, and is an expectorant, a bone builder, a brain stimulant, a thymus builder and stimulant, and a mild digestive system stimulant.

Green. Picture, if you will, a teeter-totter, and in the middle is the thing that holds it up, the fulcrum. Green is in the middle; it's the center of the visible spectrum. Everything on the side that we've just gone through — Yellow, Orange and Red — I call the ***Violet Side of the Spectrum,*** and everything on the other side — Blue, Indigo and Violet, and combinations thereof, I call the ***Blue Side of the Spectrum.*** Now we've reached the middle of the spectrum. Green is a cerebral equilibrator, a physical equilibrator, a pituitary stimulant and equilibrator. So think "equilibrium," because Green is in the middle. It's also a germicide, a disinfectant, and an antiseptic, and it stimulates the rebuilding of muscles and tissues.

Turquoise is obtained by *a combination of **Green and Blue***. Green has the governing and cleansing effect we just talked about, and Blue has the ability to reduce fever and pain. Turquoise has some of the effectiveness of each. Turquoise promotes healing in recent disorders; also it is a brain depressant. It rebuilds burned skin, which I made mention of when I was reading those quotes from Dr. Baldwin.

Blue is the color Dr. Baldwin used to treat burns. It also relieves itching, relieves irritation of abraded surfaces, encourages perspiration, reduces or removes fever and inflammation, and it is a pineal stimulant.

Indigo is a parathyroid builder and stimulant; a thyroid depressant and a respiratory depressant. It also promotes production of phagocytes, and it is a sedative. You know, when you start to feel kind of "Blue," or maybe you just get a little tired, you also get a little depressed. Blue has a sedative effect. I'm sure that if someone is too tense, he can put on a pair of Blue glasses, sit out in the sunlight for a little while, and start to feel relaxed. Indigo also is beneficial in an acute closed head injury. It reduces symptoms which can include blurred vision, double vision, and memory problems. Using Indigo Light can be very beneficial in reducing the swelling of the brain and other tissues.

Violet is a spleen builder and stimulant. It also decreases muscular activity, including the heart. It is a lymphatic gland and pancreas depressant, it promotes production of leukocytes and is a tranquilizer.

Purple induces relaxation and sleep. It is a kidney and adrenal depressant. It lowers the blood pressure; it lowers body temperature and it reduces the heart rate.

Magenta, *a combination of **Red and Violet Light,*** is an emotional equilibrator.

In 1941, Harry Riley Spitler, M.D., O.D., wrote ***The Syntonic Principle.*** As Jacob Liberman said, *Syntony* is from a Greek word which means *"to bring to balance."* What Spitler wanted to do was to balance the autonomic nervous system so that the body would function normally. His belief was that if either the sympathetic nervous system, which is responsible for the fight-or-flight response, or if the parasympathetic nervous system, which is responsible for the balancing, restorative or maintenance functions, was too dominant, it would cause problems. **Spitler believed and proved that light administered by the way of the eyes could balance the autonomic nervous system.** Spitler also based a lot of his work on constitutional body types. These three ***Biotypes*** he called *Pycnic, Syntonic and Asthenic.* Dr. Spitler arrived at nineteen conclusions about the effects of light on the bodymind, and these appeared in the last chapter of his book.

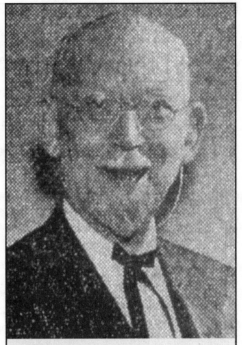

HARRY RILEY SPITLER, M.D., O.D.

The 19 Syntonic Principles

1. *There exists a closely predictable relationship between light frequency, incident into the eyes, and response.*

    This simply means that when light goes into the eyes, the eyes respond.

2. *There exists a relationship between light frequency and the rate of growth of cells and tissues, and their rate of cell division.*

    In the 1860s and the 1870s, Dr. Pleasanton did work with this principle, and he also proved it to be so. I'm pretty sure Spitler's work followed from Pleasanton's work, since he was one of his predecessors.

3. *There exists a relationship between the light in the environment and the physical development of the individual.*

    Spitler himself did research with rabbits, exposing them to different kinds of light, and they grew differently. The light had an influence on growth rate.

4. *There exists a relationship between light frequency in the eyes and the mass body potentials.*

    This has to do with the electrical charge that is carried from the eyes back to the brain.

5. *There exists a relationship between the light frequency of the environment and the development of the Biotype, modifying the hereditary tendency.*

    This is a similar idea to the previous one. Light affects how something grows, and in time, light can also affect the hereditary tendency, as things adapt to their environment, like the fish that have no eyes.

6. *There exists a relationship between light and light frequency and the action currents leaving the eye toward the brain. These action currents being both quantitatively and qualitatively altered.*

    What we're saying here is that light going into the eyes has a definite effect on the neural information that goes into the brain.

7. *There exists a relationship between the light frequency incident into the eye and the functioning power of the pituitary gland.*

8. *There exists a relationship between the reproductive cycle and the light frequency environment, probably a quantitative one, in respect to the number of individuals of any species.*

    There is work being done right now by **Dr. George Brainard in Philadelphia at Thomas Jefferson Medical School,** I believe, with hamsters. He has shown that the light environment affects the hamster's reproductive cycle, and it also affects the size of their reproductive organs. And there is much other work that he's done on this subject.

9. *There exists a relationship between the light frequency environment and the dynamic tension present between the two divisions of the autonomic nervous system.*

    So that's referring to the sympathetic and the parasympathetic nervous systems.

10. *There exists a relationship between the light frequency environment and the secretion of hormones by all of the co-acting as well as antagonistic endocrine glands, with the pituitary as the master gland.*

    Later, Dr. Shealy will give you a list of **hormones and other chemicals in the body that are affected by light.** The list that I got from Dr. Brainard included: *melatonin, prolactin, cortisone, testosterone, TS4, LH, FSH, T3, and T4 lymphocyte cells and thyroid hormones.*

    Spitler's research represented one of the first times that anyone had put down in writing the fact that we could influence the body's biochemistry with light.

11. *There exists a relationship which is largely predictable between light frequency environment and the restoration of health following departures from the normal, which are still within physiologic limits, particularly those departures which may be directly influenced by the autonomic or the endocrines toward health.*

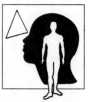

In departures from the normal, **if you're sick, you may be able to effect a cure by using light to affect the autonomic nervous system, if** the illnesses are still within physiological limits. Some of these people, like Dr. Shealy's example of the fellow who ended up dying the following August, are going to die no matter what you do; or they're going to stay sick no matter what you do. Thus, some people have been injured too badly to repair.

12. *There exists a relationship between light frequency into the eye and the degree of nerve cell irritability, thus modifying reflexes.*

13. *There exists a relationship between light frequency into the eye and bodily health.*

14. *There exists a relationship between nerve impulses from the eye, due to incident light frequency, and the state of tension in the autonomic nervous system.*

    The nerve pathways that have to do with mediating light do not just go back to the visual cortex, but to other areas of the brain, like the hypothalamus, our internal body clock, the pineal organ, and the pituitary. This principle will give you some information that you need to deal with seasonal affective disorder, sleep disorders, and so on.

15. *There exists a relationship between light frequency into the eye in either its vitamin A content or the degree of its adaptation to low degrees of illumination.*

16. *There exists a relationship between light frequency into the eye and the perception of pain.*

    When a person is in pain, headache pain for example, having them sit down at an instrument and look at a blue light can help relieve the pain.

17. *There exists a relationship between light frequency into the eye and the relative responses of both striated and smooth muscle.*

    Remember in Dinshah's color attributes we could make muscles relax; we could speed up the heartbeat or slow it down. It's the same kind of thing; Dinshah's and Spitler's work coincided a great deal.

18. *Syntony of the autonomic nervous system may be produced by light frequency into the eye.*

    This was Spitler's whole thesis, and today we are continuing to prove it to be true.

19. *The ability to continue to live depends upon syntony of the autonomic in both acute and chronic illnesses, and this attainment of syntony may be aided by light frequency into the eye.*

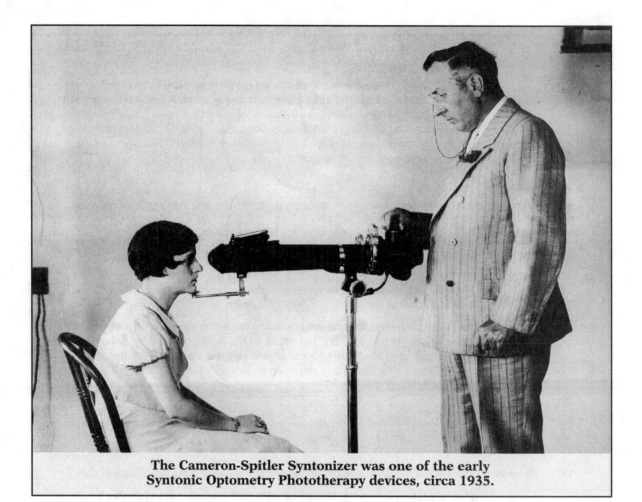

The Cameron-Spitler Syntonizer was one of the early Syntonic Optometry Phototherapy devices, circa 1935.

Dr. John Ott is one of the great pioneers in light research. He is the inventor of *The Ott-Lite*™ and a pioneer in time-lapse (stop-action) photography for the Walt Disney Studios. Ott's proof that both the type of light and the type of electromagnetic radiation surrounding plants and animals (not just visible light), including other forms of electromagnetic radiation, have a very important influence on how plants and animals respond and grow.

John Nash Ott, presently retired, wrote and lectured extensively in the field of photobiology, beginning in the 1950s. His books include: *Health and Light* and *My Ivory Cellar*. After twenty years as a successful Chicago banker, he turned his lifelong interest in time-lapse photography into a full-time investigation of the ecology of light. Ott's research has brought him citations and awards from horticultural, scientific, and medical societies, including an honorary doctor of science degree from Loyola University at Chicago.

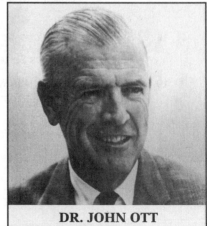

DR. JOHN OTT

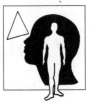

In contrast to light through the eyes, Dinshah, preceded by Babbitt and others, applied light directly to the body. We have people today at this conference, such as Dr. Ward Lamb,[3] who also work with light on the body. **Spitler took a unique approach, applying light to the body by the way of the eyes.** You can see that all of this makes sense when you think about what the sympathetic nervous system is designed to do. It gets us ready to decide if we're going to fight or get out of there.

Thus, when we want *to calm or to slow someone down*, we tend to stimulate the parasympathetic, which means using the blue end of the light spectrum. On the other hand, if we feel we need *to speed the nervous system up*, or to bring it up from *depression, fatigue*, or *lethargy*, we might use the red end. Every individual needs to respond differently. So there's going to be a learning curve and use a certain amount of intuition, some trial and error, and empathy with our clients, so that we can hear exactly what they're experiencing. This is how you get into what they really need in order to help them find the road to health and healing.

The sympathetic nervous system is the stress-producing part of the nervous system and activates the thyroid, the adrenal medulla, the pituitary, the gonads, and muscles.

The parasympathetic nervous system is opposite and activates the parathyroids, the adrenal cortex, the digestive tract, liver, pancreas, and spleen. Its functions are maintenance and restoration.

So, if you feel that you have underactive organs, Dinshah and Spitler recommend that these are places for you to start your research on learning how to apply light to people in order to help them, not to mention to help yourself get better.

Aaron's Law of Physiology states, "Mild stimuli will excite physiological action; moderate stimuli will favor it, but strong ones will retard the action or abolish it altogether." In other words, **more is not better, light treatment should always be as gentle as possible.** You don't necessarily want to hit somebody who needs a little bit of stimulation on the sympathetic side with a bright red light. It might be too much for them. They might, for example, do a lot better if you use a yellow-green light. On the other side of the coin, if someone needs blue, you might not want to give them a real strong blue. It might be too much and too depressing for them; instead, as an alternative, use turquoise. **It is blue-green and the other colors closest to green that are the filter combinations that tend to be used most frequently in healing. Moving out into the farther reaches of the spectrum achieves a more profound effect. Remember: You really have to be careful with that so that you don't give people too much light.** You are not going to "kill them," but you can certainly overstimulate them and get yourself into a place where you have to back up and start over again.

Back to *The Bible* one more time. In Matthew: The Sermon on the Mount, one of the things Jesus said to his disciples, and I think it's prophetic, no pun intended, "Neither do men light a candle and put it under a bushel, but on a candlestick; and it giveth light unto all that are in the house." Remember that this sermon was delivered by Jesus to his disciples and not to the masses, so it wasn't meant for everybody. I say this because people

---

3. See *Chapter Nine*, "One Man's Journey Into Light: The Use of Colored Light in Chiropractic."

like you, who have an interest in enlightenment, (or in "being enlightened," or "being illumined," as Jacob Liberman said earlier), you people here today are probably more ready to sit down and listen to this "voodoo stuff" that I have just been talking about — this "weird science"— than most of the masses out there.

Those of us who are doing this work with light feel that we are on a bit of a "mission." I don't want to stand up here and say, "You've got to do this, and when you do it everything will be okay." But this is work that needs to be publicized in a positive way, as Dr. Liberman is doing with his book, and as I hope all of us will be doing in our practices.

In closing, I want to mention that at the top of my light book list is: ***Light: Medicine of the Future,* Jacob Liberman's book.** You must read this book! It has an extensive bibliography that's very important. You can use it as a reference to find other sources of information that affect you and your practice, be it psychology, chiropractic, nursing, medicine, optometry, or whatever. Also on the list is **Dinshah's book, *Let There be Light.*** This book describes how to create the specific frequencies of color and how and where to use them on the body, as opposed to through the eyes.[4]

The one remains, the many change and pass; Heaven's light forever shines, earth shadow's fly; Life, like a dome of many coloured glass stains the white radiance of eternity.

— P.B. Shelley

---

4. For more information on the history of light, you can contact Betsy Hancock, the Librarian for the College of Syntonic Optometry, Bloomsburg, Pennsylvania. See *Resource List: Section Fourteen, page 380, Referrals and Educational Information.* Also see *Bibliography* for many additional sources under the *"History of Phototherapy," page 387.*

SECTION II
Light in Psychotherapy

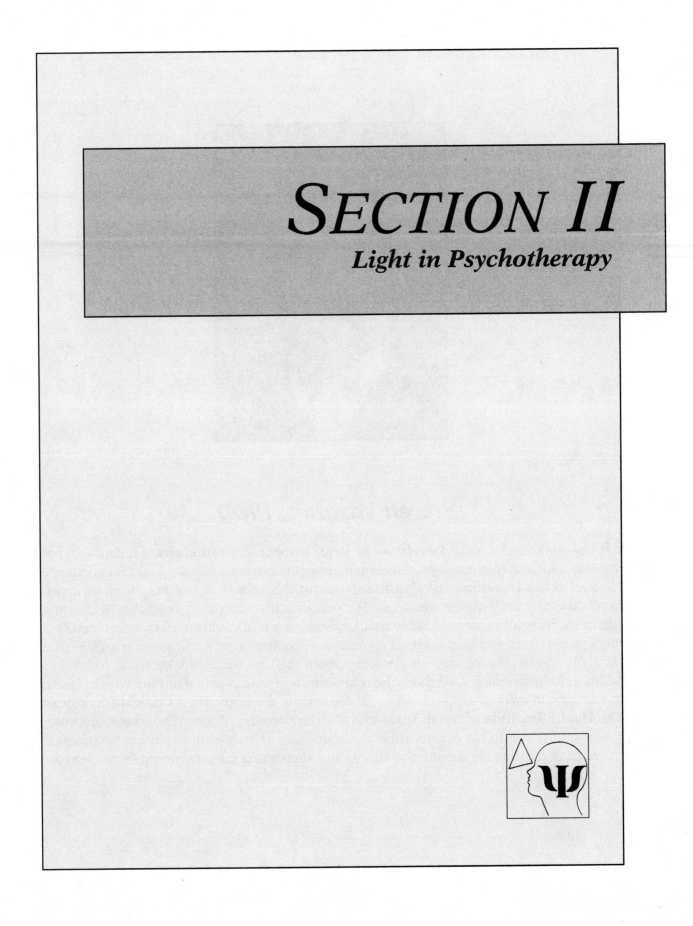

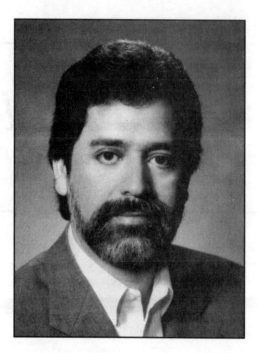

Steven Vazquez, Ph.D.

Dr. Steven Vazquez is the **Developer of Brief Strobic Phototherapy,** a technique that involves color and rhythmic light stimulation, using the Lumatron Ocular Light Stimulator™. He is also the **Developer of Confluent Somatic Therapy,** a unique blend of depth psychotherapy and energy medicine. He presents his acclaimed methods in training seminars for health care professionals all over the world. Dr. Vazquez is a board-certified medical psychotherapist, a licensed professional counselor, and a licensed marriage and family therapist. He received his doctorate from the University of Western Colorado. In addition to his training workshops, he maintains a private practice in Fort Worth, Texas, specializing in medical psychotherapy and dissociative disorders. He is **Clinical Director of The Health Institute of North Texas** and also the **Founder of The Wholeness Institute,** a non-profit, charitable organization that conducts research into non-pharmaelogical methods of treating life threatening illness and supporting the attainment of wholeness.

CHAPTER THREE

Brief Strobic Phototherapy: Synthesis of the Future

Steven Vazquez, Ph.D.

I'm going to be sharing with you some ideas about what I call **Brief Strobic Photo-therapy.** I first discovered light therapy in a speech by Jacob Liberman some time ago. Then, at one point, a colleague in my psychotherapy practice and I decided to pool our funds to send her to experience **Dr. John Downing's** and **Dr. Jacob Liberman's work.** She brought back lots of information, and we shared and talked about the different ideas she got from both of these practitioners. Ever since then I've been trying to integrate their light therapy ideas into a form to be used psychotherapeutically, within a form of psychotherapy I founded, called *Confluent Somatic Therapy.*

Approximately 80% of the people I see fit into two basic categories. One is *behavioral medicine*; this refers to people who are recovering from injury, or who have *pain syndromes,* or who have *life-threatening illnesses.* The other category has to do with what some would refer to as *chronic trauma patients*, many of whom have *multiple personality disorder,* and some of whom my colleagues might refer to as *schizophrenic.* Of these, there are those who have *psychotic* episodes quite often. So these are the types of disorders and the populations with which I work. The other 20% is anyone who comes in the door. I also work with couples or families. For the most part, I don't work with children, although the people I work with tell me that I work with their "inner children" very well, so in that way, I do work with children a lot.

We've been hearing the word "paradigm" used quite a bit at this *Light Years Ahead Conference.* So I want to take some time to define this word as I see it and use it. My background, my orientation is scientific. But today there is controversy within that particular paradigm.

Paradigm Perspectives — Old vs. New

The Older Traditional Healing Paradigm

Scientific	Other
Reductionistic	Wholes, Integrative
Materialistic, Tangible	Transpersonal
Measurable	Qualitative
Restorative	Transformative
Exclusive	Inclusive

The New Alternative and Integrative Healing Paradigm

Reductionistic	Holistic
Materialistic	Transpersonal
Sometimes Measurable	Always Qualitative in Purpose
Restorative	Transformative
Inclusive	Integrated

Reductionistic refers to the concept that says, if I can reduce something to its smallest parts, I can gain an infinitely wiser understanding of how the whole works. This perspective is basic to both the scientific method and to medical science. The reductionist position is in conflict with another vantage point that views people, things, diseases, or whatever, as wholes. This is an integrative approach.

Some time ago, when the scientific community discovered certain microbes were involved in people's physical pathology, it was really exciting, because we got down to the basic unit. We really thought we had found the culprit; microbes were the cause of illness. Ever since that discovery, there has been a tremendous movement in the use of penicillin and other antibiotics to cure illness. However, there are still a lot of practitioners who talk about seeing a person as a whole, and looking at their thoughts, their feelings, their physical sensations, and the way they operate within their families as clues to their pathologies and health. These are some of the major conflicts I see in this paradigm clash.

Another aspect of the old, let's say the "traditional view," is that it is *materialistic and tangible*. It has to do with the idea that if you can't see it, if it's not observable, and you can't touch it, then essentially, it is not real. In a system like this, when taken to its logical extreme, there's no room for the kind of *transpersonal* experiences which might include those referred to as spiritual union with the universe, or out-of-body experiences, or telepathy and things of that nature. There's just no room for such considerations in a system that demands that science must be limited to materialistic and tangible events.

Next, you have the concept of *measurability*. According to the traditional scientific ethic in its most rigorous form, if something cannot be measured, it isn't real. This mode of thought is in conflict with some people's view that what we're really after is *qualitative* changes in people, rather than quantitatively measurable ones. Along with measurability comes the idea that in medicine and psychology the focus is to restore a person. If you think in linear terms, something is broken, you fix it, and it's okay.

Another vantage point is that of the *transformative*. Now, this is a little bit different. To transform means to change at a very fundamental level. Most of the people I work with who come in with a physical illness seem to have experiences in life that have affected them far beyond what they ever felt before they got sick in the first place. So, the transformation happens when the patient actually becomes a different person and begins to live a dramatically healthier lifestyle. Transformative indicates that something larger is changing, rather than just being restored to the way it was.

The next facet of the paradigm model has to do with *exclusive* and/or *inclusive*. In other words, most scientists take a view which is reductionistic, materialistic, measurable, or restorative; they believe that is the exclusive domain of truth, that's where the answers are, that's how the world really works. Then there are the other people, like artists of various types, who think the "holistic approach" is the truth. And this is "where it's at." So now I'll show you what I think this shift is all about.

My perspective is that I invite the wonderful information we can get from reductionistic ways of thinking to combine together with the holistic. I believe that I don't have to choose one or the other. There are powerful pieces of information given to me when I'm told that a person has multiple sclerosis, or has major depression. To me, that means something. Although it's a diagnostic category, it helps me understand something about that individual. But at the same time, it's important not to get lost in that category; that's not all there is. The only problem with something that's reductionistic is that it's incomplete. It's just a part of the total picture.

Another aspect to my approach is that I believe in both the materialistic and the transpersonal. I like to help the client work toward physical change that's observable. That's wonderful! I have no problem with that. Only this alone is incomplete; I know there is much more.

I also think there's a lot more than the transpersonal realm. As far as this third category is concerned, oftentimes in my treatment things are measurable, and the important thing is that they're always qualitative in purpose. As far as the restorative aspect is concerned, yes, I like to have clients who come in with pain and then have that pain change for them. But that's not all there is in life, to change their pain; there is much more to a person's experience in life than that.

So, I'm in favor of restoring what is broken, but I'm also in favor of going far beyond that. In fact, this is the basis of the paradigm shift as I see it. In this sense **I think that illness, injury, pain, and psychological distress give us an opportunity to make a jump in our evolution, a jump in our transformation, to become bigger and better, and stronger, and still more.** When an accident or an injury, or some type of physical illness or psychological distress occurs, I see this as an opportunity to put together the parts of that individual in a new and better way than they've ever experienced before. If you've ever had a debilitating illness, you will probably notice that it is one of the things in life that shakes your system up the most. And when your system is shaken up, you have the opportunity to become greater than you've ever been before, should you process that debilitating crisis.

Finally, my theoretical approach is *inclusive*. All these things are valuable. I'm not at war with scientists. I read a lot of scientific journals, but I don't think that's the "end-all" of knowledge.

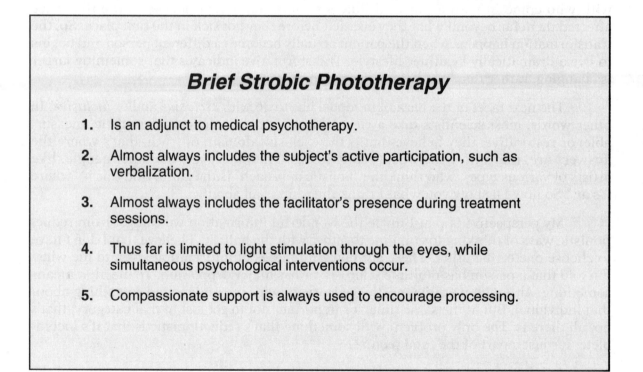

Brief Strobic Phototherapy

1. Is an adjunct to medical psychotherapy.

2. Almost always includes the subject's active participation, such as verbalization.

3. Almost always includes the facilitator's presence during treatment sessions.

4. Thus far is limited to light stimulation through the eyes, while simultaneous psychological interventions occur.

5. Compassionate support is always used to encourage processing.

I see light therapy as an adjunct to the medical psychotherapy that I do. **I would say that 90% of what I do in Brief Strobic Phototherapy can be achieved without light. However, the light work seems to offer a catalyst that allows me to do things more easily and more quickly than I can without light as an adjunct. There are some things that come up with the light that I'm not sure I could have made happen without the light.**

Another thing about my approach is that I almost always include the client's active participation, such as their verbalization, during light stimulation. The way I work with people, I'd say about 95% of the time I'm working with them at the same time while they are talking. I think talking is valuable. Of course, as a psychotherapist, I'm biased. Our magic is, you talk to people, you listen to people and tremendous things happen just by listening. So, I'm trying to integrate this approach with the light stimulation. The facilitator is present at almost all treatment sessions.

Thus far, my use of light stimulation is through the eyes only; I haven't yet done what some people are doing, applying lights to different parts of the body. One of the key ingredients to this work is that compassionate support is encouraged to assist the patient to go through their processing. I believe this is a critical ingredient in the whole treatment. In fact, as Dr. Liberman was saying earlier, it may be all there really is. These other techniques that therapists do may just be peripheral activities employed to make some kind of contact with the person.

What I find valuable in psychotherapy and in changing medical symptoms is that **in utilizing light stimulation, unconscious material surfaces. The light acts as a catalyst to bring unconscious material to the surface, and in psychotherapy we're trying to do that all the time.** For example, say a person comes in and wants to quit smoking. They may cognitively know they want to quit smoking and know how that works, but they can't do it. There's usually some unconscious activity that blocks them from doing it. What we do in psychotherapy is help them become aware of some of the things that are going on unconsciously, and then we can have a much better chance of making those changes occur.

In the chart at the right, the line is drawn through this person vertically, because usually, **I generally find that symptoms in the back portion of the body are more difficult for people to be aware of. Those back symptoms tend to be more unconscious, while the symptoms experienced on the front portion of the body tend to be more conscious and easily accessible to most people.**

About six months ago I began to tally up what's been taking place in my work with Brief Strobic Phototherapy. I realized, when I talked to Dr. John Downing, that I really work with a different population than many other practitioners. I have here, for means of linguistic communication, breakdowns in psychological and medical terms my patients' presenting complaints.

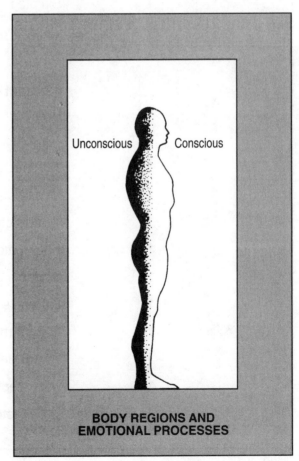

BODY REGIONS AND EMOTIONAL PROCESSES

Diagnoses of Populations Studied with Brief Strobic Phototherapy

Number of cases treated with Light	Psychological Diagnoses
8	Dysthymic Disorder
7	Cyclothymic Disorder
5	Multiple Personality Disorder (MPD)
2	Gender Identity Disorder
2	Psychogenic Amnesia
2	Generalized Anxiety Disorder
2	Dependent Personality Disorder
1	Anorexia Nervosa
1	Simple Phobia
1	Obsessive Compulsive Disorder
	Medical Conditions
4	Cancer in Remission (patients currently stabilized)
2	Multiple Sclerosis (MS)
1	Acquired Immune Deficiency Syndrome (AIDS)
1	Myocardial Infarction in Recovery
1	Temporomandibular Joint Pain (TMJ)
1	Rheumatoid Arthritis
1	Migraine Headache
1	Sjögren's Syndrome
1	Amenorrhea
1	Partial Hearing Impairment
1	Hydrocephalus
1	Hashimoto's Disease (Autoimmune)

For those of you who aren't psychotherapists, I'll interpret. *Dysthymia* is a form of depression; *multiple personality disorder (MPD)* is, of course, a very severe disorder that is in response to multiple severe trauma experiences. With *psychogenic amnesia* people can't remember big portions of their life history, or even what occurred yesterday. As for *generalized anxiety disorder* and *gender identity disorder* I think these sort of speak for themselves, as do the rest here: *dependent personality disorder, anorexia nervosa, simple phobia,* and *obsessive compulsive disorder*.

I also took about thirty people and categorized their medical conditions. Four of them were *cancer in remission*; two of them had *multiple sclerosis*; one had *acquired immune deficiency syndrome*; one had a *myocardial infarction*; one was in recovery from a *heart attack*; one had *temporomandibular joint pain (TMJ)*; one had *rheumatoid arthritis*; one had *migraine headaches*; one had *Sjögren's Syndrome*; one other had *amenorrhea, partial hearing impairment, hydrocephalus,* and *Hashimoto's disease (autoimmune)*. As you can see here, my patient population is in deep trouble. I'm usually the end of the line; they've tried everything else in the typical medical regimen; and then, lastly, they send them to me, "the shrink."

Spectrums . . . some were colors of rain, some for healing in loss,
others for strength in gain, always true was the hue . . .

Some were not nameable in mere words;
they were from beyond what mere sight can see.
I let the colors enter me.

— *Bethany ArgIsle*

I want to show you some of the *psychological outcomes* (see following chart) that I've observed. The following is from about six months ago, and I want you to know that since then, my procedures and protocols have improved, and we are getting even better responses at this point by far.

Psychological Outcomes of Brief Strobic Phototherapy

1. Depression was resolved in most cases after several sessions.

2. Panic attacks subsided in almost all cases.

3. Rage became manageable in many cases.

4. Dependent behavior became autonomous in a dramatic way in most cases.

5. Grief concluded in most cases.

6. Anxiety is relinquished in almost all cases.

7. Traumatic experiences abreacted and concluded in a high proportion of cases.

8. Shame and guilt transformed into self-esteem in the majority of cases.

9. Obsessive thoughts diminished in many cases.

10. In multiple personality disorder — discovery of the diagnosis, uncovering new personalities, reversal of dissociative phenomena occurred dramatically.

To do right is to be faithful to the light within.

— Oliver Wendel Holmes

Here are the psychological outcomes of the thirty people we tracked:

Physiological Outcomes of Brief Strobic Phototherapy

1. Migraine headaches were eliminated during several sessions.

2. Severe arthritic pain that previously existed over 15 years was eliminated in one case.

3. A viral skin condition in an AIDS patient had a rapid remission.

4. Irritable bowel syndrome was reduced in a single session.

5. A peptic ulcer was eliminated after several sessions.

6. Dramatic change in insomnia occurred in numerous cases.

7. Coughing, sore throats and other upper respiratory problems had a rapid reduction (within 3 minutes).

8. Major decreases in sinusitis during sessions for several cases.

9. Amenorrhea was reversed after a series of five sessions.

Thus, in the majority of cases in which there was a presenting symptom, these dramatically changed. The above results are from an academic journal article I tried to submit. The reviewers said to me, "Well, how do you know these results really took place and are accurate?" In this particular case it didn't take a physician to observe the visible changes. For example, have you ever had the kind of cough that with every breath you take, you cough again? How many of you have had those coughs? Well, there was a person I treated who was having a repeated cough, virtually every breath, and within a couple of minutes it was extinguished. Now, I'm not a physician, but I can tell the cough was gone, and it was pretty bad to start with. Also, there were significant observable decreases in *sinusitis* during sessions of several cases. *Amenorrhea* was reversed after a series of five sessions, in one case, since then it's happened in several other cases. I just want to give you an idea of some of the possible outcomes using light in psychotherapy.

I find that one of the very best ways to make sense of Brief Strobic Phototherapy for people is for me to do a demonstration. So I'm going to be up here working the Luma-tron™. The way I operate demands that my clients have an equal participation in what takes place, 'cause it's *their* life. So, I want to do a demonstration with a person from the audience to show you the efficacy of it. I think the system I've developed at this point is pretty consistent as far as responses are concerned. Otherwise, I wouldn't be volunteering to do this. I estimate it's taken probably a thousand sessions in the last year to figure out this system.

What I want to do now is have some volunteers. Can you tell me what is your current difficulty? Okay, we're going to solve that today. Do you feel any symptoms with it? She has an active cancerous tumor. She has a headache — the "old right-side-of-the-head syndrome." Trouble walking on your heels? Okay. Every time I do this I hear a new symptom I have never worked with. Lower back pain, okay. If I kept on, I think everybody would have something. Arthritic little finger. This room is in bad shape; I'd better go home!

Probably, one of the things I'm most concerned about when I do this, as I travel around the world and teach and do workshops, is that I don't want to be a person who "zips" through town, "zaps" somebody and just leaves them. That's why I would like to hold off on working with the volunteer who has the tumor. I think that would probably need a little more attention and might not be best in this circumstance.

Do you have something? What do you have? What's wrong with you? Numbness in your left hand? What do you have? PMS? Okay. Headache? You had a headache? It makes people feel good just to talk about what's wrong. What do you have over here? Oh, the "old root canal problem." I've done lots of "teeth things" with this. Stiff neck, okay. Anything else, while we're asking? A bone spur? Sinuses? I better stop here. I think we have enough. I wanted to hear you out, because I know those things are uncomfortable for you, and you deserve to at least get a little bit of attention.

Let me just start with the headache. You want to come up here? We will have microphones on, and you may not be able to see everything, but we will discuss it afterwards. You know, it's great to talk theory, but if I can get one person to feel better by the time we leave through this kind of light therapy process, I'll feel like a success. I always like to do at least one demonstration.

For those of you who are unfamiliar with this machine, let me familiarize you. What we have here on the **Lumatron Ocular Light Stimulator**™ is a lot of dials. This dial here changes the color. You see the "v" here? V is violet, and the "i" stands for indigo. Now, this is not very complicated, in that you turn it and it has a first letter that signifies one of the different colors. This one is blue. Now, this other dial regulates the flicker rate — the frequency of light flashing off and on — and we can regulate it from 1 to 60 cycles per second. Right here you will see numbers that come up that will tell you the exact flicker rate I'm using at the time. You will need to watch this meter, because I use the flicker rate quite a bit in this process.

Now, let me tell you something else about my orientation. Your name is what? Margaret, okay. Every time I start working with someone personally, I view this individual as the most precious being on the planet. This person is brave enough to come up here and to divulge whatever she might have related to her condition. Since she's going to be sharing with us publicly, my first task is to let her know, and to let you, the audience, know that Margaret is my very first priority. I don't care if the audience gets anything out of this; if you get better, Margaret, it's going to be worth it. So, it's going to be up to all of you in the audience to move around and see, whatever you need to do, because once I start working with Margaret, mentally, I'll leave you. I'm going to be over here between the machine and Margaret, okay?

Brief Strobic Phototherapy Demonstration

DR. VAZQUEZ: Can you describe to us a little bit more about the symptom, your headache?

MARGARET: There's like a line that starts here and comes up across the top of my head and comes down. There's a real sore spot right at the base of my skull; goes down the right side of my neck; comes down to the right of my spine and then kind of comes out to my shoulder.

DR. VAZQUEZ: Can you tell me something about that? Have you had this for very long, or is it just today?

MARGARET: I get headaches. I didn't have one yesterday. I had a really loud night at the Marriott last night, where I could feel a lot of tension and anger about the people having a party and not quieting down. And I woke up with it.

DR. VAZQUEZ: And if you had to designate a number as to its magnitude, from one to ten, ten is the worst, would you say it's about a six right now? Do you have any idea what it's about? Have you ever experienced this before?

MARGARET: Yes, I have. I do have two discs in my neck that are compacted, and it seems like when I get in an anxious situation, it puts pressures on that area and . . .

DR. VAZQUEZ: Which discs are they? Do you happen to know?

MARGARET: They're right above the knot. I'm trying to think of what that number would be.

DR. VAZQUEZ: Cervical, all right. If I were the greatest therapist on earth, what would you want to happen? If we could do anything?

MARGARET: Oh, I'd love never to have that pain again.

DR. VAZQUEZ: Now, you can ask for anything, who knows? What I'd like for you to do, Margaret, is to move your chair up here. Take your glasses off, if you would. The chair can be regulated so that your eyesight is equal to that circle where the light is coming out. So you scoot under there. You can hear me okay?

MARGARET: Uh huh.

DR. VAZQUEZ: Now if you had to guess about this headache, you have any ideas you can share? Do you have any guesses about this? Do you want to say anything about it?

MARGARET: It's a sick feeling that even goes to my stomach. It's like negativity.

DR. VAZQUEZ: A sick feeling, negative, that's okay. You don't have to worry about that. You just do what you need to do. Do you feel anything else?

MARGARET: Uh, suppression!

DR. VAZQUEZ: Suppression, of? Can you say some more about that?

MARGARET: Not being able to relax into a situation or control it so that it shifts and changes.

DR. VAZQUEZ: Okay, all right. So, I tell you what we're going to do, Margaret. I'm going to turn this light on, and I'm going to take a few minutes here adjusting the flash rate to exactly what's best for you. Now I want you to tell me, because the way I work is with your feedback; you're the one who is important here. I'm just going to be your helper, okay? I'm going to turn the light on, and it's going to be a violet light, and it's going to be flashing. So what I'd like for you to do as soon as I turn it on, is to tell me any reactions that you have to this.

MARGARET: My heart's beating faster.

DR. VAZQUEZ: Your heart's beating faster? Okay.

MARGARET: My throat and my chest.

DR. VAZQUEZ: And you feel it in your chest and your throat? Okay.

MARGARET: And my right ear.

DR. VAZQUEZ: Your right ear? Okay. What I'm going to do is, turn this flash rate up, and I'd like for you to share with me how you react when I do this, okay?

MARGARET: I just got a shudder all through my body.

DR. VAZQUEZ: You got a shudder through your body?

MARGARET: And now I can feel the crown of my head.

DR. VAZQUEZ: You feel the crown of your head? Is that good? Do you have a designation for that? Is it comfortable or uncomfortable?

MARGARET:	It's comfortable, very soothing.
DR. VAZQUEZ:	Okay, the flash rate is about 49 right here. And what about physically, what are you noticing?
MARGARET:	I feel pain towards the front part of my head.
DR. VAZQUEZ:	Pain towards the front part of your head? Okay. Now, I'm going to beg your permission to try something that might be a little bit uncomfortable to you. But it might be part of a process that will lead to you feeling better. Are you willing to try that?
MARGARET:	Yes.
DR. VAZQUEZ:	I'm going to turn it down; it's going to start flashing more slowly, but it might be a little uncomfortable for you. So I'm going to turn it down to about 5 per second. Do you have any reaction to that you can share with me?
MARGARET:	It feels depressing.
DR. VAZQUEZ:	It feels depressing? Okay.
MARGARET:	And I can feel the energy go down more towards my stomach and lower body.
DR. VAZQUEZ:	Okay, you can feel the energy go down more towards your stomach and lower body. Let me ask you... It was more comfortable going faster than it was going slow, right? So, what I want to look for is something that's "custom-tailored" just for you. And I want to find the border between comfort and discomfort as far as the flashing rate. So will you help me do that? If I speed it up, will you tell me when to stop? I want you to tell me when it's a little bit uncomfortable, but not too much. Would that be okay? I'm speeding it up, and you just let me know whenever it's a little bit uncomfortable but not too much. See, there's a value in it being somewhat uncomfortable, but I don't want it to be too much.
MARGARET:	Yeah, there.
DR. VAZQUEZ:	About there? Okay, you like that? It's 11.9 per second. Okay, so what happens when you look at this light, with it flashing at this rate?
MARGARET:	I feel the energy more between, like, about my third eye.
DR. VAZQUEZ:	Okay, you feel the energy in your third eye. What about the headache?
MARGARET:	The headache is much better. I can still feel the line of pain right between my shoulder blades.
DR. VAZQUEZ:	Let me ask you to elaborate on something you said a few minutes

	ago. You said something about difficulty controlling situations. Can you talk about that a little bit while you look at this light? What was that about? I didn't quite understand.
MARGARET:	That was about... (flood of tears)
DR. VAZQUEZ:	I want you to know I'm right here with you; and if you need my hand, it is right here, okay? And you can talk about it or you can not talk about it. Either way is fine with me.
MARGARET:	It's about being sexually abused as a child.
DR. VAZQUEZ:	It's about being sexually abused as a child. Okay, so let me ask you — take a few deep breaths — so, that's related to the controlling attempts that you feel?
MARGARET:	I'm trying to, but I'm not being able to.
DR. VAZQUEZ:	Oh, trying to but not being able to, okay. So when you think about that, what happens as you look at this light?
MARGARET:	My headache gets worse.
DR. VAZQUEZ:	Your headache gets worse. Where exactly does it get worse?
MARGARET:	The front part of my head.
DR. VAZQUEZ:	Okay, Margaret, the front part of your head. Okay, let me ask you, can you say just a little bit more, so I can help you with it. Because you were sexually abused, you attempt to control and fail often, and that's frustrating; is that what you're saying?
MARGARET:	Sometimes I become paralyzed and unable to act.
DR. VAZQUEZ:	Sometimes you become paralyzed and unable to act. When you're paralyzed, where do you feel it in your body?
MARGARET:	In my stomach and my liver.
DR. VAZQUEZ:	Okay, your stomach and your liver. Why don't you try to breathe right into those parts of your body? I want you just to breathe deeply, because, you know, when we get scared, we tend to hold our breath and not breathe. So, if you just look at that light, what I'd like for you to do is squeeze my hand any time you get scared, and I'm right here, so you know I'm here, okay? And what I'd like for you to do is to breathe out some of that fear and breathe in that violet light as you look at it and as you think about that fear you have. That's enough to frighten anybody. So stay right with it, you're doing very well, and tell me what happens. What does the light look like at this point?
MARGARET:	It kind of split. It has more red on the right side.

DR. VAZQUEZ: Okay, it has more red on the right side.

MARGARET: More blue on the left.

DR. VAZQUEZ: More blue on the left. So let me ask you . . . and you're still feeling the strain of this controlling and inability to control?

MARGARET: Not since we're not talking about it.

DR. VAZQUEZ: Okay, since we're not talking about it. Since I brought it up, though, it's not comfortable? Are you feeling more or less comfortable?

MARGARET: More comfortable. Feeling more comfortable.

DR. VAZQUEZ: What about the headache?

MARGARET: My headache feels much better. It feels like, now maybe because we're talking about it, it's kind of like a tenseness in my throat.

DR. VAZQUEZ: Tenseness in your throat, okay. So let's do this then; I'm going to change colors; is that okay? I'm going to let go of your hand here. I'm going to change colors to a blue color. And my hand's right here if you need it. How does this blue color affect you when you look at this?

MARGARET: I see the blue, and there's magenta around it, and then there's yellow around the outside edge.

DR. VAZQUEZ: And how do you feel physically when you look at it?

MARGARET: I like it.

DR. VAZQUEZ: You like it, okay. So, would you do this . . . I want you to, if you would, open your mouth and breathe through your mouth as you look at this color. Make sure your mouth is really stretched open as you breathe through it. And the headache, can you tell me about the headache at this point?

MARGARET: It's just like a feeling of pressure now, rather than a feeling of pain.

DR. VAZQUEZ: Feeling of pressure, okay, let's see what we can do about that pressure. Is there anything else that you feel like you need to say? If talking about it helped earlier, is there more that you could talk about that might help it a little bit more?

MARGARET: Well, I got a thing that came up . . . like I'm sick and tired of dealing with this in my life.

DR. VAZQUEZ: Could you say that again a little bit louder? I mean, I think it would be helpful just for you to actually say it.

MARGARET: I'm sick and tired of dealing with this in my life!

DR. VAZQUEZ: Okay, now, I think it's valuable to you to say it again; I think you might even feel better; but could you say it louder please, one more time?

MARGARET: I'm sick and tired of dealing with this in my life!

DR. VAZQUEZ: Okay. So how do you feel right now?

MARGARET: Hot.

DR. VAZQUEZ: Hot, okay. The headache, where do you feel the headache? Or is it there, or, what's left with that?

MARGARET: Well, now I feel like I'm supposed to be better.

DR. VAZQUEZ: Well, what do you feel?

MARGARET: I feel it's back to the original place, but more as a pressure, not pain.

DR. VAZQUEZ: Pressure. You say it's gone back to the original place, but more as a pressure, not pain? I wonder if there's any pressure that you feel, emotional pressure? Is there pressure you put on yourself, or anything of that nature?

MARGARET: I feel definite pressure to be able to survive and take care of myself, and not believing in that ability.

DR. VAZQUEZ: And what is it like after you say that? Does that make sense to you? Do you want to have this pressure? Is it valuable to you?

MARGARET: It forces action.

DR. VAZQUEZ: It forces action. Okay, so it has some good value. So as long as you listen and you take the action that's appropriate, then maybe it's not necessary to put quite so much pressure on yourself. Does that make sense to you?

MARGARET: Yeah.

DR. VAZQUEZ: So what's happening in your body right now?

MARGARET: My left leg is kind of tingling.

DR. VAZQUEZ: Hmm, "the old left leg tingling." That's a good sign. Is it uncomfortable tingling, or is it comfortable? So you like that? Everybody should have their left leg tingle, okay? So how are you doing generally right now, as compared to when we started?

MARGARET: I feel a lot lighter.

DR. VAZQUEZ: You feel a lot lighter, okay. How about let me let go of your hand here. I'm going to change the flicker rate just a little bit, and I want you to report to me what you're experiencing as I do this. Can you talk to me about this?

MARGARET: Well, it changes the dimension, the light is no longer sitting on the flat surface, or the surface is no longer flat. And it's like losing my place in space.

DR. VAZQUEZ: Well, how does it affect you?

MARGARET: It's disorienting.

DR. VAZQUEZ: Okay, would you like me to keep it still? Would that make it easier?

MARGARET: It's easier, but this is interesting.

DR. VAZQUEZ: Easier, but interesting. So a little disorientation is an adventure. That's exactly what you said was the problem with controlling and now you see disorientation as an adventure. And that's pretty good. So how are you feeling now?

MARGARET: Like I had an "aha!"

DR. VAZQUEZ: Okay. I think we need to stop there. I'm going to turn it off. Are you okay? Let's talk a little bit about what happened procedurally here. The headache?

MARGARET: Oh, my back just popped.

DR. VAZQUEZ: Back popped, headache changed, she went through some emotional experience, and she had a tingle and "aha," okay. Margaret, let me thank you for volunteering.

DR. VAZQUEZ: Any questions about how this took place?

QUESTION: Why did you start with the violet light?

DR. VAZQUEZ: I'm going to explain why I start with any particular color. There's a whole regimen I've come up with, but basically the words she said about controlling were a key for me to choose the violet, because I've found that, as far as the content of what people talk about, violet is often times associated with trust and mistrust issues. So in Margaret's case, I started with this.

As a psychotherapist, what I'm interested in, is — what do these colors mean to people? I really listen to the content of what they've said. I think **I've given somewhere near a thousand sessions in the last year and I've tried to come up with themes of what each color means or evokes. What are the themes people talk about when they see these particular colors?** This is what I've come up with. Now, everyone doesn't fit this model, but generally, it fits pretty well.

Colored Light and Inherent Meanings in Brief Strobic Phototherapy

Unresolved Issues ⟫ ⟫ ⟫ ⟫ ⟫ Potential Experience

RUBY: *The Color of the Life Instinct*

death wish	existential issues	desire to live
survival, insecurity	safety issues	stability, rootedness
numbness, shock	sensory issues	sensory awareness

RED: *The Color of Passion*

sexual depravity or omission	sexual issues	sexual pleasure
primitive rage	anger issues	euphoria
danger	risk issues	purpose in life

RED/ORANGE: *The Color of Freedom*

guilt, shame	issues of conscience	spontaneity
inhibition	issues of inner child	creativity
excessive sense of responsibility	issues of interpersonal boundaries	playfulness

ORANGE: *The Color of Self-Esteem*

ego distortion	issues of identity	self-concept
passivity	issues of disclosure	assertiveness
inferiority	issues of confidence	self-love

YELLOW: *The Color of Hope*

corrupted power	issues of power	flexibility
helplessness, panic	issues of control	empowerment
resentment, frustration	issues of letting go	optimism

YELLOW/GREEN: *The Color of Peace*

adversarial relationships	love, hate issues	compatibility
jealousy, envy	issues of hurt	acceptance of love
abandonment	issues of separation	union with others

GREEN: *The Color of Love*

deprivation of affection	issues of needing affection	fulfilled affection
destructive affection	issues of distorted affection	appropriate affection
loneliness, loss	issues of grief	inspiration

BLUE/GREEN: *The Color of Wholeness*

extreme intellectualization	issues of emotion vs. thought	confluence
detachment, impersonal	issues of mind vs. body	harmony
unawareness of self	issues of somatic awareness	self-awareness

BLUE: *The Color of Joy*

introversion, inarticulate	issues of verbalization	expression
distortion of communication	communication issues	healthy contact w/others
dependency	issues of bonding contact	independence

INDIGO: *The Color of Understanding*

confusion	issues of logic and philosophy	clarity
inner conflict	issues of inner search	insight
overwhelmed	issues of ordered thinking	inner peace

VIOLET: *The Color of Faith*

mistrust	trust issues	trust
worry	issues of letting go	contact w/spirit
aberrant spirituality	religious issues	vision

Colored Light and Associated Anatomy and Psychological Issues in Brief Strobic Phototherapy

	Anatomy	Primary Site	Secondary Site	Issues
RUBY	Coccyx Sacrum 5th lumbar	rectum, anus hip, bones, buttocks lower legs, ankles, feet	head heart stomach	existential safety sensory awareness
RED	4th lumbar 3rd lumbar	prostate, lower back muscles, sciatic sex organs, uterus, bladder, knees	back of neck stomach	sexual anger risk
RED ORANGE	2nd lumbar 1st lumbar	appendix, abdomen, upper leg large intestines, inguinal rings	trapezius shoulders	conscience inner child
ORANGE	12th thoracic 11th thoracic 10th thoracic	small intestines, lymph circulation kidneys, ureters kidneys	heart throat	interpersonal boundaries identity disclosure confidence
YELLOW	9th thoracic 8th thoracic 7th thoracic 6th thoracic	adrenal, supra-adrenal glands spleen pancreas, duodenum stomach	back of neck arms hands upper legs	power control letting go
YELLOW GREEN	5th thoracic 4th thoracic	liver, solar plexus, blood gall bladder, common duct	top of head feet	love, hate hurt, separation
GREEN	3rd thoracic 2nd thoracic	lungs, bronchial tubes, breast heart, coronary arteries	sacrum 3rd lumbar	needing affection distorted affection grief
BLUE GREEN	1st thoracic 7th cervical	esophagus, trachea, forearms, hands, wrists, fingers thyroid gland, bursae in shoulders		emotion vs. thought mind vs. body somatic awareness
BLUE	6th cervical 5th cervical 4th cervical 3rd cervical	neck muscles, shoulders, tonsils vocal chords, neck gland, pharynx nose, lips, mouth, eustachian tube cheeks, outer ear, face bones, teeth		verbalization communication bonding contact
INDIGO	2nd cervical 1st cervical	sinuses, mastoid bones, tongue, forehead, eyes, optic nerves, auditory nerves pituitary gland, bones of the face, brain, inner and middle ear		logic and philosophy inner search ordered thinking
VIOLET	top of skull	organ, hypothalamus, cerebrospinal fluid	coccyx	trust letting go religious

So, as you can see, with Margaret, I identified by listening to several recurring themes, the issue of controlling, which ultimately has to do with a lot of mistrust in her environment. If she was abused by those people closest to her, then of course she's going to mistrust people around her later on, and a lot of times, she's not clear why that's a problem. And the struggle itself manifests in the headache.

When we needed to go a little bit further, talking about it helped. Margaret next described a constriction in her throat, so I went to the blue region and encouraged her to talk about it some more. This gave her the resolution she needed. Now, in a private session, in all likelihood, I would go much further than this, but mainly, I wanted to show you all a little of the dynamics of how we can change things relatively consistently and easily with Brief Strobic Phototherapy.

Criteria for Selecting the Color for Initiation of Treatment with a New Subject

VIOLET	When subject exhibits tension, intensity, or mistrust as in an excessive need to control; when head symptoms such as pain predominate.
INDIGO	When the subject exhibits confusion or expressing overwhelming emotion or cognition, such as obsessive thinking; when initial symptoms of the forehead or eyes are reported.
BLUE	When inhibited verbal expression and introversion predominate; when symptoms of ears, nose, and throat predominate.
BLUE/GREEN	When the subject appears intellectual or otherwise unaware of emotions; when release of and or amnesia of repressed experiences is sought.
YELLOW	When the subject experiences extreme fatigue and unresponsiveness.
RUBY	When the subject reports physical numbness and detached awareness of sensory experience.

These are just the rudimentary beginning points, and these are merely a few of the reasons. My rationale comes from how do I start with this person? Where can I find a rapport for the journey itself? This isn't the endpoint usually, but sometimes it is. **My preference is to try to start as far at the top of the blue range as I can. If I'm fuzzy about the patient's particular issue, I'll start with violet, and I'll get a sense of**

what's going on with violet, and then from there I'll move to other regions. Generally, what I try to do is start with attempting to develop rapport and trust or get them to be able to talk. **Next, I'll go toward the symptom areas a little bit more, and ultimately in the same session I'll move to a color where they will deal with the actual *key conflict*, what I sense is the root cause of the problem.**

Sometimes people I work with are very fragile and sensitive, and I want to be really careful not to just "dive in" initially, because I've seen some very strong negative reactions to that, but I eventually do get to deeper material. I think it's important, and I usually wouldn't end with blue, but in this case she had relief at that point.

In the demonstration, after the flicker rate was altered, did you notice that I changed it again after Margaret had pretty much completed the work? I began to raise the flicker rate; this was when she experienced what she termed "disorientation." This was to her, an "adventure" and was "fun." Notably, this was in complete contrast to what she said when she started.

About 60% of the people tested, according to Penrey and his coauthor in their book on photosensitive seizures, seem to respond to flickering light in a trancelike manner. This whole idea of flickering light contributing to trance phenomena is really pretty old. I found a text that showed **in 1898, a hypnotherapist in London, named Saxtus, who was already using flickering candlelight as a hypnotic induction technique.** So, for those of us who are familiar with hypnosis, a flickering light is a familiar tool.

Before I do Brief Strobic Phototherapy, I generally go through a *disclaimer*. Since this is a non-medical device, I talk to my clients about this procedure being experimental. I usually check to see if they have a history of *photosensitive seizures*. Then I'll ask a series of questions like: "Are you on any medications? What is your marital status? Do you have any medical conditions?" I get some background information and ask what symptoms they're experiencing and what positive change they want to happen. I always start with what they want to happen. It's their agenda, not mine. Maybe I want something big to take place for them, but I have to start with what they want.

Margaret dictated what we did by her responses. So, before I started I was careful to explain what was going to happen first, second, and third. This really comforts the "inner child" in a person, to go through these steps. I remember when I was a kid and went to the doctor's office, and they said, "Now we're going to do this, and then we're going to do this, and then somebody's going to do such and such," and all those little things really helped when you were kids. So you find they help when you're adults too.

Life is an opportunity so that we may become better people, wiser, more loving and illuminated as we progress in evolution.

— *Pir Vilayat Inayat Khan*

The Chakra System as it Relates to Lumatron™ Colors

Next, let's consider the effects of different colors on different body regions. These are approximate dividing lines indicating which colors affect which regions of the body. They aren't precise. For example, if orange affects the shoulders, there are often "referred" issues here. If there's tension in the lower abdomen, often there is also increased tension in the shoulder region between the neck and the deltoid. **So by utilizing the light to affect several body parts, I think I gradually get to the core of the issue. The assessment I do is dynamic in nature. I found it was tedious to go through the whole color spectrum on the Lumatron™ and find out how a person responded, because some people had pretty strong responses initially.** I use my criteria to decide where to start, and then I ask for feedback from the subject. "What is your reaction?" Just a generalized, open-ended question suffices: "How do you react to this?" Next, I check the flicker rate reaction: "What's happening in your body?" and, "Where is it happening in your body? What emotional reaction do you have to this light? What occurs when you view this light?"

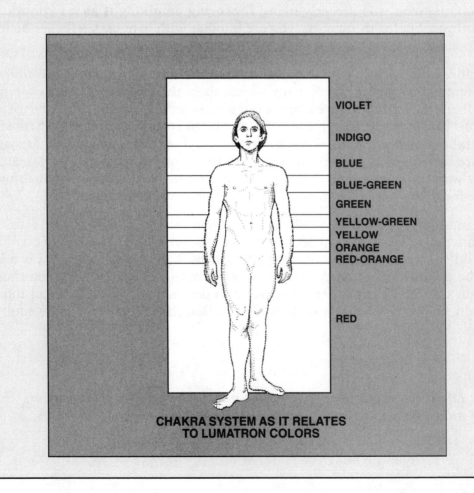

VIOLET

INDIGO

BLUE

BLUE-GREEN

GREEN

YELLOW-GREEN

YELLOW

ORANGE

RED-ORANGE

RED

**CHAKRA SYSTEM AS IT RELATES
TO LUMATRON COLORS**

The Chakra System and Its Relationship to the Autonomic Nervous System and Time

What we have here are a few basic principles. The further you go down *the chakra system,* **the more patients talk about things that relate to their past.** The areas of the chakra regions around the **blue-green** to **blue** to even **indigo** tend to deal more with **present day experiences.** When you get to **violet,** sometimes you have experiences dealing with things **beyond time, or in the future.** The colors **red, orange, yellow** tend to relate to issues in the client's **past.** So, in Margaret's case she had a memory of something that was related to control, and that came up even in the upper chakra levels, where I was working. Generally, the division of *colors from yellow on down (orange and red) tend to activate the sympathetic nervous system,* and the *colors above that point (yellow-green, green, blue-green, blue, indigo, violet) tend to activate the parasympathetic nervous system.*

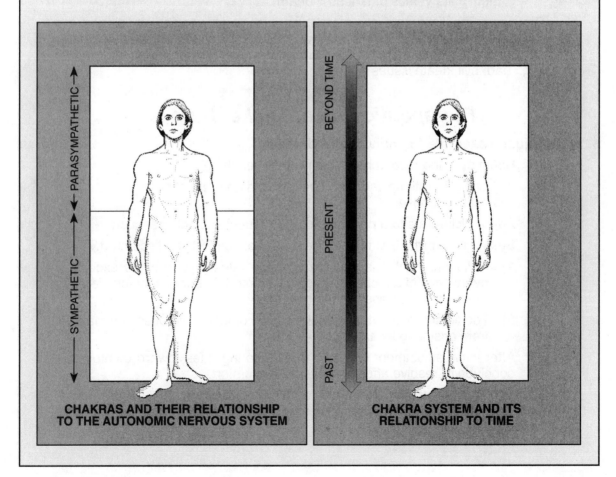

**CHAKRAS AND THEIR RELATIONSHIP
TO THE AUTONOMIC NERVOUS SYSTEM**

**CHAKRA SYSTEM AND ITS
RELATIONSHIP TO TIME**

Considerations for Choosing Flicker Rate

- Slower flicker rates are more likely to cause delayed reactions and interfere with the subject's ability to retrieve or grasp the meanings or the content of their experience.

- When working with issues like extreme depression, suicidal tendencies, and panic attacks, keep it at a higher flicker rate as the subject reports verbally. This helps to diminish the intensity of the experience.

- Verbal reporting elicits beta-theta states in which unconscious material can be integrated into normal waking states, thus encouraging awareness and empowerment.

- The experience of viewing rapid sequences of light and then the absence of light is often seen as a contrast of meanings about light versus darkness.

  Light = good versus darkness = bad

  Light = conscious mind versus darkness = unconscious mind

  Light = God versus darkness = evil

  Light = life versus darkness = death

- The slower the flicker rate, the more the subject is able to actually discern the dark part of the strobe. This often allows subjects to become aware of a greater proportion of their "shadow" in the form of previously unconscious information (e.g., bad, evil, death issues).

Therapeutic Use of Flicker Rate

I. **Adjust flicker rate for individualized needs.**

   A. Begin by using researched flicker rate for each color.

   B. Adjust flicker rate upward to 50 per second and request subject's response.

   C. Adjust flicker rate to 5 per second and request subject's reaction.

   D. Seek a flicker rate that is near the border of comfort vs. discomfort.

      1) Rationale for this is that too aversive rates may provoke excessive overwhelm of affect or physical discomfort. In some subjects defense mechanisms of dissociation may occur.

      2) Too comfortable rates may slow down or inhibit unconscious material from arising to awareness.

   E. After initial adjustment of flicker rates, altering rates toward comfort can conclude or resolve affect or physical discomfort.

II. **Flicker rates induce entrainment or trance in about 60% of subjects, therefore allowing them to become amenable to a wide range of hypnotic techniques.**

Dynamic Assessment

I. Initial orientation and feedback from the subject.

    A.   What reaction do you have to this light?

    B.   How do you react to each flicker rate?

    C.   Notify me when the flicker rate is mildly uncomfortable but not too uncomfortable.

    D.   What reaction do you feel in your body? Where?

    E.   What emotional reaction do you have?

    F.   What thoughts occur when you view this light?

II. Increased discomfort exhibited by one or more of the following:

    A.   Emotional reaction

    B.   Physical discomfort

    C.   Perceptual distortion

    D.   Uncomfortable thoughts such as images, memories or negativity

    E.   Increase in galvanic skin response (GSR), decrease in skin temperature, increase in muscular tension

As to the *Therapeutic Use of Flicker Rate,* here are some of the principles I've come up with. I adjust the flicker rate for individualized needs. Some people think everybody should fit a certain flicker rate. But as you saw, I began by using the researched flicker rates, something very close to **Gerard's**[1] research, that Dr. John Downing shared with me. Often I try to start at this rate, and then I move up to ascertain how they respond to a faster flicker rate and then ascertain how they respond to a slower one. From there we can find a range that fits their particular needs. The idea being, **I want to stimulate unconscious material to come up. Usually the patient is a little bit uncomfortable if we do that, and I don't want it to be overwhelming, so I look for that border between comfort and discomfort. I adjust the flicker rate upward and then I go down to a slower rate until we find this border**. Basically, what happens with rates that are too comfortable is the progress is too slow, and I like to try to get something happening, as you saw, in a single session. I like to get some change to take place that is significant.

---

1. The reference for Gerard's research monograph can be found in the *Bibliography: Section Two, page 389, Light in Optometry.*

The first and foremost *intervention technique* is giving the person a chance to talk. Did you notice when Margaret was upset at one point, I encouraged her to say it again, and to say it even louder? *Verbal catharsis* all by itself is probably the number one mode of release these days, and more and more people are being healed by it. Talking is vital.

I can use a much more extensive variety of treatment approaches in a session to accommodate an extensive variety of situations. Some of them I borrowed from **Dr. Francine Shapiro's** work, ***Eye Movement Desensitization and Reprocessing (EMDR)***[2], as well as some others, in order to help alleviate traumatic symptoms. Sometimes I use *eye movement techniques*. You also saw me use some *breath work* with Margaret, and sometimes I use *alteration of the flicker rate*. All these techniques were evolved to actually transform a person from a state of disruption and chaos to a state of relief. Sometimes I change to another color. In Margaret's case there was still some discomfort I thought could be alleviated if we changed to a different color. And it did work. It's up to the patient to tell me when they feel better; this dictates when I stop, at least during demonstrations. So, I eased the flicker rate at the end of the demonstration as I often do, and that seems to promote a surge of well-being, as you saw with Margaret.

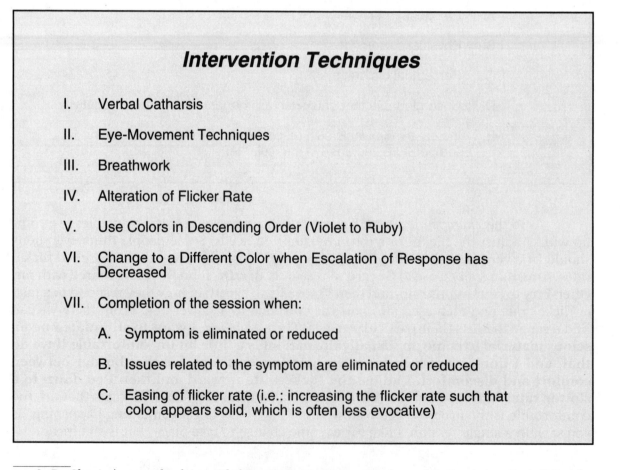

Intervention Techniques

I.   Verbal Catharsis

II. Eye-Movement Techniques

III. Breathwork

IV. Alteration of Flicker Rate

V.   Use Colors in Descending Order (Violet to Ruby)

VI. Change to a Different Color when Escalation of Response has Decreased

VII. Completion of the session when:

    A. Symptom is eliminated or reduced

    B. Issues related to the symptom are eliminated or reduced

    C. Easing of flicker rate (i.e.: increasing the flicker rate such that color appears solid, which is often less evocative)

---

2. Dr. Shapiro's recent book is entitled *Eye Movement Desensitization and Reprocessing: Basic Principles, Protocols and Procedures*, New York, N.Y. Guilford Press, 1995.

Patterns of Psychoemotional Energy Movement In the Body

Looking at this diagram about the *psychoemotional energy movement in the body,* I realize I am working on a radically different paradigm than that of the Western medical model. What I have here is a diagram that shows how I perceive the *psychoemotional energy* to move through the body. This model is very crucial for me and the way I work with people. I have three different movements here: *primary movement* is from the bottom chakra upward through the crown chakra; the *secondary movement* is from the back of the chakras to the front, and outward; and the *tertiary movement* is toward the back, and down. What this tells me is that you may have, let's say, a traumatic emotional experience, and you feel tension in your lower abdomen. Initially, you may feel it in the lower abdomen, and then you'll feel it in the chest, maybe the throat, wherever the blocks are. But **generally you'll notice a movement upwards as the person processes the trauma and works it through. Sometimes you'll notice a movement from the front to the back.** So these are the things I'm paying attention to when **I'm listening to a client's description of physical reactions to particular things like colors, thoughts, feelings**. There are even more movements than these; however, these are just some basic ones to which I pay attention. When clients are giving me their feedback, this is vital information to me. **I'll know you're getting better when I see a movement upward of the tension.**

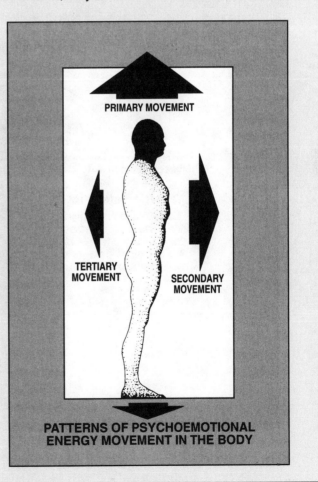

PATTERNS OF PSYCHOEMOTIONAL ENERGY MOVEMENT IN THE BODY

The Qualitative Experience of a Typical Brief Strobic Phototherapy Session

What I see happen when I change colors is an *increase in tension,* which manifests as *strong emotion, physical discomfort, behavioral movement, verbalization, rapid thoughts, temperature change, EMG, GSR changes,* etc. As I work with a person there is often an escalation of tension; then I use the *intervention techniques* to transform the experience when it is at its peak. After there is a reduction of that tension, I change the color. This is the procedure when I use multiple colors within a given session. So, this gives you an idea of the Light Assisted Therapeutic process and the kinds of choices made between shifting colors and intervention strategies.

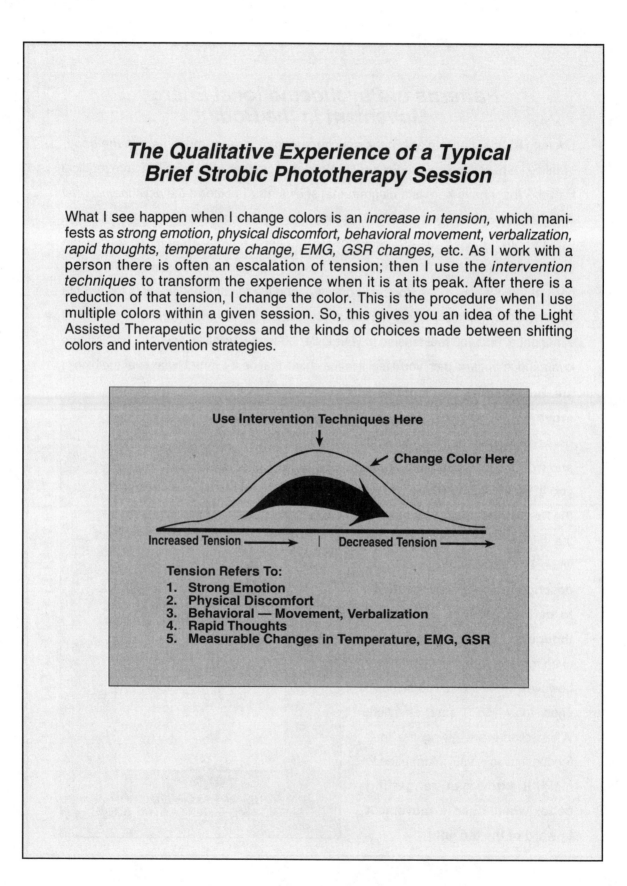

Use Intervention Techniques Here

Change Color Here

Increased Tension ———→ | Decreased Tension ———→

Tension Refers To:
1. **Strong Emotion**
2. **Physical Discomfort**
3. **Behavioral — Movement, Verbalization**
4. **Rapid Thoughts**
5. **Measurable Changes in Temperature, EMG, GSR**

Body Regions and Gender Issues

I notice that some people talk about **issues related to women or their mothers with the colors that move from green upward to violet.** Conversely, they talk about **men or father issues downward from yellow through red.** Another schemata has to do with **masculine issues, or issues with father. These are often connected to symptoms or sensations on the right side of the body, and the issues related to mother or relationships with females are often found on the left side of the body.** Now, I've seen it happen both ways, and I just have to listen very carefully, but these are guiding principles I've seen take place time and again.

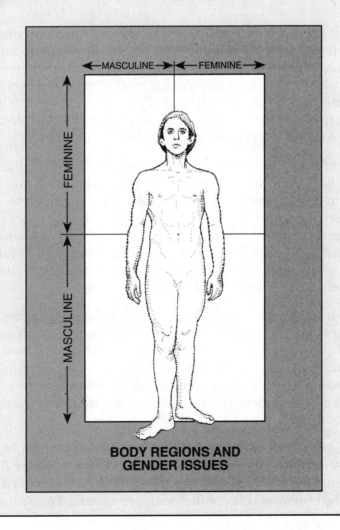

**BODY REGIONS AND
GENDER ISSUES**

Dr. John Downing and Dr. Jacob Liberman talked about using the more *"homeopathic approach" to light treatment.* I want to correct that. I have presented my own approach to light treatment, and I'm not yet exactly sure which words to use other than my own. **There is one approach that says if a person is basically tense, you want to use the upper frequency colors at the blue end of the spectrum to relax them. The point is to balance them, so if they are too relaxed or fatigued, sometimes you want to use stimulating colors from the red to yellow range. That's one approach. The other approach is the homeopathic, in which you go for the bottom line cause, and actually use the colors that are most uncomfortable for them. What I do is an integration of both of these strategies.** I've known of Dr. John Downing's work and of Dr. Jacob Liberman's work for some time, and it's always amazed me that **both methods are equally effective,** yet the two approaches are completely opposite to each other. I have been intrigued with their work for some time, and have finally figured out an integration that I can use.

Example of a Brief Strobic Phototherapy Session

This is how it goes, process-wise: Client is nervous upon entering the session; basic procedures are explained, and a disclaimer is given; background about client is obtained; client identifies goals as relief of depression and lower gastrointestinal discomfort; client is directed to view *violet light;* client reports discomfort with flickering, but comfort with violet color. This case is actually a composite of several people with whom I've worked. After the flicker rate is adjusted, client discloses a conflict with her spouse; she then reports physical relaxation, except for tension in her lower chest.

So, what happens is there's been a reduction of the tension; then I change color to *yellow-green.* After the flicker rate is adjusted, client reports seeing numerous other colors; and as she begins to talk more about her conflict with her spouse, she begins to cry. Compassion and verbal support are given; confluent breathing techniques are instructed. After the breathing techniques, client reports relief of sadness, and the client's color perception changes to a true yellow-green. The next thing that usually happens, along with relief of the chest tension, is an awareness of lower abdominal tension as she reflects on conflicts with her father during childhood.

Next, we change the color to *red-orange.* This light is perceived to contain numerous colors colliding in conflict, and she reports irritation from viewing it; client remembers an incident of sexual and physical abuse by her father; she then talks as if she is a little girl, and the incident is in present tense; compassion and empathy are given and her options are explained; client chooses to pursue relief; physical tension escalates; the fear is expressed; lateral eye movement is directed; and the emotional trauma subsides within minutes as the body relaxes.

Again, as tension comes down, I go back up the spectrum again to *indigo.* The change of colors is initially uncomfortable, and the color appears distorted. As client reviews her experience of the event with her father, it is viewed in past-tense perspective, and she sees how she re-enacts this conflict with her spouse. Then all physical symptoms dissipate, and the light now appears to be a true indigo color. She then experiences peace and understanding, and the light stimulation is stopped.

So, what I do is **generally to start at the top with violet, indigo, or blue, depending on what that person needs initially. Then I'll work with the symptom;** in this case, depression was the primary symptom she talked about, which was located in the green/yellow-green region, but I knew that wasn't the cause. It wasn't the bottom line of what her discomfort was about. Then the next step in this particular case would be to go to red-orange, and the action really occurs. **Here I see what I call the *latent cause* of this particular symptom. We work through that, and then, in order to bring the session to a proper conclusion, we bring the light back up the spectrum,** in this case, to indigo. Most of what I do works in a loop formation. **There's a time and a place to provoke memories and unconscious material, and then there's a time and a place to assist a person in experiencing a sense of peace and a new clarity of understanding.**

QUESTION: Can you tell me more about using this technique with *multiple personality disorder* patients? Aren't there some potential dangers with this technique?

DR. VAZQUEZ: I suspect that you might be referring to *ritualistic abuse victims*, as well, who had been programmed by colors. I work with a lot of multiples, and I've been doing this for some time. I have a supervision group teaching other therapists about the diagnosis and treatment of *multiple personality disorder (MPD)*. So I've been doing that extensively for many years. It's very difficult to work with them; you have to work with them very carefully, especially with the Lumatron™. The problem with people who dissociate is that they're likely not to feel anything and not to give me much verbal response at all. This is very important to me, especially if their defense mechanism is to dissociate and not feel anything. MPD clients are generally not able to tell me very well where the proper flicker rate is. They err in thinking that they can handle it, when, in fact, their fear turns into dissociation so quickly that they don't feel anything. So, I have to presume that initially, they are not skilled in estimating how they feel. Thus, I have to err on the side of being "extra safe" and particularly slow, because I don't want them to dissociate. If they're not present, nothing happens. I find that the Lumatron™ does work well with these patients, and I've used it with them a lot. But I have to be very careful, just as any therapist would, in any treatment with them. These people have been through horrendous trauma and they're difficult for everybody. However, with regard to the client's color programming, Brief Strobic Phototherapy can provide an opportunity to work through that programming. You can change colors and you can change flicker rates, which will alter their programming with colors in many cases. It is a slow and careful process that you have to work up to and prepare them for. You have to be aware that it's really easy to overwhelm them.

As far as *the chakras and their relationships to Lumatron™ colors* I talked about earlier, when I first started working with this, I was familiar with the chakra system. But I honestly wasn't sure that the Lumatron™ colors would match my previous understanding of the chakra colors. I observed for many months, and I found that naive subjects would spontaneously describe things, both physiologically and psychologically, that matched the chakra system. I recommend that you explore for yourself. That's what I did initially. In fact, some of the ways in which I describe the meanings associated with color differ with some of the more traditional ideas about how the chakra system is supposed to work.

What's different about light stimulation as opposed to some other forms of therapy is that the effects of light do linger, sometimes for 24 hours or longer. If I were to see you in another session, I'd want to know what had taken place 24 hours after the session, because I think we've stimulated a change, and you had an "aha." These things affect the entire system. Everybody's a little bit different, so I just observe and get feedback, and according to how you respond, I operate differently than with the next person. Some people have much more delayed responses, while others are more spontaneous. With Margaret's example today, we just saw the tip of the iceberg, and it could be the beginning of a whole number of changes for her.

QUESTION: Tell me what you make of the client perceiving the light as multicolored versus monochrome.

DR. VAZQUEZ: **Basically, I use color perception as important feedback. When people see numerous colors, it can be for one of two reasons: first, the misperception of color; and secondly, what's going on with them emotionally can also cause this situation. I find that when emotional catharsis takes place, true color perception clears up, and it looks like one clear, unmuddled color. It looks like the true color again.** In fact, most of the time, when people have a lot of unconscious emotional disturbance, they see all kinds of colors. They don't see the pure color that is actually there at all. **Lumatron™ work is quite beautiful, like a "moving Rorschach,"** a projective psychological test, and I just tell them **what they're seeing in the light is their unconscious material projected before them.** It's like you put your unconscious on the screen so now you can look at it.

One woman I worked with in Chicago just recently was working through a birth incident, and she saw a vagina in the Lumatron™, so I went over there to look inside and see if I could see it! Of course I didn't see it; it's her projection! Anyway, I thought, "Well, maybe it's there; I don't know. People see all kinds of things in there." They see with tremendous clarity, their unconscious material coming forward. I haven't seen a vagina in there yet, but I'm still working on it!

How does it affect me to have the machine come between me and the client? I think the *medicine of the future* is to marry all these machines that we've created with a very compassionate, personal contact. Some therapists do one or the other. They either use machines, or they're personal, like a massage therapist. Why not use the best of both worlds? I think this kind of an integration works quite well.

Now in Margaret's case, if you remember, I held her hand through much of the process, and I was talking to her. There was a lot of rapport happening. But it actually changes the transference when the client begins to transfer thoughts and feelings onto the therapist. In this case, she's transferring them more to what she sees in the light. It actually puts a little bit of a partition up, so that the transference doesn't get quite so confusing. I was teaching in a massage therapy school not too long ago, and they were talking about transference issues. I was saying that when virtually any woman gives me a massage, I fall in love with that woman while she's giving me that massage. That's transference "big time." I just love it! So there are great things that can happen there in transference; depending on how you handle it, it can be very good or very toxic. Working with the Lumatron™ as a tool just gives me a little bit of distance from the patient, so that I can direct things more easily.

So, I'm not giving up traditional therapy, and there are many times that I don't even use the machines. I use the Lumatron™ when and if I think it's appropriate. These days it's most of the time. Margaret, I don't mean to put you on the spot too much, but did you feel like there was some contact between us? She said that the sound of my voice, the way I was holding her hand, that I was really there. There are always ways you can do that. That's one of the things that I want to demonstrate — that you can really be with a person and use a machine too. I have to tell you that I'm not a machine-person. I have problems with all kinds of machines. I don't like them. This is the first machine I became friends with; this one feels like an extension of me.

My view is that therapy starts with establishing safety. I don't think you're going to get anywhere if you're not establishing safety; that has to be first. I want you to notice how we started this process. Do you remember how we started it? I set up exactly how important she was in this process and how I was going to go about this. I made her, as she said, feel protected. I do that first and foremost, and it's amazing what you can do once you get that sense of safety. Then you can do anything.

Do I have a Lumatron™? Yes. It's in a room that . . . it all depends on the time of day . . . how bright it is . . . usually we put a curtain over it. So, it's not completely darkened; but I do want to move it into a darkened room. But that's how I've worked with it so far.

The people with whom I work are often very fragile, and I feel far more comfortable being there right in the room with them. I depend on my judgment to establish what's "safe" in a particular situation. **The Lumatron™ and other light instruments are not toys to me. The colors can elicit very profound responses.** A person just recently told me about someone who was stimulated with yellow light and the next day the person committed suicide. Now, we don't know whether these incidents are connected or not, but I do think you have to be careful. I've had people who have gotten very suicidal when I would use certain colors early on, when I was exploring how to use these techniques, so I know that it can be dangerous.

Now, regarding *Light Assisted Dream Interpretation,* I developed a method for Dream Interpretation through use of the Lumatron™. I discovered it serendipitously while working with a woman who, at one point during a session, began to tell me about her dream. So I listened to the dream, and so forth, and I thought that was interesting, and then I thought, I wonder what would happen if I'd put her on a different color? So I put her on a different color and asked her to repeat the same dream. Then we got a different story and there was more information. So then I thought, okay, I'll put her on another color. Tell me the dream again, and she gave even more in-depth information about it. So then I really went wild. We did all the colors, and she got the total meaning of the dream. So then I began to explore this dream stuff more and more. It's kind of cumbersome to go through every single color, but essentially, the whole interpretation comes out, and I don't have to do anything but support the client.

The technique I finally came up with is extraordinary, and I have to make one disclaimer about it. Here again, **one must be very careful, because dreams are disguised for a reason, and that reason is that most of us are not ready to handle the unconscious information.** Quite often one outcome that was really a problem here was people were overwhelmed and emotionally distraught when they got the material from their dream interpretations. So I've developed a protocol which I use after trying out several different approaches. It is a system of four colors. *First color I start them with is the bluegreen light,* but before this occurs they tell me the dream without light stimulation. *The dream information is either talked out or written out.* When I ask them to repeat the dream, they tell me under blue-green light stimulation. They always get some new awareness that they didn't have before. I use *blue-green,* then *yellow-green,* then *orange,* and then *red.* If they're in trouble at that point, which they usually are with this kind of work, I will go back to *indigo* or *violet,* to re-establish a sense of stability with them, so that we can bring this dream interpretation to a conclusion. *The color selection is altered* if a specific color stands out when the person reports the dream; then I'll include that color.

Light Spectrum Assisted Dream Work

I. **Extraordinary dream interpretation can occur by having the subject report the same dream while viewing different colors, one at a time.**

II. **Vazquez procedures for dream work.**

    A. *1st—Blue-Green, 2nd—Yellow-Green, 3rd—Orange, 4th—Red*

    B. Color selection is altered if a specific color stands out in the reporting of a dream.

    C. Color selection is altered if the dominant dream theme is associated with colors.

    D. Color may be altered if the subject reports a strong intuition that a certain color needs to be used.

III. **Psychotherapy processes include the following:**

    A. The subject reports a written or typed copy of the dream to the therapist.

    B. The subject verbally repeats the same dream over on each color.

    C. During the reporting, compassionate empathy is provided and any deviations from the initial report are noted.

    D. After each of the four reports, the subject is encouraged to verbalize insights.

    E. Dreams are often disguised to defend against extreme reactions such as shock, overwhelm, etc. Therefore, discomfort may be expected.

IV. **If major discomfort occurs, light work can help conclude it.**

    A. If *stifled verbalization* occurs, repeating a dream while viewing *Blue* can bring relief.

    B. If *confusion or conflict* about the dream occurs, concluding by repeating it in *Indigo* can bring clarity.

    C. If *tension* related to *an inability to let go* occurs, repeating the dream in *Violet* can bring relief.

Dream Agents

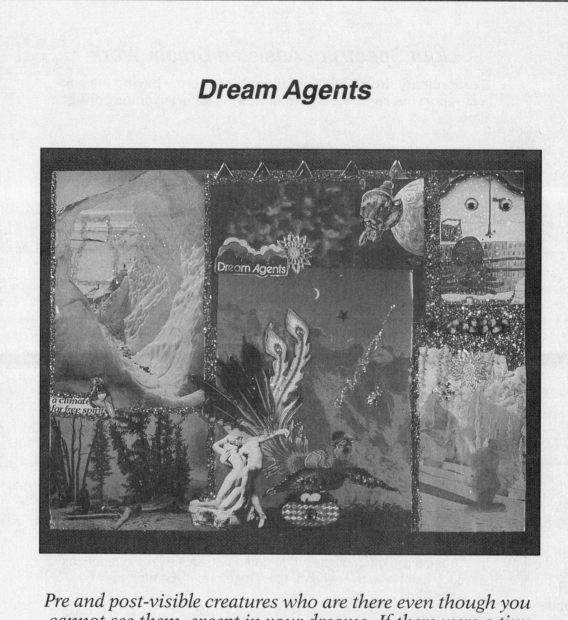

Pre and post-visible creatures who are there even though you cannot see them, except in your dreams. If there were a tiny silver hammer in your dreams — in case of emergence, you could break the glass and plant the blue corn. Bodies rub up against life to keep the spark of dream passion aglow.

Collage art by Bethany ArgIsle.

The color choice is also altered if the dominant dream theme is associated with particular colors, like the themes that I shared with you earlier. *Color may also be altered if the subject reports a strong intuition that a certain color needs to be used.* The colors I choose vary, but if I'm not treating any of these problems associated with other colors, **I'll just go with the four basic colors which affect the four major regions of the body, head, heart, solar plexus, and the pelvic and perineum areas. I've found this to be the most efficient way to get to all the dream information rapidly.**

Case History – Incest

Now I'd like to tell you about one person I worked with. By the time we got to the second color, she wasn't even talking about the same dream. She was definitely talking about the *latent experience*, which was a case of *incest*. At that point she was definitely remembering it; whereas, before, the dream disguised this information. So again, **I warn you when you use this process, you better be ready to handle what might come up. That means occasionally having some pretty distraught people. That is why I usually conclude the session with indigo, or violet, to bring their process to a conclusion so it makes sense to them, and they can integrate it into what they already know.** I'll ask them if they have any insights and what do they think their dream means? I'll ask them that while they're looking at a particular color, and **they usually get a different insight with each different color.** Sometimes you may get defensive reactions, so you may want to offer them choices about whether to go deeper or not. For example, do you want to find out more about it, or would you prefer to stop?

Finally, let's turn to the *law of disruption and reintegration*. This model comes from **Dr. Frederic Flach's** book, *Resilience*.[3] It explains how people are able to have *exceptional healing experiences* take place after some trauma has occurred in their lives. For example, a car wreck or whatever, and their whole system is shaken. And then they have some options about how they're going to respond to that. What I consider to be the most successful response is this *process of renewal*, where a person allows themselves to be disrupted, to descend into chaos, and that's when they need us, as therapists, to help them through their process. The *structure*, or the mindbody structure, relates to such issues as family or job. In trauma this structure gets disrupted. In a *resilient response* the patient bounces back up again toward *reintegration* and develops a whole new structure. This is what I mean by a *transformative response:* A person with a whole new homeostatic structure may be a totally different person. For example, let's say a person has a heart attack. Okay, he goes to the hospital; he cries; he tells his family; there is a family upheaval and all kinds of chaos; and then he begins to get a new meaning to his life. He may change his lifestyle and his relationship with his wife, and he has a whole new structure at that point. He is clearly not the same person as he was before. I discovered a long time ago that **changing symptoms, physical or psychological, is wonderful, but there's so much more to the process of true mindbody healing. I think that the acquisition of wholeness should be considered a basic function. By wholeness I mean an integration of thoughts, feelings, and behaviors — all those things that make us who we are.**

---

3. See *Bibliography* under *Resilience: Discovering a New Strength at Times of Stress*, (New York, NY: Fawcett Columbine, 1988).

Before closing, I'd like to share that I am currently doing training seminars and am in the process of developing a manual for psychotherapists or anyone else who might be interested in the use of Brief Strobic Phototherapy[4,5].

The light of the body is the eye: If therefore thine eye be single, the whole body shall be full of light. But if thine eye be evil, thy whole body shall be full of darkness. If therefore the light in thee be of darkness, how great is this darkness.

— Matthew 6:22-23

Our whole business this life is to restore to health the eye of the heart whereby God may be seen.

— St. Augustine

---

4. In 1995, Dr. Vazquez published a comprehensive 50 page manual on Brief Strobic Phototherapy that is available from the Health Institute of North Texas, in Hurst, Texas. See *Resource List* for Dr. Vazquez's address under Light Years Ahead Authors and *Bibliography* under Light in Psychology and Education.

5. For training opportunities with Dr. Vazquez, contact either **Light Years Ahead Productions** or Dr. Vazquez directly. Dr. Vasquez also has a non-profit foundation dedicated to the study of exceptional mindbody healing and the use of light therapy, called the Wholeness Institute for Research and Therapy.

Photosensitivity Assessment[6]

Subject Name_____ Date_____

Objective:

To assess the subject's individual response to various wavelengths of strobic light.

Instructions:

1. Seat the subject in front of the Lumatron™ with their eyes about 18 inches from the light.

2. Ask the subject to close his/her eyes.

3. Set the flicker rate of 14 for the entire assessment.

4. Turn on the Lumatron™.

5. Set the color to white.

6. For each of the eleven colors:

   a. Ask the subject to open his/her eyes.

   b. Say, "This color is called _____."

   c. Ask the subject the following five questions and briefly record response.

      Do not spend more than 1 to 2 minutes on each color, or the results could be adversely affected.

      1. What is your reaction to this color?

      2. What does it look like in term of colors seen, movement, and other appearances?

      3. What is your bodily experience while looking at this color and where do you feel it?

      4. What thoughts and emotions do you have when you look at this color?

      5. On a scale of 1 to 10, with 10 being most preferable, how would you rate this color?

   d. Ask the subject to close their eyes.

   e. Set Lumatron™ for the next color and repeat Step 6.

---

6. The last three pages of this chapter, page 97-99, include the Photosensitivity Assessment form and Six Important Questions Before Beginning Brief Strobic Phototherapy, used by Dr. Vazquez to determine a treatment regimen with the therapeutic colors most consistent with his patients' physical and emotional conditions and goals. This can also be used as a form of self-assessment for the need of particular colors. You may wish to do this many times and observe how your colors may shift and change.

Photosensitivity Assessment

WHITE:

Reaction	1. _____
Visual Appearance	2. _____
Bodily Experience	3. _____
Thoughts/Emotions	4. _____
Preference	5. _____

RUBY:

Reaction	1. _____
Visual Appearance	2. _____
Bodily Experience	3. _____
Thoughts/Emotions	4. _____
Preference	5. _____

RED:

Reaction	1. _____
Visual Appearance	2. _____
Bodily Experience	3. _____
Thoughts/Emotions	4. _____
Preference	5. _____

RED ORANGE:

Reaction	1. _____
Visual Appearance	2. _____
Bodily Experience	3. _____
Thoughts/Emotions	4. _____
Preference	5. _____

ORANGE:

Reaction	1. _____
Visual Appearance	2. _____
Bodily Experience	3. _____
Thoughts/Emotions	4. _____
Preference	5. _____

YELLOW:

Reaction	1. _____
Visual Appearance	2. _____
Bodily Experience	3. _____
Thoughts/Emotions	4. _____
Preference	5. _____

Photosensitivity Assessment

YELLOW GREEN:

Reaction	1.	_____
Visual Appearance	2.	_____
Bodily Experience	3.	_____
Thoughts/Emotions	4.	_____
Preference	5.	_____

GREEN:

Reaction	1.	_____
Visual Appearance	2.	_____
Bodily Experience	3.	_____
Thoughts/Emotions	4.	_____
Preference	5.	_____

BLUE GREEN:

Reaction	1.	_____
Visual Appearance	2.	_____
Bodily Experience	3.	_____
Thoughts/Emotions	4.	_____
Preference	5.	_____

BLUE:

Reaction	1.	_____
Visual Appearance	2.	_____
Bodily Experience	3.	_____
Thoughts/Emotions	4.	_____
Preference	5.	_____

INDIGO:

Reaction	1.	_____
Visual Appearance	2.	_____
Bodily Experience	3.	_____
Thoughts/Emotions	4.	_____
Preference	5.	_____

VIOLET

Reaction	1.	_____
Visual Appearance	2.	_____
Bodily Experience	3.	_____
Thoughts/Emotions	4.	_____
Preference	5.	_____

Photosensitivity Assessment Summary

Most Therapeutic Potential *(colors in priority order):*

1._____
2._____
3._____
4._____
5._____
6._____

Least Therapeutic Potential *(colors in priority order):*

1._____
2._____
3._____
4._____
5._____
6._____

Treatment Objective:

_____
_____
_____
_____
_____

Colors chosen to address subject's goals and issues:

_____
_____
_____

Six Important Intake Questions Before Beginning Brief Strobic Phototherapy

Considering the aforementioned list of cautions regarding this type of photo-therapy, Dr. Vazquez asks these questions:

1. Do you have medical conditions that are important to disclose here? If so, what? ☐ Yes ☐ No

_____
_____
_____.

2. Do you have cancer? If so, explain: ☐ Yes ☐ No

_____
_____
_____.

3. Do you have a history of photosensitive seizures? ☐ Yes ☐ No

4. Are you taking medications that are known to have photosensitive side-effects. If so, what medications: ☐ Yes ☐ No

_____
_____
_____.

(Check with your physician to determine if these side-effects are significant enough to recommend avoiding low-brightness light stimulation.)

5. Do you have suicidal thoughts or are you deeply depressed? If so, explain: ☐ Yes ☐ No

_____
_____
_____.

6. Do you feel prone to violence or homicide? If so, explain: ☐ Yes ☐ No

_____
_____
_____.

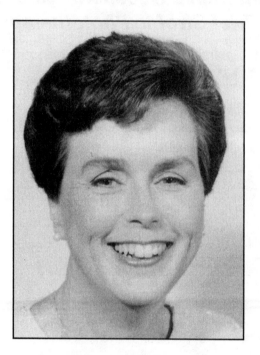

Lee Hartley, Ed.D.

*D*r. Lee Hartley is a licensed Marriage, Family and Child Therapist and a pioneer in the therapeutic combination of clinical hypnosis and light therapy. Her unique skills have brought her acclaim with clients who have travelled from all over the country to work with her at her former clinic in San Jose, California. Dr. Hartley holds a doctorate in counseling psychology from the University of San Francisco. She was the ***Director of The Light Years Ahead Conference,*** and currently she is ***Coordinator of Education at Light Years Ahead Productions,*** in Tiburon, California, a company that develops programs (conferences, seminars and workshops) and materials (audio tapes, video tapes, and this book), designed to help people understand the interplay of the mind and body and how it affects physical health and psychospiritual well-being.

CHAPTER FOUR

Make Those Blues Go Away:
The Effect of Light on Seasonal Affective Disorder (SAD) and Premenstrual Syndrome (PMS)

Lee Hartley, Ed.D.

I'm talking to you today about both **Premenstrual Syndrome (PMS)** and **Seasonal Affective Disorder (SAD).** Over the years in my practice, I have had a number of clients who have had symptoms of SAD and PMS; women who have come in with PMS, and both men and women who have come in with symptoms of SAD. When I started working as a therapist about fifteen years ago, I certainly didn't understand anything about seasonal depression. Seasonal affective disorder (also referred to as **Winter Depression**) had not been identified and wasn't something that was out there in the literature; in fact, it has been researched only in the last ten years.

Now, I want to give you a bit of an idea about some of the clients that I have worked with who have had these two problems, but first a story . . . One day I was driving to work, and in front of me there was a car sitting at the signal. On the license plate bracket there was the message . . . "I have PMS and I have a gun." Ironically, I just happened to be going to my office to work with a woman who had severe PMS, and I thought it was so appropriate. I just loved it!

I'm going to tell you about another client who presented me with a dramatic series of problems. She came into my office saying that her physician had told her that she was an *alcoholic* because she drank before she went to bed. For years she had trouble falling asleep. As I did the history, I heard this incredible series of physical and emotional problems that came up for her every month. She said, "I am on the verge of being fired at work; I have been written up every month. I get so upset, usually I find one of the men that I'm working with who says something to me, and then I just blast him. So I get in this big argument and other people in the department get sucked into it." Then she reported that she would be very irritable and would lapse into crying spells for three to four days. After work she would go home and not be able to sleep at all. Notably, her insomnia problem had occurred since early childhood, so she had this long list of problems which included a lot of *anger, verbal aggression, crying jags, and insomnia.*

Along with the psychotherapy, she also did *phototherapy*. I initially started doing psychotherapy with her in the few months before I came across the light treatment. **Dr. Sam Pesner** arranged for me to borrow one of the old *Syntonic Optometry Light Instruments.* It is a long "tube-like" instrument with an internal light source, in which you can insert color filters. (See *Chapter Two* for picture of **Cameron-Spitler Syntonizer**.) I had been trying to get this woman to go into hypnotic trance, and she couldn't at all; and that doesn't happen very often in my practice. I brought this instrument in and said, "Well, let me show you." I sat her down in front of it. I thought she needed red light from other pieces of information that I had read. Not much emotional content came up previously. She instantaneously and spontaneously regressed back to a time that I had suspected had occurred. She had been *sexually abused*; and it had happened repeatedly in the middle of the night. Someone had come into her room. So her pattern was to try to stay awake to prevent the abuse from occurring.

During the initial exposure to the Syntonic Light Instrument she spontaneously regressed to one of the sexual abuse memories. Thus, I started working with her regularly with the syntonic instrument. During every session she would go into a deep trance; and one day I said, "I wonder what the difference is? Before, I couldn't get you to go into a trance." The next session I tried to do hypnosis with her again. I usually have the client in a recliner chair. I put a sleeping mask over their eyes and then do the hypnotic induction. I do this partially because when a person is in a trance and they have some image come up, they often will open their eyes and then sometimes lose the image. It helps many people to just feel like they are a bit "hidden." That gives them a sense of a "safe space." And she said, "Oh well, with the light instrument I didn't have to close my eyes." **Not only was she ready to do this, because her eyes were open and she felt safer, but the red light brought up some of the somatic memories we were able to reframe.**

Then within a couple of months, I discovered the ***Ott-Lite*®, a full spectrum fluorescent light box,** and I started using it myself. During the next session, I told her, "Well, I've ordered one of these, and I'm going to try it. If I think it'll be a good thing for you, I'll recommend it to you." She said, "No, order me one right now!" Although the client knew she was getting better, some of the information I had been sharing with her about the Ott-Lite® had to do with being able to sleep better and its potential to alleviate some of the *PMS problems* and so on. I ordered it for her. She took it home and started to use it. **Within that first month she reported that her PMS symptoms were diminished by about 70%. Remember, this is only within the first month of daily use**.

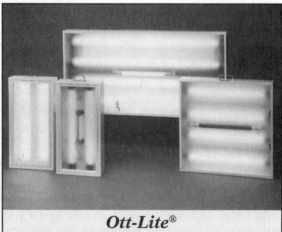

Ott-Lite®
Full spectrum fluorescent light boxes

Alleviating PMS Symptoms with Light

Dr. Barbara Parry of University of California San Diego's Department of Psychiatry[1] has conducted several studies addressing light's effects on PMS. PMS is currently called "premenstrual dysphoric disorder," and affects women seven to fourteen days before their period. During winter's low-light conditions, symptoms of premenstrual tension are frequently worse than other seasons. These include such *psychological symptoms* as depression, anxiety, mood changes, irritability, *sleep problems, appetite changes,* and low energy levels, and such *physical symptoms* as feeling bloated, breast swelling and tenderness, and pain in the joints.

Two hours of *Bright Full Spectrum Light* administered either in the mornings or evenings and dim red light are all equally effective in reversing PMS symptoms when used on an ongoing consistent basis. More recently, Dr. Parry recommends two hours of 2,500 lux bright light full spectrum phototherapy one to two weeks before menstruation. Morning bright light also eliminates *menopausal hot flashes.*

---

1. For information about Dr. Parry's research, See *Resource List: Section 3, page 344: "Medical Phototherapy and Light Research."*

The client's therapy continued. The psychotherapy included regression work, using the light equipment in each session; she also continued using the Ott-Lite® on a daily basis. She reported that **she had more energy, was less depressed, and that the irritability had diminished** a great deal; and during that month, she had not gotten into one argument with anybody at work. **During the second month of combined light-assisted psychotherapy and home Ott-Lite® treatments, she indicated that there was a 90% improvement in her symptoms. By the third month she reported that she was virtually symptom-free**.

Then she decided to take a winter vacation in Oregon. Did she take her Ott-Lite® with her? No, she went up there for about ten days and stayed with her family, then came back, went back to work, and sure enough, within about three or four days, she "blasted" somebody at work again. The next day she phoned me, and she sounded really upset. I asked her, "Well, did you take the light with you?" She said, "No." So I suggested that she start using it the very next morning. She followed my advice, and the next month she once again went back to being symptom-free. When she came in, she said, "I learned my lesson; I'm using that thing for the rest of my life!"

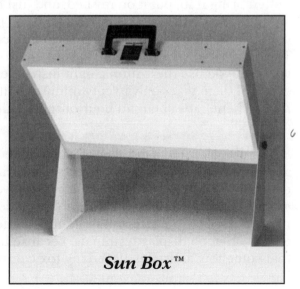

***Sun Box*™**

So, there's a part of her that at this point in time, is actually a little bit afraid not to use it because of the negative results she got when she didn't use it. The full spectrum white light had been a very positive thing for her. She also indicated that **her sleep pattern gradually shifted back to normal.** Now part of this result may come about through alleviation of a lot of the sexual abuse trauma. Yet at the same time, there's an aspect of using the Ott-Lite® or the **Sunbox**™ or the various other light instruments that allow the person to begin shifting some of their mindbody patterns. **Notably, every woman with PMS I've treated who used the Ott-Lite® had a reduction in symptoms.**

I know when I first tried full spectrum light, I noticed within a very short period of time that I started getting up earlier; I just woke up earlier. Up to that point I had always been the kind of person who would naturally wake up around 7:00 a.m. or 7:30 a.m. And over the period of one to two months, that shifted down to about 5:00 to 5:30 a.m. This also worked better in my schedule, because I've been trying to do more positive self-care. So, now I do a light treatment in the morning, and I also go for a morning walk. Getting up earlier can really add up in "new found" time. I noticed a shift in my daily rhythm to getting up earlier, and I would also get tired and go to bed about an hour or two earlier. I also noticed much more energy for myself within just three days' time, and the first Ott-Lite® panel that I got my husband and I used for five consecutive days, and I then gave it to one of my clients to use. I had ordered another panel but it hadn't arrived yet. About the fourth day my husband said, "If I drive to Santa Barbara, can I pick up one of those things so I can use it tomorrow?" I said, "No, they don't store them there. It'll be here in another couple of days." We had both felt such a large increase in energy that when we stopped using it, there was a noticeable effect of decreased energy.

All of the scientific literature I have read indicates that **the length of Ott-Lite® panel exposure time is very individual, and you need to try it yourself to find your optimal "dose."** I always tell people to start with an hour, although some people may need an hour and a half, and others may need only thirty to forty-five minutes. You can set the Ott-Lite® up in an area where you're sitting, and you can read or do whatever. I often do affirmations or write in my journal, or I read while I'm sitting by the Ott-Lite®. I often bring it in, put it on my bed, and just crawl back under the covers and sit there for an hour. You can also watch television, or put it in the kitchen and have it there while you're fixing breakfast; so you aren't chained to a specific spot just looking at the light. The light panel is merely there in your environment, and you don't have to use it the same way that you use the syntonic light instrument or the Lumatron™. Doing a treatment on either of them takes only twenty minutes, but if you're also doing psychotherapy and talking to clients, it's about an hour of time, guiding the client through a psychotherapeutic process.

I've also had a number of women who have taken the full spectrum lights to work and put them on their desks. My daughter has one. She works with visual display terminals all the time. Some of the research I have read indicates that many women have had *miscarriages* and other physical problems develop by sitting in front of computer terminals all day long. I believe the light is something that may be a deterrent to the toxic effects of video display terminals, because it may serve as an electromagnetic "diffuser" that somehow assists in dispersing toxic energy in one's field.

QUESTION: Do you use it in just the winter months?

DR. HARTLEY: No, I use it all year round. Most people will need to diminish the length of time that they use it to twenty or thirty minutes a day in the summer, but then they will increase it again in the winter.

QUESTION: Do you get the same benefit if you put it in the ceiling?

DR. HARTLEY: I work under an Ott-Lite® and have for years, and I spend about eight hours a day under it. Yes, it is possible for you to do that. A lot of people are not necessarily in an environment that they can control like that. Some people can put it in the ceiling if it's in their own home. Or if it's in their own office, they can have a small one set up by their computer. My daughter has already moved two different times in her work environment, and that's one of the things that she takes with her. So it really depends on the person and the environment where you're going to spend your time.

I want to read you a quote from **Dr. Katherina Dalton's** book, *Once A Month,* (Alameda, CA: Hunter House, 1990):

> *It is not surprising that **pre-menstrual tension,** with its irritability and confusion, frequently leads to problems with the law. There are those cases of aggression where, in a sudden fit of temper, a woman makes an unjustified assault on her neighbor or boss, or violently attacks a police officer. There are cases of baby-battering, husband-beating, and homicide. Becoming drunk and disorderly when under the influence of alcohol or drugs may also lead to charges.*

Not all women become violent when they have PMS, but there are certainly a number of violent cases in which PMS has been used as part of the legal defense. Many women have been acquitted because they have been under some kind of medical or psychological treatment. I would say that a lot of women, though certainly not all women, suffer from varying intensities of PMS symptoms.

Women come to see me for psychotherapy for emotional reasons; these same reasons also happen to coincide with symptoms of PMS. (See the following list.)

If there is a hell upon Earth, it is to be found in a melancholy heart.

— *Robert Burton*

Presenting Problems for Psychotherapy Referral that Coincide with Symptoms of PMS

- Nervous tension

- Mood swings

- Irritability

- Anxiety

- Depression

- Forgetfulness

- Crying

- Sleeplessness

- Problems with alcohol or drugs

- Physical problems associated with PMS leading to physician referrals: Headaches, cravings for sweets, increased appetite, pounding hearts, fatigue, tremulousness, weight gain, swelling of extremities, breast tenderness, cramps in the lower abdominal area, backache and skin problems.

In my opinion there's also another set of conditions that can contribute to a woman having PMS, and these are far beyond the everyday stresses of life. **These contributing factors to PMS may have to do with various types of traumatic incidents, such as: incest, rape, abortion, putting a child up for adoption, miscarriage, or having a stillborn child. Dr. Shealy**[1] says very often women experience some abnormal bleeding each month, and it frequently relates to an old experience of having had an abortion.

In my practice I often do psychotherapy using hypnosis and the Lumatron™ concurrently, and I find that some of this information eventually surfaces. In session we will usually cover these incidents, and at the same time I will suggest that they work with the light at home on a daily basis. I find that these two different light treatment approaches are a wonderful combination. I've always appreciated using hypnosis, because it speeds up the therapeutic process. It is something that you can use to assist clients to get to the cause of the problem much more readily, and you are also able to

---

1. See Dr. Shealy's presentations in *Chapters Seven, page 165, and Eight, page 185,* entitled "The Reality of EEG and Neurochemical Responses to Photostimulation," Parts I and II.

accomplish much more in a shorter length of time. **So what I find when using the Lumatron™ is that it speeds up the therapeutic process even more; and by having clients use a light panel at home, it begins to also assist them to get their body back into balance.**

Dr. Susan Lark, **a physician** who formerly practiced in Los Altos, California, is now focused primarily on writing women's health books. One of her books is called *The PMS Self-Help Book* (Berkeley, CA: Celestial Arts, 1989). In her practice she discovered what is charted below:

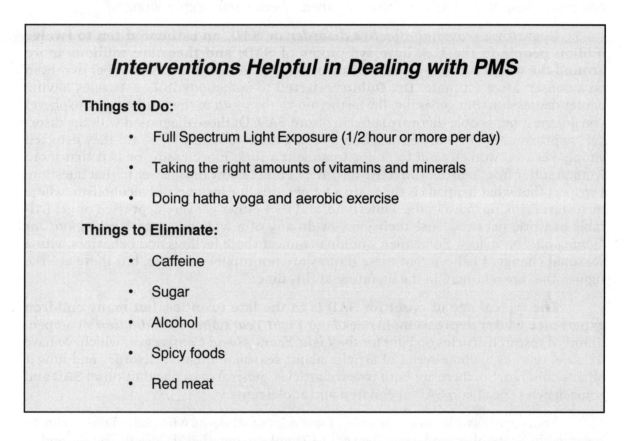

Interventions Helpful in Dealing with PMS

Things to Do:

- Full Spectrum Light Exposure (1/2 hour or more per day)
- Taking the right amounts of vitamins and minerals
- Doing hatha yoga and aerobic exercise

Things to Eliminate:

- Caffeine
- Sugar
- Alcohol
- Spicy foods
- Red meat

She has also put together a whole program that includes a detailed analysis of the effects of vitamin and mineral supplements. When I went to her home to have a discussion with her, I was surprised to see right there, sitting in her family room, a *Light Bed,* a bed-like structure that had a built-in light over it. I asked her, "Is this something you use every day?" Dr. Lark said, "Yes, we have this in our home all the time."

Dr. Lark first started using a full spectrum white light and then did some experimenting with red light. **She has recently been involved with an AIDS research project and found that AIDS patients were getting such positive results with phototherapy that many of the staff people involved in the study began coming in and using the Light Bed on a daily basis.** The researchers were so thrilled that they were vying for time on this piece of equipment! When this project was over, she ended up taking it home, and now her family uses it daily.

Dr. Kristine Green, **an obstetrician/gynecologist** who practices in Palo Alto, California, talked to me about using Ott-Lite® Panels for SAD. I also talked with her regarding using light with PMS. She told me, "Well, you know that **these two conditions, PMS and SAD, always go hand-in-hand.**" And I said, "No, I didn't know that." She went on to say that whenever she has a woman come in who's expressing symptoms of PMS, she talks to them about how they feel in the winter and whether or not they get more depressed, more lethargic, and so on. I thought that this was an extremely interesting piece of data that she had put together. If somebody comes in during the winter saying that they are very depressed, she talks to them about PMS as well. Likewise, if her patients come in talking about PMS, she also asks them about winter depression.

Regarding *seasonal affective disorder* **or** *SAD*, **an estimated ten to twelve million people in the U.S. have symptoms of SAD; and there are millions more around the world suffering from this disorder.** My sense is that this number may even be a conservative estimate. **Dr. Dubin**[2] referred to somebody in Los Angeles having winter depression. But generally, the farther north (or south in the southern hemisphere) you go, the more people there are suffering from SAD. Of those diagnosed with the disorder, approximately 70% are female and 30% are male. Of those 70%, are they detected simply because women tend to go for treatment a little more easily, or is it that more women suffer from seasonal affective disorder? I don't know the answer to that question. I suspect that what happens is there are a lot of cases, for instance, of alcoholism, where men start drinking more in the wintertime, and they either get very depressed or get irritable at work, get fired, lose their jobs, or do any of a wide range of *"striking-out" or "zoning-out" behaviors.* Some men wouldn't connect these feelings and behaviors with a seasonal change. I believe that these figures are not totally accurate, but these are the figures that are out there in the literature at this time.

The typical age of onset for SAD is in the late twenties, but many children experience winter depression. In one of our *Light Years Ahead Production's* compendiums of research articles on light for the *Light Years Ahead Conference,* which we have for sale, there is a whole series of articles about seasonal affective disorder and how it affects children. So, there are both types of articles, general ones on adult-onset SAD and some articles specific to SAD in children and adolescents.

Years ago, as a classroom teacher, I saw a lot of students who started out performing great in September, and when they got to Thanksgiving, they'd "lose it." By the end of the first semester they were getting terrible grades, having difficulty getting up in the morning, getting sick more often, not doing well in their school work, and beginning to really develop a dislike for being at school, because they were being criticized and told that they were lazy. **These symptoms of SAD really affect children's self-confidence and self-esteem, as well as their enjoyment of learning**. By the time the days start to lengthen in March, they begin to feel better, and come June, they get better grades. It's funny that teachers and parents often take credit for this great improvement, and it really doesn't have anything to do with them. It has to do with the child feeling better because of increased light exposure.

---

2. See Dr. Bob Dubin's two chapters entitled "Post Traumatic Stress Syndrome: Something Can Be Done With Light," *Chapter Five, page 119;* and "Downing Technique, Ocular Light Therapy and Cranial Sacral Therapy in a Chiropractic Setting," *Chapter Ten, page 227.*

SAD Symptoms with November Onset

As the days get shorter in November there's an increase in the number of:

- Prescriptions for anti-depressants

- Hospitalizations for depression

- Attempted suicides

- Successful suicides

- Domestic violence

- Use/abuse of drugs and alcohol

- Alcohol-related accidents and injuries

I'd like to talk about the symptoms and treatment of seasonal affective disorder. Next I'd like to describe the symptoms assessed in three questionnaires routinely used in the clinical evaluations of SAD. The first is the ***Hamilton Psychiatric Rating Scale for Depression (HRSD),*** and the second and third are the ***Seasonal Pattern Assessment Questionnaire (SPAQ),*** and the ***Weekly Mood Inventory (WMI).***

Truly the light is sweet, and a pleasant thing is for the eyes to behold the sun.

— Ecclesiastes 11:7

The SAD Facts

SAD is a severe depressive illness that regularly manifests in late fall (precipitated by light deprivation) and subsides with the longer, sunnier days of spring.

The severity and incidence of SAD symptoms increase the farther away from the equator's longer and brighter days.

Anyone deprived of regular sunlight exposure can suffer from SAD. Symptoms are similar to other forms of depressive illness:

- Lethargy

- Fatigue

- Decreased energy and activity level

- Anxiety

- Irritability

- Lowered sex drive

- Avoidance of social activities

- Sadness and depressed mood

- Concentration difficulties

- Interpersonal difficulties

SAD symptoms differ from other depressive illnesses in: the time of year of onset and the sufferer's unusually intense desire for sleep (sometimes beyond 16 hours a day), craving for sweets and carbohydrates (especially in the late afternoon and evening), and increased appetite and weight gain.

Scientists speculate that these symptoms may be due to an increased production of the hormone melatonin (melatonin has a sedative effect on the body, and the body releases more melatonin at night). Winter's long nights lead to increased melatonin production and an even greater sedative effect.

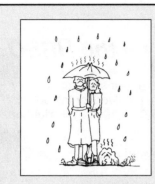

From SAD to GLAD: Treating SAD

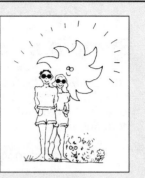

CONSULT an experienced and licensed light therapy practitioner as found in *Resource List.* All mood disorders should be evaluated by a licensed mental health professional.

DOSAGE: At an intensity of 2,500 to 10,000 lux (1 lux is the power of illumination of one candle at a distance of 3 feet away). 2500 lux suppresses melatonin production and is roughly equivalent to the amount of light coming through your windows on a bright summer day.

TREATMENT: **Bright Artificial Full Spectrum Lights**[1]

ADDITIONAL TREATMENTS: **Dawn Simulation.** Full spectrum lights that gradually increase in intensity from 4 a.m. until awakening at a brightness of only 250 lux were as effective as bright light phototherapy. This treatment has the advantage of being effective while the SAD sufferer slept, and did not produce side effects.

Light Visor: Preliminary results for this portable phototherapy unit are positive.

EXPOSURE TIME: Begin with 1-2 hours per day in late fall mornings between 6-8 a.m. and taper off during spring. SAD symptoms tend to return once light therapy is stopped, so continue treatments till your symptoms go away, usually in springtime.

If SAD symptoms don't decrease within four days, **increase exposure time** and/or switch to an additional early evening exposure time.

Although phototherapy is generally safe, side effects may occasionally occur; such as, redness or eye irritation, eyestrain, headaches, insomnia, or hyperactivity. If any of these occur, **decrease exposure time.**

EXERCISE: Take a daily one hour walk in normal winter sunlight.

---

1. See *Resource Lists: Sections Six through Thirteen, pages 373-380,* for manufacturers and distributors of Light and Phototherapy products.

Symptoms of Depression Assessed by the HRSD

The Hamilton Depression Rating Scale is a list of symptoms that are assessed for severity by a clinician on the basis of a brief structured interview. Guidelines are provided for the behavior to be considered under each symptom and for the severity ratings (0 = absent, 1 = slight or doubtful, and 2 = clearly present).

1. **Depressed mood**

2. **Feelings of guilt**

3. **Suicide** (has client ever attempted or threatened?)

4. **Insomnia — Initial or early**, meaning client can't fall asleep very easily in the evening.

5. **Insomnia — middle**. Does client wake up in the middle of the night?

6. **Insomnia — delayed**. Does client wake up near the end of sleep cycle and is client then unable to go back to sleep?

7. **Work and Interests**. How is client's work and activity level affected?

8. **Retardation** — slowness of thought and speech, impaired ability to concentrate. (These symptoms **sound a lot like chronic fatigue syndrome.)**

9. **Agitation.** Some clients will be very slow and lethargic, while others will be agitated.

10. **Anxiety-psychic.** This could be fear or emotional anxiety.

11. **Anxiety-somatic.** Is the client feeling anxious physically in their body?

12. **Somatic symptoms, gastrointestinal**

13. **Somatic symptoms, general**

14. **Sexual Symptoms**. Loss of libido, or sexual interest.

15. **Hypochondriasis**

16. **Loss of weight**

17. **Loss of insight.** Acknowledges being depressed and ill, may attribute it to bad food; clients may have an illogical reason why they're not feeling well.

18. **Other depressive symptoms** this scale examines include:

    a) **Diurnal variation —** is the depression worse in the evening or morning?

    b) **Paranoid and obsessive-compulsive symptoms**

    c) **Depersonalization and feelings of unreality**

As for the last symptom — depersonalization — a woman I'm working with right now experiences *feelings of unreality*. What I've discovered about this particular symptom is that this client had been constantly feeling *anxious* because she was holding, or stopping her breathing, or was breathing very shallowly; her lack of breathing precipitated her moving into a sense of unreality much of the time. As I worked with her to breathe more fully and more frequently, she began to get more grounded and more in touch with reality.

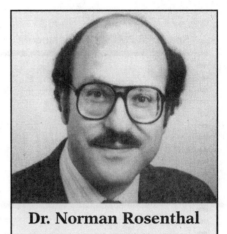

Dr. Norman Rosenthal

I want to introduce you briefly to ***The Seasonal Pattern Assessment Questionnaire* (SPAQ)** that was prepared by several SAD researchers: **Drs. Norman Rosenthal,**[3] **Gary Bradt, and Thomas Wehr**. Dr. Rosenthal is from the **National Institute of Mental Health's (NIMH) Department of Psychobiology,**[4] which is one of the places that has done much of the pioneering research on SAD. Two other research institutions I'm familiar with are **Thomas Jefferson Medical School in Philadelphia** and the **University of Oregon Health Sciences Research Group in Portland.**

In looking over the SPAQ, I see that there are a large number of questions to help people figure out when they may have experienced *seasonal affective disorder* or a *subclinical seasonal pattern.* It lists each question and the months to fill in. (For example: When do you feel better? When do you gain weight? When do you socialize the most? When do you sleep the least? Eat the most? Lose the most weight?. . . and so forth.)

This same group at NIMH also developed the ***Weekly Mood Inventory.*** On this inventory there are a series of choices: I have experienced bad feelings; I feel guilty; I have been efficient at work; I describe myself as energetic, and so forth. A rating scale goes from 1 to 7, so that the person can rate him or herself as to how many SAD symptoms were experienced during the week.

These questionnaires can be very useful in determining if the individual is experiencing seasonal affective disorder. I urge you to use them.

---

3. Norman E. Rosenthal, M.D., is Director of Seasonal Studies at the National Institutes of Mental Health, where he led the team that described the syndrome of seasonal affective disorder (SAD) and conducted the first controlled treatment of light therapy for this condition. He is past president of the Society for Light Therapy and Biological Rhythms and the recipient of the prestigious international Anna-Monika Award for research in depression. He is the author of over a hundred scientific publications, co-editor of *Seasonal Affective Disorders and Phototherapy* (New York: Guilford, 1989), author of *Winter Blues: Seasonal Affective Disorder: What It Is and How To Overcome It* (New York: Guilford, 1993), and co-author of *How to Beat Jet Lag: A Practical Guide for Air Travelers* (New York: Holt, 1993).

4. To contact Dr. Rosenthal or Dr. Wehr, See *Resource List: Section Three, page 344, "Medical Phototherapy and Light Research."* If you're interested in participating in the Clinical Research Program at NIMH, contact Ronald L. Barnett, Ph.D., or Todd Hardin at (301) 496-0500.

Seasonal Pattern Assessment Questionnaire ■ ■ (SPAQ)

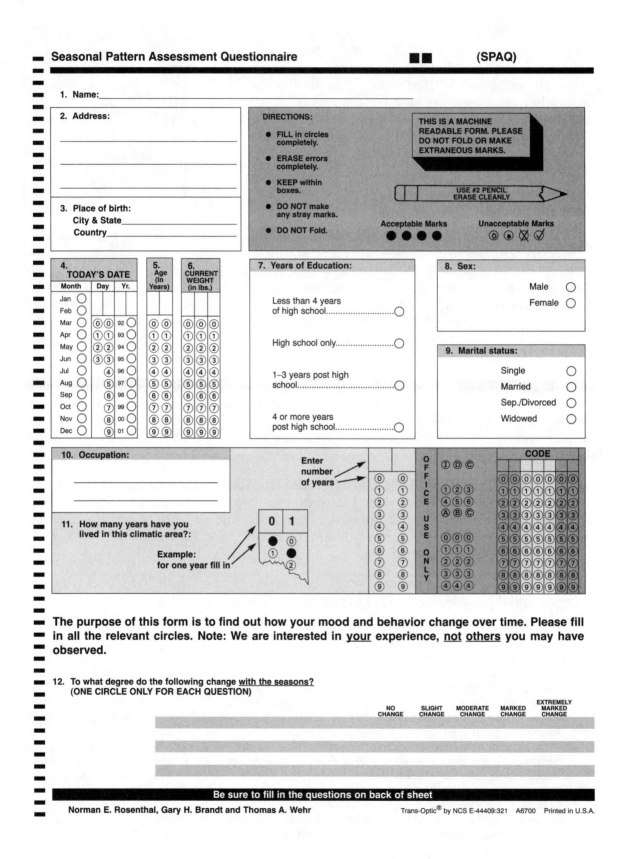

1. Name:_____

2. Address:
   _____
   _____
   _____

DIRECTIONS:

- FILL in circles completely.
- ERASE errors completely.
- KEEP within boxes.
- DO NOT make any stray marks.
- DO NOT Fold.

THIS IS A MACHINE READABLE FORM. PLEASE DO NOT FOLD OR MAKE EXTRANEOUS MARKS.

USE #2 PENCIL ERASE CLEANLY

Acceptable Marks ● ● ● ●

Unacceptable Marks

3. Place of birth:
   City & State_____
   Country_____

4. **TODAY'S DATE**

Month	Day	Yr.
Jan		
Feb		
Mar	0 0	92
Apr	1 1	93
May	2 2	94
Jun	3 3	95
Jul	4	96
Aug	5	97
Sep	6	98
Oct	7	99
Nov	8	00
Dec	9	01

5. Age (in Years)

6. CURRENT WEIGHT (in lbs.)

7. **Years of Education:**

Less than 4 years of high school..........................○

High school only......................○

1–3 years post high school......................................○

4 or more years post high school.......................○

8. **Sex:**

Male ○
Female ○

9. **Marital status:**

Single ○
Married ○
Sep./Divorced ○
Widowed ○

10. **Occupation:**
    _____
    _____

11. How many years have you lived in this climatic area?:

Example: for one year fill in

Enter number of years →

CODE

OFFICE USE ONLY

The purpose of this form is to find out how your mood and behavior change over time. Please fill in all the relevant circles. Note: We are interested in **your** experience, **not others** you may have observed.

12. To what degree do the following change **with the seasons?**
    (ONE CIRCLE ONLY FOR EACH QUESTION)

	NO CHANGE	SLIGHT CHANGE	MODERATE CHANGE	MARKED CHANGE	EXTREMELY MARKED CHANGE

Be sure to fill in the questions on back of sheet

Norman E. Rosenthal, Gary H. Brandt and Thomas A. Wehr   Trans-Optic® by NCS E-44409:321   A6700   Printed in U.S.A.

13. In the following questions, fill in circles for all applicable months. This may be a single month ●, a cluster of months, E.G., ● ● ●, or any other grouping.
At what time of year do you . . .

	Jan	Feb	Mar	Apr	May	Jun	Jul	Aug	Sep	Oct	Nov	Dec		
A. Feel best	○	○	○	○	○	○	○	○	○	○	○	○		○
B. Tend to gain most weight	○	○	○	○	○	○	○	○	○	○	○	○		○
C. Socialize most	○	○	○	○	○	○	○	○	○	○	○	○		○
D. Sleep least	○	○	○	○	○	○	○	○	○	○	○	○		○
E. Eat most	○	○	○	○	○	○	○	○	○	○	○	○	OR	○
F. Lose most weight	○	○	○	○	○	○	○	○	○	○	○	○		○
G. Socialize least	○	○	○	○	○	○	○	○	○	○	○	○		○
H. Feel worst	○	○	○	○	○	○	○	○	○	○	○	○		○
I. Eat least	○	○	○	○	○	○	○	○	○	○	○	○		○
J. Sleep most	○	○	○	○	○	○	○	○	○	○	○	○		○

} No particular month(s) stand out as extreme on a regular basis

14. Using the scale below, indicate how the following weather changes make you feel. (ONE CIRCLE ONLY FOR EACH QUESTION)

−3 = In very low spirits or markedly slowed down
−2 = Moderately low/slowed down
−1 = Mildly low/slowed down
 0 = Moderately low/slowed down
+1 = Slightly improves your mood or energy level
+2 = Moderately improves your mood or energy level
+3 = Markedly improves your mood or energy level

	−3	−2	−1	0	+1	+2	+3		DON'T KNOW
A. Cold weather	○	○	○	○	○	○	○		○
B. Hot weather	○	○	○	○	○	○	○		○
C. Humid weather	○	○	○	○	○	○	○		○
D. Sunny days	○	○	○	○	○	○	○		○
E. Dry days	○	○	○	○	○	○	○	OR	○
F. Grey cloudy days	○	○	○	○	○	○	○		○
G. Long days	○	○	○	○	○	○	○		○
H. High pollen count	○	○	○	○	○	○	○		○
I. Foggy, smoggy days	○	○	○	○	○	○	○		○
J. Short days	○	○	○	○	○	○	○		○

DO NOT WRITE

IN THIS SPACE

15. By how much does your weight fluctuate during the course of the year?
○ 0–3 lbs.
○ 4–7 lbs.
○ 8–11 lbs.
○ 12–15 lbs.
○ 16–20 lbs.
○ Over 20 lbs.

16. Approximately how many hours of each 24-hour day do you sleep during each season? (Include naps)

		Hours slept per day	OVER 18 HOURS
WINTER (Dec 21 - Mar 20)		⓪ ① ② ③ ④ ⑤ ⑥ ⑦ ⑧ ⑨ ⑩ ⑪ ⑫ ⑬ ⑭ ⑮ ⑯ ⑰ ⑱	○
SPRING (Mar 21 - June 20)		⓪ ① ② ③ ④ ⑤ ⑥ ⑦ ⑧ ⑨ ⑩ ⑪ ⑫ ⑬ ⑭ ⑮ ⑯ ⑰ ⑱	○
SUMMER (June 21 - Sept 20)		⓪ ① ② ③ ④ ⑤ ⑥ ⑦ ⑧ ⑨ ⑩ ⑪ ⑫ ⑬ ⑭ ⑮ ⑯ ⑰ ⑱	○
FALL (Sept 21 - Dec 20)		⓪ ① ② ③ ④ ⑤ ⑥ ⑦ ⑧ ⑨ ⑩ ⑪ ⑫ ⑬ ⑭ ⑮ ⑯ ⑰ ⑱	○

17. Do you notice a change in food preference during the different seasons? . . . .
○ No
○ Yes →

Please specify:
_____
_____
_____
_____

18. If you experience changes with the seasons, do you feel that these are a problem for you? . . . .
○ No
○ Yes

MILD	MODERATE	MARKED	SEVERE	DISABLING
If yes, is this problem . . . . ○ | ○ | ○ | ○ | ○

Thank you for completing this questionnaire.

Trans-Optic® by NCS E-444010:32   A6700   Printed in U.S.A.

Weekly Mood Inventory

For Office Use Only

DIRECTIONS

This form is designed to find out how you have been feeling and functioning *during the past week.* After answering the questions on this side, please answer the scaled questions on the other side.

THIS IS A MACHINE READABLE FORM. PLEASE DO NOT FOLD OR MAKE EXTRANEOUS MARKS.

USE #2 PENCIL
ERASE CLEANLY

Acceptable Marks   **Unacceptable Marks**

Name:_____

DATE

Month	Day	Yr.
Jan ○		
Feb ○		
Mar ○	⓪⓪	92 ○
Apr ○	①①	93 ○
May ○	②②	94 ○
Jun ○	③③	95 ○
Jul ○	④	96 ○
Aug ○	⑤	97 ○
Sep ○	⑥	98 ○
Oct ○	⑦	99 ○
Nov ○	⑧	00 ○
Dec ○	⑨	01 ○

CURRENT WEIGHT

CODE

During The Past Week:

1. **Have you taken any medications or had light therapy?**

   ○ No

   ○ Yes, no changes since previous week

   ○ Yes, changes since previous week →

   Medication (or lights) & dosage:
   _____
   _____
   _____

2. **Have you had a cold, flu or any illness?**

   ○ No

   ○ Yes →

   Please specify:
   _____
   _____
   _____

3. **Has anything happened during the past week which might have affected your feelings of functioning?**

   ○ No

   ○ Yes →

   Please specify:
   _____
   _____
   _____

4. *For menstruating females only:* **Have you menstruated this week?**

   ○ No

   ○ Yes →

   Date began:_____

   Date ended:_____

Be sure to fill in the questions on back of sheet

Norman E. Rosenthal, Gary H. Brandt and Thomas A. Wehr

Weekly Mood Inventory
Page 2

Please read the following items carefully and fill in the circle that best describes how you have been feeling in the past week.

		NOT AT ALL						VERY MUCH

1. I have experienced sad feelings . . . . ① ② ③ ④ ⑤ ⑥ ⑦
2. I have felt hopeful about the future . . . . ① ② ③ ④ ⑤ ⑥ ⑦
3. I have felt like crying . . . . ① ② ③ ④ ⑤ ⑥ ⑦
4. I have experienced sleep interruptions . . . . ① ② ③ ④ ⑤ ⑥ ⑦
5. I have felt gulty . . . . ① ② ③ ④ ⑤ ⑥ ⑦
6. I have felt happy or elated . . . . ① ② ③ ④ ⑤ ⑥ ⑦
7. I have been sleeping less than usual . . . . ① ② ③ ④ ⑤ ⑥ ⑦
8. I have waking in the early hours of the morning . . . . ① ② ③ ④ ⑤ ⑥ ⑦
9. I have been efficient at work . . . . ① ② ③ ④ ⑤ ⑥ ⑦
10. I have had a great need for sleep. . . . . ① ② ③ ④ ⑤ ⑥ ⑦
11. I have felt energetic . . . . ① ② ③ ④ ⑤ ⑥ ⑦
12. I have felt that life is not worth living. . . . . ① ② ③ ④ ⑤ ⑥ ⑦
13. I have had a desire for sweets and starches . . . . ① ② ③ ④ ⑤ ⑥ ⑦
14. I have wanted to socialize with others . . . . ① ② ③ ④ ⑤ ⑥ ⑦
15. I have been gaining weight . . . . ① ② ③ ④ ⑤ ⑥ ⑦
16. I feel I have been looking good . . . . ① ② ③ ④ ⑤ ⑥ ⑦
17. I have had difficulty getting to sleep . . . . ① ② ③ ④ ⑤ ⑥ ⑦
18. I have felt creative . . . . ① ② ③ ④ ⑤ ⑥ ⑦
19. I have felt disappointed in myself . . . . ① ② ③ ④ ⑤ ⑥ ⑦
20. I have had a large appetite . . . . ① ② ③ ④ ⑤ ⑥ ⑦
21. I have had an interest in sex . . . . ① ② ③ ④ ⑤ ⑥ ⑦
22. I have been able to think quickly . . . . ① ② ③ ④ ⑤ ⑥ ⑦
23. I have been losing weight . . . . ① ② ③ ④ ⑤ ⑥ ⑦
24. I have been sleeping more than usual . . . . ① ② ③ ④ ⑤ ⑥ ⑦
25. I have had a hard time making decisions . . . . ① ② ③ ④ ⑤ ⑥ ⑦
26. I have been able to enjoy things. . . . . ① ② ③ ④ ⑤ ⑥ ⑦

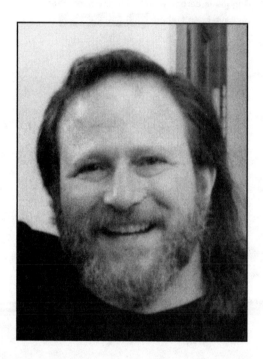

Robert Dubin, D.C.

Dr. Robert Dubin is a chiropractor who has been using "Flashing Light Therapy" in his office in Petaluma, California, since 1985. Using the Lumatron Ocular Light Stimulator™, he has successfully treated a wide variety of patients, including Vietnam veterans suffering from post- traumatic stress disorder, as well as those individuals suffering from chronic pain, neurological handicaps, and seasonal depression. **He has successfully integrated light therapy and cranial sacral therapy into his private practice.** As an expert witness in court, Dr. Dubin has introduced light treatment to the legal community. He is a frequent lecturer at **Life Chiropractic** and **Palmer West,** two San Francisco Bay Area chiropractic colleges, and he has also lectured at Sonoma State University and Santa Rosa Community College. For over nine years Dr. Dubin has hosted radio programs on non-drug and alternative health care on San Francisco's KEST-AM, KTOB in Petaluma, and KATD-AM in Concord.

CHAPTER FIVE

Post Traumatic Stress Syndrome:
Something Can Be Done With Light

Robert Dubin, D.C.

I originally learned the therapeutic use of light from Dr. John Downing himself; and it's taken me a long way and in a lot of different directions from where I was going in my chiropractic practice.

What I want you to really get is the sense that light is not only important; light is not only critical; light is not only nourishing; **light is actually the fundamental physical basis of the universe. All matter in the universe is based on light!**

Five years ago, theoretical physicists who subscribed to the *big bang theory* decided that they had a serious problem, which was that immediately following, in one to the fiftieth power microseconds after the big bang took place, there was a tremendous scattering of matter throughout the universe. This matter was not scattered in very even sheets, but it was scattered in lumps. The very particles that made up this matter were so small and had so little mass, gravity could not be an active force. You have to remember that gravity is the weakest physical force known in the universe. It operates at a tremendously high level of matter and interaction, so it does have tremendous power, but in itself, it's a much weaker force than magnetism or electricity.[1]

If you have doubts, go back to your high school chemistry text, or to even your college chemistry text, and remember that in every chemical reaction whenever an electron jumps an orbital ring inside the atom, whenever an electron jumps from one level to another, a photon of light is released. Now that photon couldn't be released unless it was there, because matter cannot be created or destroyed. So that photon is sitting there and is, in some way, creating the "glue," or the substance or the underlying power that holds

---

1. So initially, these particles did not have enough mass to attract each other gravitationally, and it wasn't until photons started colliding with larger particles that the mass necessary to allow gravity to "kick in" as a force began to form. Thus, light is the fundamental basis of all matter.

that atom together. Light is where we're starting from. Even though I had an appreciation for this before I met John Downing, I didn't know how profoundly it would impact both my life and my clinical experience in providing health care.

I literally became a chiropractor "by accident." I hurt myself; I went to see a physician who told me that I needed surgery. Then a friend of mine, who is a lay person in the health food business, took me to see a chiropractor who said, "I don't think you need surgery." He fixed me in less than five minutes for a total cost of seven dollars. Needless to say, based on that experience, I had my doubts about what medical people knew about lower back problems and about the efficacy or propriety of surgical procedures. Having my foundation shaken so profoundly in my mid-twenties put me on a completely different path. I was almost finished with a degree at U.C.L.A., and I just dropped all my classes and enrolled in chiropractic college. So it was a complete accident that I got into chiropractic.

It was also by complete accident that I met **Dr. John Downing**. I was running a radio program in San Francisco for the **Bay Area Chiropractic Society**, co-hosted by **Dr. Irene Lamberti**.[2] She has an exercise video that's just incredible! We were doing our weekly radio show, interviewing people from health-related professions. Our show's selection criteria were that they had to be practicing non-drug, non-surgical approaches. We had a chiropractically-based radio program. So we combed through the practitioners who were available and who were willing to come in and talk in the "Chiropractic Forum." Dr. John Downing was on the list, and he was a well-known figure in the area. When he came on the program, we talked about *soft visual correction* versus very *crisp visual correction*. He is not only a brilliant speaker and on top of his craft, but he is also a very nice man. We became friends immediately. He was the first optometrist who said he would try to fit my wife for contact lenses. My wife has what's called "a grade seven" or a 7-dioptor *astigmatism*, and contact lenses for her were next to impossible. But John was willing to try.

During the time that I took my wife to Dr. Downing's office to investigate the application of these contact lenses, he discovered from her profile that there were signs of *allergy, headache, phobia* — and other things in her history that he thought Lumatron Ocular Light Therapy™ could help. That was my introduction to the Lumatron™. He tested my wife, who hated it! Not just didn't like it, she hated it! She thought he was crazy. Thought the whole thing was insane; and she was never going back, under any circumstance. Well, I knew I'd been married long enough to this nice lady that when she reacted like that, something "good was happening," and it probably required a life change of some kind which she was not willing to commit to at that point in time.[3]

---

2. For information regarding Dr. Irene Lamberti's excellent product line, refer to Spectrum Sports Research Institute, *Resource List: Section Sixteen, page 383, Luminaries.*

3. At this writing, Mrs. Dubin has had several hundred sessions on the Lumatron™ and she is my chief consultant on appropriate color usage and flicker rate. However, she still has doubts about it.

Knowing that, I went ahead and took a course from John; and then I bought a Lumatron™. And you wouldn't believe what I went through, not only at home, but in the office as well, because my wife works in the office. Well, I was able to tell her, "Look, we need it as a tax write-off. We haven't bought equipment for awhile, so shhh! Even if I don't need it, it'll save us some money in taxes even if I never use it again!"

Case – SAD – *Winter Depression*

I got the machine in December 1985, the beginning of winter. The first patient who came through is an old friend of mine, and even though he was born and raised in Los Angeles, he suffered from seasonal affective disorder. I thought that the closer you got to the equator the less the incidence of this disease or problem existed, but apparently my friend Michael was one of the "odd ones." He went into hibernation from late October until April. He wasn't heard from. He wouldn't move out of his bedroom. He wouldn't work. He wouldn't eat. All he would do is sit around and drink tequila, yes — and that's not good for anybody! Let me tell you this man is also a very talented artist, a very dynamic individual who's done some amazing things in his life. He was painting almost exclusively in monochrome (black and white), was known for that. So he came into the office with a bad sciatica problem, and he was a 50-mile-a-day runner for a long time. It's been said of him that he's obsessed and he's driven. When I first met him, I said, "You know, running 50-miles a day if someone's chasing you is a good idea, but...". And we talked about it. He had a problem with *sciatica,* which is not uncommon for people who run 50-mile races. I mean if you beat yourself up like that, you can expect a negative response from your body!

So he'd been a regular chiropractic patient, and this was, as I said, in the very beginning of the winter depression in December of 1985. Michael dragged himself into the office because he was hurting really bad. He couldn't do anything. He and his wife were in the middle of redesigning and remodelling their house, and he shut down in the middle of the project, went into his room, closed the door and wouldn't come out. He wouldn't talk to anybody except to get a bottle of tequila. So he came in, and I saw that he was just miserable. You know, I could handle the mechanical aspect of his problem. It wasn't any big deal — a quick, easy chiropractic adjustment, and he had relief. But this psychological component, this *depression!* He was a beautiful human being when he was functioning. He was funny; he was up; he was happy; he was great to be around. Then in the winter he became like a bear! He'd go hibernate.

So I said, "You know, I have this new machine . . .". John Downing had brought it over that morning, if I'm not mistaken, or the day before. I said, "I think I can help you with this depression that you're having." You know, people with depression don't react very much. So he'd mumble something. Then I took him by the ear, and I led him into the room where I set up the Lumatron™, and I sat him down. I didn't test him, because he was totally antagonistic and not "with it" at all. I just said, "Here, you're depressed, try some **red light." I flipped the machine on. I set it at fifteen blinks, and I walked out of the room for twenty minutes.** When I came back he was screaming at me, "What did you do to me?" I said, "It looks like you woke up!"

He stormed out of the office, went home, and about three hours later his wife called and said, "Bob, what did you do to him?" I said, "What do you mean?" She said, "He's tearing the walls down." I said, "So?" She said, "He's doing it by hand!" I said, "Well, I guess his depression's broken." And all this, with just that one session with the Lumatron™ and I could never get him back on the Lumatron™ again. He still comes in for adjustments, but I could never get him back into the Lumatron™ room, no way, under no circumstance — because the depression broke, and it never came back.

That was one session in 1985. It is now 1992. The winter's coming, and Michael is now the illustrator for the magazine *Electronic Arts*. Anybody here familiar with the computer games? See, all of these trick machine guns and airplanes and tanks and flying saucers and aliens that go along with these computer programs? My friend Michael is drawing them now in vivid color. He doesn't do monochrome work anymore. He doesn't own India inks anymore. He's got airbrushes now that he uses to blend pastel colors that are not to be believed. Just one session!

So certainly, that's an isolated case, but it just happened to be very serendipitous, because I could say to my wife, "Look what happened to Michael." She scratched her head and said, "I still think John Downing is nuts." I said, "Be that as it may, he's got a good machine. He may be crazy — so what?" There has never been a person who has stepped beyond normal, beyond acceptable, beyond the average, that hasn't been considered "off-the-wall crazy," or at least eccentric. So I don't know what else to tell you. I have found in my interaction with John that's he's probably one of the sanest people I know. In any event, my experience with the Lumatron™ has been almost overwhelmingly positive.

Of course there's always the patient who says, "Big deal, flashing lights." To give you an example, since we're into case histories now, this lady I saw about three-and-a-half years ago was the catalyst for introducing the legal community in the North Bay to Lumatron Ocular Light Therapy™. Now, you go into a deposition, or into court testifying about flashing lights and ohhh boy! Good luck to you! But the research is there. The woman had headaches. Fortunately there had been an article in the journal *Headache* that talked about the use of **stroboscopic light therapy for migraine**[4]. I brought it to the deposition with me, and I said, "Excuse me, but here." And in the last deposition I went to, they talked about the **blinking light therapy** like they knew what it was about. So, a little bit of an educational process has taken place, and it's not being questioned anymore — at least in the personal injury legal arena up in Sonoma County, California. I assume it will be spreading throughout the state and across the country pretty soon, because lawyers like to talk. They tell each other this kind of stuff; it'll be disseminated.

Anyway, Lisa, the lady who was my headache patient, was a designer of underwear and lingerie. She had her own business in Marin County. But when she had a car accident, she became very dysfunctional and had to quit the business and move out of the area. She couldn't afford to live there anymore. So she moved to Petaluma and took a job as an interior designer, working for one of the furniture houses. She was miserable! She was not doing what she wanted to do, but she couldn't function to the point where she was able to get back to her work, to do what she really wanted to do. So I suggested doing Lumatron Ocular Light Therapy™ with her, and she looked at me like I was crazy.

---

4. See *Bibliography Section*.

But she went for it, because she didn't know what else to do. After the twentieth session, she said, "You know, this is stupid. It's the biggest waste of time that ever happened in my life. I don't know why I ever went for this, and I think you're crazy; you're a nice guy; you're a good chiropractor, but this is crazy! I don't know what happened and I can't imagine any good coming from this." A week later she reopened her business, and she's now selling lingerie. Whether it was the light therapy or not, who cares. She's back to full functioning.

I'm not here to tell you that the light therapy is going to solve every problem for every person who comes to your office, because it probably won't. But in your hands this device, this concept, is such a powerful tool. It works! And there's a positive effect and a positive response. **You couldn't ask for two more separate or disparate approaches to the light work than those of John Downing and Jacob Liberman. Yet both have phenomenal clinical experience with it, and definite positive results for their patients.**

So, what I'm trying to tell you is that this therapy is powerful; this therapy is real; and this therapy has a positive effect on people, if your intention is clear. I think **Dr. Shealy** talked about that yesterday. If you go into a health care practice without clear intention to help people, sell stereos, because all you're doing is a disservice to your fellow man and you're making a bad name for the health professions at the same time! It's not only your intention, but the physical, psychological, and endocrinological changes that occur as a result of the light infusing, filling up, changing . . . whatever.

Let's leave it to the scientists to figure out on what atomic or submolecular level this stuff works. I really don't care. I'm a chiropractor; my main focus in practice and in business is to get that person back to full function, whatever it takes. To break it down to the finest little point of science and the finest little hormone kicking in over here, that's not my focus. How many people here could go into a biochemical laboratory and make a tuna fish sandwich into adrenaline? How many people could go into a biochemical laboratory and make white bread into testosterone? Yet, I want you to know that everyone of you in this room does that when you eat tuna fish and white bread; you do that every day without thinking about it, from the time you wake up to the time you go to sleep, and from the time you're born until the time you die. A lot of these processes cannot be repeated in the laboratory, and they never will be repeated in the laboratory, because there is something other than a strictly physical phenomenon that takes place, which has to do with what chiropractors call *innate intelligence* — what the acupuncturists call *"chi" energy* — what the holistic practitioners call *life force* — I don't care what you call it. If you're religious, you'll call it *God*. That's okay. It exists within us, this force makes things happen, and that cannot be replicated in the laboratory.

Now, let's go back to where we started in this talk. **If the fundamental basis of all matter in the universe is light, and somehow sickness or dysfunction is a shortage or a lack of or improper utilization of light**, **then the two go hand-in-hand.** When you put the two together, you get fabulous clinical results, no matter what approach you take to light treatment. Unfortunately, with a therapy as powerful as this, you're going to have a downside to it. For example, in **Dr. Vazquez's** talk he mentioned the person who was exposed to yellow light and went out and committed suicide. That is a definite problem for me as a chiropractor. I'm not a psychotherapist, and in the years that I've been doing this work, I have run across a lot of people who have psychotic breaks, or who went through recollections of sexual abuse, and other traumatic memories. I don't know how to deal with these problems, and I refer them for the appropriate psychological or psychiatric treatment.

To tell you the truth, I never was abused. How lucky can I be? I was raised in New York City by a father who was, by all recollection and by all measurements, an alcoholic, but he wasn't really an abusive man. I never heard of sexual abuse until Oprah Winfrey started talking about it. I mean really, that's just so far beyond my own personal experience! I have a daughter, and her friends come over to the house; they sleep over; they walk around the house "half naked." It's like they're still children. I can't imagine how somebody could have such a twisted mind to feel sexual attraction for children, but I don't doubt that it happens.

When abuse *does* happen, and somebody comes up and says, "Well, this happened to me," I say, "What am I supposed to do now?" Thank God, I know a good shrink right down the street. **So when you're in practice, like I am, if you're not a psychotherapist, if you're a lay practitioner, or if you're an M.D. or a chiropractor, or any other practitioner who doesn't specialize in psychotherapy, it's a real good idea to have allies in the field**. If you're going to do this kind of work, all kinds of painful affect is going to come up, because *post traumatic stress disorder (PTSD)* manifests not only from physical trauma, but from emotional and psychogenic trauma as well.

Somebody can be screamed at their whole life and manifest all the symptoms and signs of post traumatic stress disorder. In looking over the current literature about PTSD, one thing is agreed upon, and that is what the symptoms are, while the treatment protocols and modalities seem to differ according to the author. But everybody recognizes the same set of symptoms. If you're dealing with people who have been traumatized, you'll most likely see the following symptoms in everybody who's had trauma.

Post Traumatic Stress Disorder (PTSD) Symptoms

1. **Recollection of the event that's intrusive** — They can't get it out of their mind; they can't shake it.

2. **Bad dreams** — Maybe of the event, maybe not, but bad and disturbing dreams.

3. **Sleep problems**

4. **Increased Startle Response — The Key Symptom** is agitation, and, an acceleration of the nervous system.

5. **Severe Anxiety**

I found it really fascinating that every patient who had overt manifestations of PTSD were blue light responders; they needed blue light stimulation, according to John Downing's concepts. I've never gone beyond that. I figured John did the work; I'll follow it if it works well enough. If it stops working I'll probably have to invent some other protocol, or go in another direction. But as it stands now, **the results have been very consistent, very predictable — over 90%.** So why fight with something that works? Anyway, **blue light seems to be the key to treating the symptoms of traumatic stress**, at least in the patients that I have seen who had it.

Dr. Steven Vazquez was talking about the patient population that he sees, and it's really true that in any kind of health care practice each practitioner will attract a certain type of person that nobody else will attract. This is why you can have twenty-five offices on a block, and everybody can be busy. Because not everybody is going to be the right person, the right practitioner for every person that comes through. In my patient selection apparently I attract a lot of crazy people. What can I say? My own history is one of multiple trauma. I fell out of a car when I was three-and-a-half. I fell off a four-story building when I was ten. I've had eleven car accidents and as many severe head injuries. Some people I know say that I'm a Type A personality. Do you know what a Type A personality is? It's a risk taker. I'm most comfortable driving on the autobahn in Germany at 250 kilometers per hour. I'm in heaven, absolute heaven while my wife is hiding under the dashboard, and my daughter is in the backseat saying, "Faster!" So, the people who come in to see me are typically agitated, artistic types, for some reason. I don't know why, but I seem to attract people who have a bent toward the arts, and I interact with them very well. I have lots of rapport.

Lately, I have been seeing a tremendous number of Vietnam veterans. They're coming out of the woodwork. Now it's not a stigma to have been in Vietnam. In the past these men were considered "babykillers," and then we went to the Persian Gulf, and the American people changed their minds about the military. The people who were in Vietnam are "victims" of whatever happened; they're not babykillers or murderers anymore, which is a really tremendous shift for these guys, because they went through hell! They went to the bush and they were murdered, maimed and abused, and they came back here and they got abused by their fellow citizens. You talk about traumatic stress; you talk about mindsets and screwing over people's psyches — these guys had it the worst, absolutely the worst! That's why today you see a lot of them represented among the homeless population, and you also see them disproportionately represented in mental health clinics. This wasn't true for World War II veterans, and it wasn't true for Korean War veterans, and it certainly wasn't true for veterans of the Persian Gulf. It had largely to do with the response of the people here, which really created an important part of the trauma that drove most of them off the edge.

I met a lady who is the resident psychotherapist for the **Vietnam Veterans of California**. Her daughter was in a car accident, and she brought her in to see me. I helped her out and fixed her up in six weeks, after she had experienced six months of discomfort. We talked about this. I told her about the Lumatron™ and how I would really like to be able to help some of these guys, the Vietnam veterans. So she said, "Well, this is a very esoteric thing that you're doing, and I have to run it by the authorities and whatever. Let's get some test projects done first."

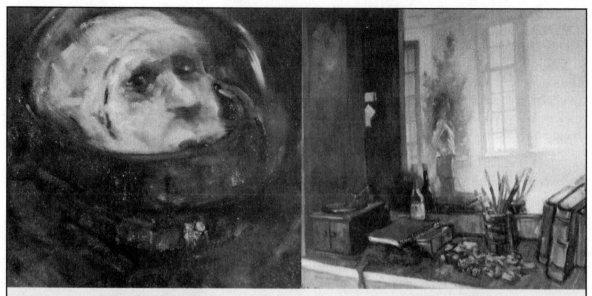

SPACE PERIOD
Before Lumatron™ Treatments

STILL LIFE
After Lumatron™ Treatments

Example of PTSD patient's (Art's) paintings before and after Lumatron™ light therapy, showing shift from monochromatic and dark isolation to increased perception of colors and relatedness.

Case – PTSD – Vietnam Veteran

Fortunately, the first test project was Art. Art was the actual name of the soulmate, or significant other if you will, of this lady Susan whom I'm talking about. Art was a Vietnam veteran who still showed significant signs of PTSD. This is his art. Arthur is an artist, a painter. The above is an oil painting from the period of his life he calls his "Space Period." Now I don't exactly see outer space in there. What do you see in this picture?

RESPONSE: Despair, terror, deep depression.

DR. DUBIN: That's right. **So after thirty sessions on the Lumatron™, look at what he's painting now. I don't know any better way to look into a person's psyche than through their artwork.** Just after he finished the sessions, I wanted to put him through ten to thirty more light therapy sessions. But unfortunately, after thirty sessions he got tired of coming in. I don't know what happened; he just said, "Look, I'm better. I don't need this any more. I love you. You're beautiful. You helped me. Thank you very much." Which was fine, you know. That's all you really could ever ask for in a health care practice. Somebody knows you helped them, that's great! And then about a month later, he came in with this new painting. And he said, "Look at this." Before we started with the Lumatron™ therapy, he gave me that "Space Period painting." I said, "Art, I want this other painting to be entitled *Still Life*." And he said, "Well, that's why I brought it over here, it's for you." This was only the beginning of it. **His work now is lighter; it's brighter; it's more beautiful; it's more hopeful; and it's much more open. And you know what? He doesn't have nightmares any more. He doesn't want to kill everybody who talks to him. He doesn't want to kill himself, and he doesn't really care that he left dead people behind in Vietnam. He's not suffering the guilt anymore!**

Case – PTSD – *Auto Accident*

The next case is a lady named Diana who came to see me several months ago. She was a registered nurse, and she had been in an *automobile accident* five years earlier, where her head went through the windshield. Miraculously there were no cuts, no lacerations — even though her head went through the windshield. One of her only symptoms was that she couldn't think straight, and the people around her thought she was just indulging herself. She was a registered nurse in charge of obstetrics at Marin General Hospital — she was *not* a flake; she was not just indulging herself!

What I had here was a highly active woman who was fully capable and who had been functioning at a high level for the last five years and was not able to work. She was not able to function; *she was not able to focus; and she was unable to remember things.* She could barely drag herself out of bed. Somebody, somehow — again by accident — sent her to see me because I was doing *cranial sacral therapy*. **Light therapy and cranial sacral therapy together are a wonderful combination! And they are powerful tools to use as adjuncts to whatever you're doing.** So I started doing the cranial sacral work with her, and I realized she really needed Ocular Light Therapy, big time, more than anybody I'd ever seen to date, because her nervous system was shut down, even worse than Art's had been.

As a matter of fact, Diana was shut down worse than any of the Vietnam veterans that I've seen, so much so that her husband and her kids were ready to leave her. She was on the verge of becoming homeless, because she was so seriously dysfunctional. **To date she's had over one hundred Lumatron™ sessions.** When we started she was so depressed she could barely get angry or raise her voice at anybody. Also, she was having a problem with her attorney. She thought that he wasn't representing her properly, but she didn't have the nerve to fire him. So I said, "Well, I know a good attorney. Why don't you go see this guy?" So, she went to see this other attorney, and the other attorney fired the attorney that she didn't want to fire. She didn't have the nerve to fire him.

To give you an idea of her changes, he took her to a deposition to talk about this thing, and he asked some questions she didn't like, and she fired him on the spot — at the deposition! Now I think that's a really significant action for somebody who was so severely depressed she couldn't fire somebody over the telephone or get up the nerve to write a letter. She sat in on that deposition, and she got so angry at what her attorney said that she said, "You're fired. Get out." This was the first big step that Diana had taken in five years, of her own volition. Now, her litigation is being settled. And she's planning on re-entering the work force. Please note that I was the third cranial sacral therapist she saw, and certainly not the best one, because the two people she saw before me had in excess of fifteen years experience each doing that kind of work. So I'm not going to tell you that my working on her cranium made the difference; I'm telling you the Lumatron™ did! And for this lady, she was so far "out to lunch" **it took one hundred sessions before she started to come back to normal.** It was only after the sixtieth session that she fired her attorney. And when she called to tell me that, she was hysterical, she was crying. I said, "You shouldn't be crying; you should be tickled pink." She said, "Why?" "Because your depression broke." She said, "What do you mean?" I said, "Could you fire the last person? Well, you fired this guy on the spot, didn't you?" Diana replied, "Yeah, I guess I did." I said, "I think that means you're doing better now. At least you're able to say what's on your mind without worrying about what somebody's going to think about you."

As I was learning to do this work, **Dr. John Downing** gave us the theoretical constructs of **Lumatron Ocular Light Therapy**™. He told us about **congestion of the optic nerve at the optic foramen as the result of intraocular or intraneural pressure. This pressure is generated by the cerebrospinal fluid that bathes the nerves, and under stress the cerebrospinal fluid pressure increases.** It seemed to me that if it really was physical, **then anybody who was doing the Lumatron Ocular Light Therapy**™ **could probably accelerate healing by opening up the optic foramen.** To those of you who are familiar with the anatomy of the cranial vault, the orbit of the eye[5] where the optic nerve comes in is made up of twelve different bones. There are actually twelve pieces of different cranial bones that comprise the cranial vault, and any mechanical distortion or dysfunction in these bones can create an impediment to the transmission of that particular nerve, and might possibly generate pressure on the nerve at the same time. Mechanically, it all makes sense to me.

I had to change my life because of the Lumatron™. My wife was right, this guy John Downing is crazy! I buy the machine and now I have to change my life to conform to it. It's fascinating — everything in my life happens by accident!

I started a cranial sacral workshop with some people; we became very close friends and now we're doing therapy workshops with each other. This has happened over the last two years. One of the practitioners also has a Lumatron™ in his office. The best way to use a device as powerful and as positive as this is to have a clear intention about what you're going to do for the patient. When you have this kind of powerful therapy, you'll be unstoppable. You're not going to make mistakes. You're not going to screw up anybody's life. And you don't necessarily have to follow John Downing's protocol, or you don't necessarily have to follow Jacob Liberman's, or follow me, or follow Steven Vazquez. With a clear mind and a clear heart, you're going to get good results for your patients. That's what it's about. Any questions?

---

5. See Dr. Downing's *Chapter Six for "Pathways of Photocurrent illustration", page 134.*

QUESTION: If the impingement on the optic nerve is mechanical, why do we get better results with the Lumatron™ than we do with mechanical interconnectiveness, such as cranial sacral therapy or chiropractic?

DR. DUBIN: I'm not sure that it is. I have found, for whatever reason, that **those patients I have treated simultaneously under both Cranial Sacral Therapy and Lumatron Ocular Light Therapy™ get better faster**. I don't know exactly why that happens, but I have noticed it does happen regularly. Maybe one day I'll write a paper about it, or a book.

DR. DOWNING'S RESPONSE: **If the problem is mechanical, and you relieve that mechanical stress, the nerve fibers on the optic nerve are not necessarily going to automatically start firing. They need to be restimulated themselves, and the only thing that they will respond to is light, because they are hooked up to the photoreceptors in the eye that will always respond to light. So it's the light that will restimulate that process even after the mechanical pressure is relieved.**

QUESTION: I want to ask you about your patient, Art. You did thirty sessions with him, and you said earlier that if you get someone with psychological problems that you know nothing about, that you know a good "shrink" down the street?

DR. DUBIN: No, no, let me get into that. If I have the kind of response that Steven Vazquez is talking about, where people start crying or start coming off the wall or start talking about early life experience, or multiple personalities, if that happens, I'm not equipped or trained to handle that. That's when I make the referral. With Art, he had a catharsis. He felt better. **I've also never seen anybody have a break on blue light stimulation. Not yet. But with the red, red-orange and yellow, the red end of the spectrum, whew! Good luck. It's emotionally evocative and sometimes people can just come unglued! But with the blue light, all I've really seen it do is to help people integrate their experience and just get back down to normal.** With Vietnam veterans, specifically, most of their fears and disruption to their system happened from terrifying flashes of bright red light: explosions, mines, machine gun fire and with semi-automatic weapon fire.

Finally, the most important thing that I want to suggest to you about being a health care practitioner is, if you don't really *love* your trauma patients, you're not going to help them, and that's got to be unconditional, clear, unrestricted love. You have to love them or you're not going to help them.

SECTION III

Neurophysiological Effects of Lumatron™ Light Therapy

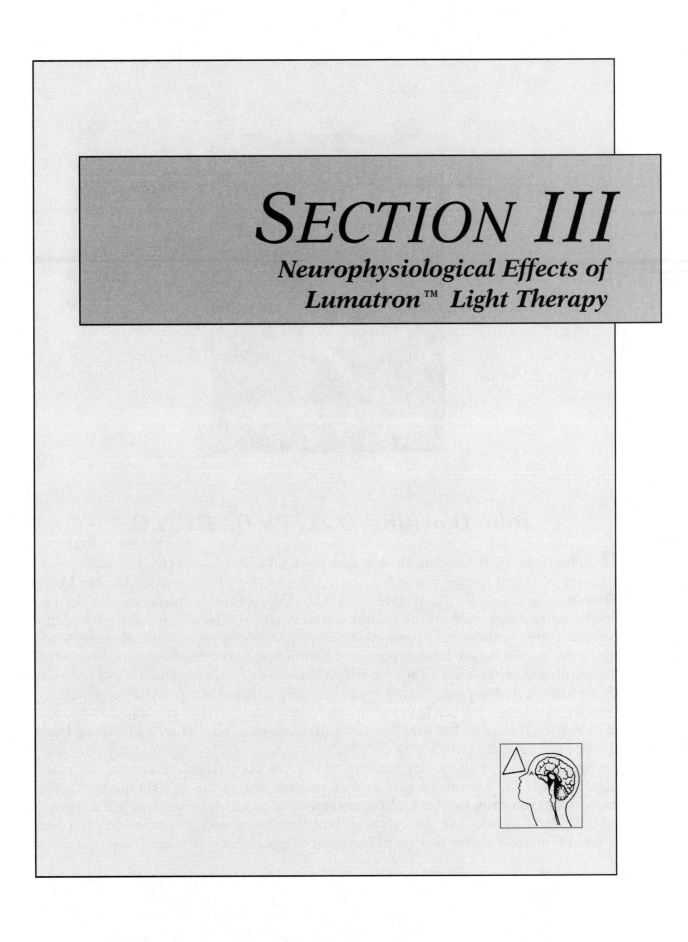

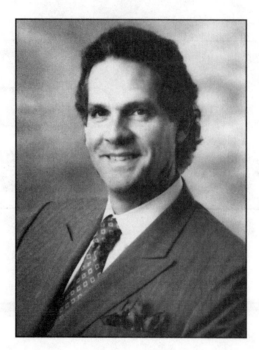

John Downing, O.D., Ph.D., F.C.S.O.

Dr. John Downing is an optometrist in Santa Rosa, California, who has conducted over 25 years of neuro-science research and clinical practice in the area of **Ocular Light Therapy**, for which he has received international professional acclaim. Among his credits is the recognition of the profound and practical effects that light has on: the cerebral cortex in stimulating motivation, learning, thinking, creativity, and memory; on the limbic system, where visually perceived light brings in the emotional impressions of the world; and on the brain stem, where light helps to provide coordination and balance. Dr. Downing's clinical research with visual field testing has also exposed a major physiological mechanism by which light therapy improves brain function. It is the phenomenon of increasing the amount of light-generated nerve current (photocurrent) traveling from the eye to the brain which acts as a necessary biological stimulus for its normal functioning. Along with his development of the first comprehensive system of Ocular Light Therapy, Dr. Downing created the first modern, state-of-the-art light therapy device called **The Lumatron Ocular Light Stimulator**™, for which he received a U.S. patent in 1990. Dr. Downing has doctorates in both optometry and vision science and has taught his method of light therapy to hundreds of practitioners in over 20 countries.

CHAPTER SIX

Clinical EEG and Neurophysiological Case Studies in Ocular Light Therapy

John Downing, O.D., Ph.D., F.C.S.O.

*L*et's do an experiment. I want everyone to stand up with your eyes open, looking straight ahead, and get in a position where you can stand on one leg without touching your neighbor. Everyone on one leg? Fairly easy to balance, right? Now close your eyes and continue to stay on one leg and try to keep your balance. *(With their eyes closed, most of the participants were unable to keep their balance and started falling over within five seconds.)*

I want to give you some physiology to start with. Let's look at the **pathways light enters and travels inside the brain.** When light strikes the *retina*[1] it's converted into nerve impulses because that's what the brain reads. The exercise we just did demonstrated the fact that light energy goes into the *brain stem* and affects our balance. *(See Photocurrent Pathway 3 on following chart.)* It is by seeing that we know where we are in space. When you shut your eyes, you started falling over, and it was because the system in the brain stem was not getting the cues as to where you were. **What I'm talking about is the method of therapeutically sending light through the eyes in order to stimulate brain function, which I call** *Ocular Light Therapy*.

---

1. When light waves strike the retina, they are converted into nerve impulses (photocurrent) that enter the brain along various tracts of nerve fibers.

The Pathways of Photocurrent

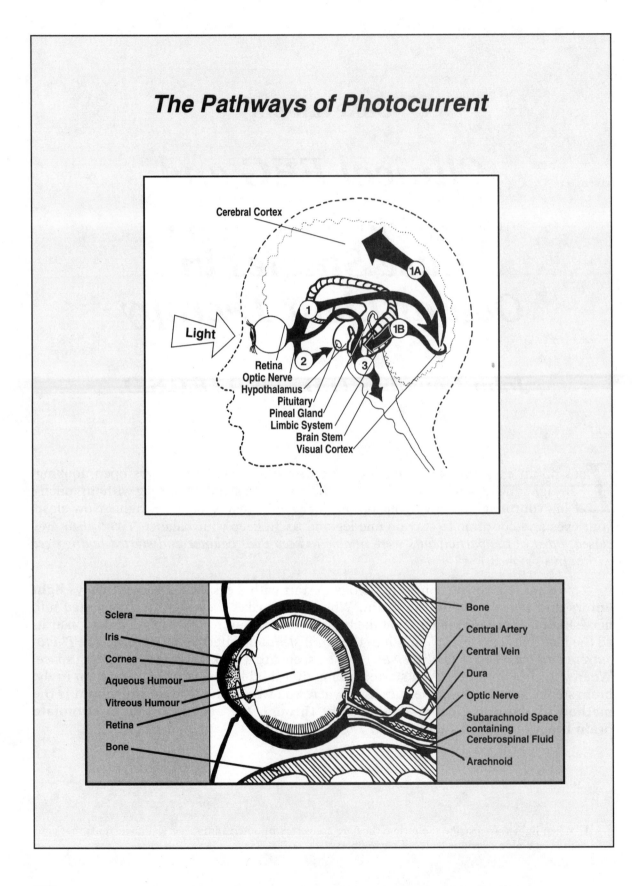

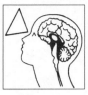

The photocurrent pathway that most light researchers base their theory of light therapy on is the **retinohypothalamic tract** *(See Photocurrent Pathway 2 on previous chart).* This pathway leads from the retina of the eye directly into the **suprachiasmatic nucleus (SCN)** of the hypothalamus. The SCN is believed to be the body's *biological clock* which sets in motion most of our daily, monthly, and annual biological rhythms.

Entrained (programmed) by photocurrent from the eye, the hypothalamus is a *brain within the brain.* It controls 75% of our life processes, including the control of the autonomic nervous system and the pituitary, the master gland, which is actually attached to the hypothalamus.

There are two very important pathways of light action that are unknown to many light researchers. The first pathway leads from the **visual cortex to the cerebral cortex** *(See Photocurrent Pathway 1-A in previous chart).* Elementary sight occurs with photocurrent's arrival at the visual cortex, bringing with it the world's impressions of form and color. However, it's not until this photocurrent passes deeper into the cerebral cortex that we can interpret what this form and color actually means to us. Here we associate it and compare it to other things we've seen, think about it, and get descriptive meanings. In addition, the abundance of photocurrent received by the cerebral cortex in excess of what is needed for vision acts as a general stimulus to our process of thinking, organizing, reasoning, memory, and overall understanding of the world around us.

The second pathway leads from the **visual cortex to the limbic system,** the primary emotional center in the brain *(See Photocurrent Pathway 1-B in previous chart).* Photocurrent brings in the emotional impressions of the world, usually creating a healthy, fleshed out emotional system, if a proper amount of photocurrent reaches the limbic system — and an apparent psychotoxic buildup of painful emotional experience; if it does not. The limbic system is also the site of smell perception and plays some role in learning, memory, and sexual behavior.

I could present hundreds of cases that would illustrate the effectiveness of Ocular Light Therapy; however, for this short presentation, I have selected only a few that will demonstrate light's effect on electroencephalography, the recording of the electric currents in the brain.

If you have knowledge, let others light their candles in it.

— Margaret Fuller

Neurological Typing

Dr. Downing has developed a unique system to determine the correct color stimulation. The full details of this comprehensive system are beyond the scope of this book. A summary of this system is as follows:

Neurological Typing utilizes a **Constitutional Profile** *(see charts at end of this chapter on page 153)* of symptoms to categorize a patient as either a *Fast Neurological Type,* which loosely corresponds to a sympathetically dominant autonomic nervous system or a *Slow Neurological Type,* which loosely corresponds to a parasympathetically dominant autonomic nervous system.

A Fast Neurological Type is usually treated with the blue side of the color spectrum in order to slow down the manifest energy and bring the nervous system into balance. **A Slow Neurological Type is usually treated with the red side of the color spectrum in order to speed up** the manifest energy and bring the nervous system into balance.

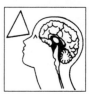

Downing Technique of Ocular Light Therapy — Colors of Associated Flash Rates

Lumatron Colors	Flash Rates	
RUBY	15Hz	
RED	15Hz	Brainwave Range Beta 13Hz and above
RED ORANGE	15Hz	
ORANGE	14Hz	
YELLOW	13Hz	
YELLOW-GREEN	11Hz	
GREEN	10.5Hz	Alpha 8–13Hz
BLUE-GREEN	10.0Hz	
BLUE	9Hz	
INDIGO	8Hz	
VIOLET	7Hz	Theta 4–8Hz
VIOLET	6Hz	
VIOLET	5Hz	
VIOLET	4Hz	
VIOLET	3Hz	Delta 0–4Hz
VIOLET	2Hz	
VIOLET	1Hz	
VIOLET	0Hz	

Flash rates above 15Hz are used with red for extremely slow neurological types.
Flash rates below 7Hz are used with violet for extremely fast neurological types.

Pre and Post-Treatment EEG

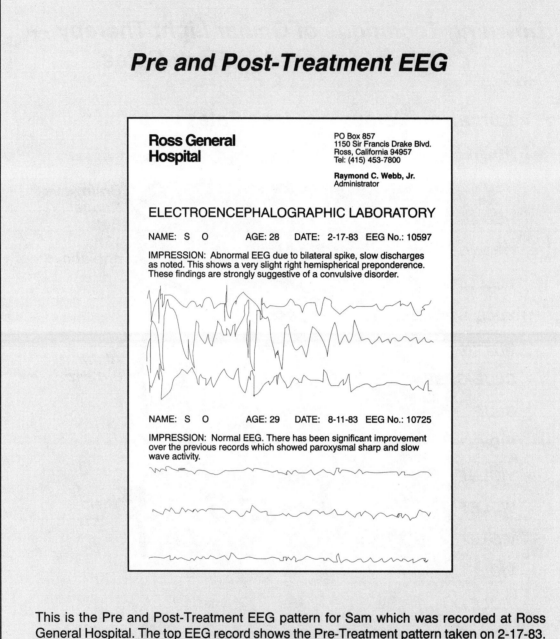

Ross General Hospital

PO Box 857
1150 Sir Francis Drake Blvd.
Ross, California 94957
Tel: (415) 453-7800

Raymond C. Webb, Jr.
Administrator

ELECTROENCEPHALOGRAPHIC LABORATORY

NAME: S O   AGE: 28   DATE: 2-17-83   EEG No.: 10597

IMPRESSION: Abnormal EEG due to bilateral spike, slow discharges as noted. This shows a very slight right hemispherical preponderence. These findings are strongly suggestive of a convulsive disorder.

NAME: S O   AGE: 29   DATE: 8-11-83   EEG No.: 10725

IMPRESSION: Normal EEG. There has been significant improvement over the previous records which showed paroxysmal sharp and slow wave activity.

This is the Pre and Post-Treatment EEG pattern for Sam which was recorded at Ross General Hospital. The top EEG record shows the Pre-Treatment pattern taken on 2-17-83. It shows a preponderance of very slow brain waves in the theta range, which is around five to seven cycles per second. The interpreting physician stated that this was an abnormal EEG due to bilateral spike and slow discharge. This EEG pattern shows a very slight right hemispheric predominance. These findings are strongly suggestive of a *convulsive disorder*. The bottom EEG record shows the Post-Treatment pattern taken on 8-11-83. The interpreting physician now states that during the six-month period corresponding to the time Sam was undergoing Ocular Light Therapy, his EEG was completely normalized.

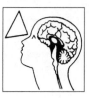

Case – Sam – *Epilepsy*

Sam, age 28, seen in 1983, was one of my first cases to have a before and after recording of the brain's electrical pattern, called a brain wave pattern or an electroencephalogram (EEG). Sam had epilepsy and was having a *grand mal seizure* every two weeks. He was developing brain damage from his numerous seizure-caused falls which produced severe blows to his head.

After examining Sam, I classified him as a **neurologically slow type** with a correspondingly slow brain wave pattern. For this type of patient, I usually suggest Ocular Stimulation with the **red side of the spectrum,** and that is what I used in this case. I started him on a series of twenty, 20-minute sessions of Lumatron™ red light stimulation through the eyes. He then received one month off, followed by a second series of twenty, 20-minute Lumatron™ orange light stimulation.

After Sam completed light therapy, he was still having seizures. However, instead of every two weeks, they were every two months. Then they decreased to three months, and after that it was a year before he had another one. The last time I saw him was seven years after light therapy, and he was having much milder seizures and only once every nine months. His success with light therapy, not only saved him from most of the future brain damage that he would have incurred, but he reported functioning much better both mentally and emotionally, with a significant reduction in the slurring of his speech.

Case – Fred – *Epilepsy*

Fred, a 32-year-old male, was observed by me in my initial examination to be *hyperactive* with a distinct aggressive *Type A personality.* He was having *petite mal seizures* every morning, which was creating much fear and emotional distress. Fred's biofeedback therapist reported that his eyes-closed brain wave pattern was locked in beta at 17 cps *(cycles per second),* and no matter what she did by way of biofeedback training, she could not get him to relax below that level into a normal eyes-closed alpha pattern.

Upon determining Fred to be a **neurologically fast type**, the **blue end of the spectrum** was chosen as the proper stimulus. After only twenty minutes of stimulation with **Lumatron™ violet light**, his biofeedback specialist retook his EEG and found that his brain wave pattern had dropped to theta at 4 cps. He was already feeling more relaxed and significantly less hyperactive. I continued light therapy with nineteen more sessions, consisting of violet for a few more days, **then indigo, and ending with blue.**

At the completion of his light therapy, Fred's closed-eye EEG showed a normal alpha pattern of approximately 10 cps and a decrease in seizures from one every morning to one every other morning. He continued to be significantly more relaxed and settled and was quite happy with the result. I suggested that he return for another series in order for him to finish what he started. He reported that he was satisfied enough with the success that he chose not to undertake the arduous long distance travel that another series would entail.

Case – Bonnie – Sleep Disorder, Fibromyositis, Panic Attacks, Anxiety, Light Sensitivity, Fatigue, Depression

Bonnie was a 64-year old woman, referred to me by her osteopathic physician who was unable to relieve her *fibromyositis,* which was causing severe muscle pain in her back. She also had a *sleep disorder.* She couldn't get to sleep until about 1 a.m. She'd wake up during the night, unrested, with an overabundance of thoughts that were keeping her from being able to sleep. She was taking Xanax to stop the *panic attacks* that had started fours years earlier. She had *fatigue* from not sleeping well, tremendous *anxiety, depression,* and was very *light sensitive.*

After examining Bonnie, I determined that she was a **neurologically fast type.** I started treating her with **Lumatron™ violet light at six cycles a second for twenty minutes each treatment.** Before she started the first session she was depressed. After one session on violet her depression lifted. After only five sessions, she reported sleeping better and not having as many thoughts before sleep onset. The pain of her fibromyositis also decreased. After fourteen sessions, she noticed less light sensitivity, and nighttime car lights didn't bother her anymore. Her back pain continued to decrease. She reported getting clearer mentally about her difficult relationship with her husband and that the light therapy was producing within her mind spontaneous insights and resolutions about other life problems.

She appeared to be much more relaxed and much less anxious. When I next saw her, I decreased the flash rate from **six to four cycles per second on the violet light.** At that time she told me she no longer needed to take Xanax for her panic attacks and anxiety. Finally in her post-treatment history she said, "No depression at all. I feel very up; had incredible dreams and much healing; experienced more energy; went to bed much earlier; was able to sleep deeply and comfortably."

Following are the results of *Bonnie's visual field tests* which show that light therapy increased the photic stimulation to her visual cortex and associated higher brain centers. This increased energy to the limbic system and cerebral cortex is suspected to be the cause of her new mental clarity and emotional rejuvenation.

Seeing light is a metaphor for seeing the invisible in the visible, for detecting the fragile imaginal garment that holds our planet and all existence together. Once we have learned to see light, surely everything else will follow.

— *Arthur Zajonc*

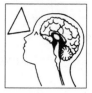

Bonnie Pre and Post-Visual Field Tests

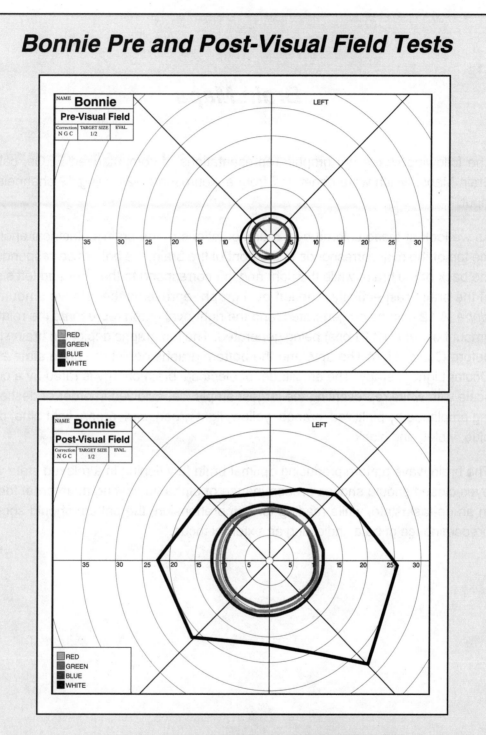

The extreme smallness of Bonnie's Pre-Treatment Visual Field (top) indicates that there is little photocurrent traveling from the eye to the visual cortex and thus not enough light energy to properly stimulate brain function. Bonnie's Post-Treatment Visual Field (bottom) has been enlarged over ten times the area of the Pre-Treatment Field, which indicates a significant increase in the amount of photocurrent energy stimulating the brain.

Brain Maps

The following charts are graphic representations of computerized EEGs, called Brain Maps, which were generated from a Neurosearch-24 using 19 channels of input.

As we look at these colored oval representations of the brain's electrical energy, the top of the oval corresponds to the front of the brain, the bottom corresponds to the back of the brain, while the right and left correspond to the right and left sides of the brain, respectively. The left oval graph represents the relative amount of *alpha* (8-12 cps) being generated, and the right oval graph represents the relative amount of *beta* (12-21 cps) being generated. The top graphs depict the brain state before Ocular Light Therapy, and the bottom graphs depict the brain state after Ocular Light Therapy. The amplitude, of electrical brain energy is rated by a color scale with white representing the largest amplitude, followed in order of descending amplitude by pink, red, orange, yellow, light green, dark green, light blue, dark blue, violet, and black.

The brain wave pattern producing optimal brain functioning in a relaxed state with eyes closed should show a predominance of alpha, indicating an internal focus. In an on-task state, while reading for comprehension, the pattern should show a predominance of beta, indicating an external focus.

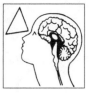

Bonnie Brain Maps Relaxed with Eyes Closed

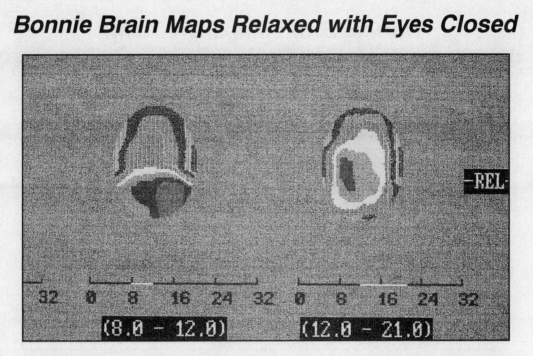

In a relaxed state with eyes closed, a comparison of Bonnie's Pre-Treatment Brain Map (top) with her Post-Treatment Brain Map (bottom) shows that light therapy has significantly increased her alpha and decreased her beta, signifying an improved brain state. This pattern change is consistent with the decrease in her symptoms of anxiety, muscle tension, back pain, and with the diminishing of her panic syndrome. The pre-therapy state of higher beta in Wernicke's area, the site of language comprehension, mirrors the obsessive thinking that kept her awake at night. The post-therapy state suggests the ability to sleep much better with Wernicke's area showing lower beta and the rest of the brain showing more alpha.

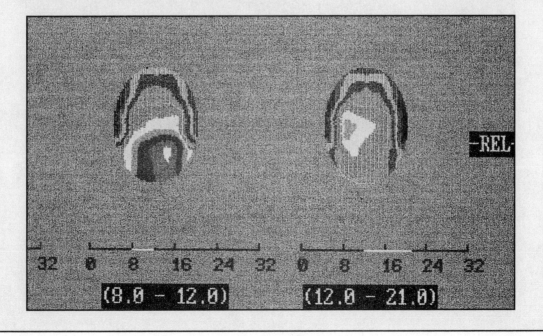

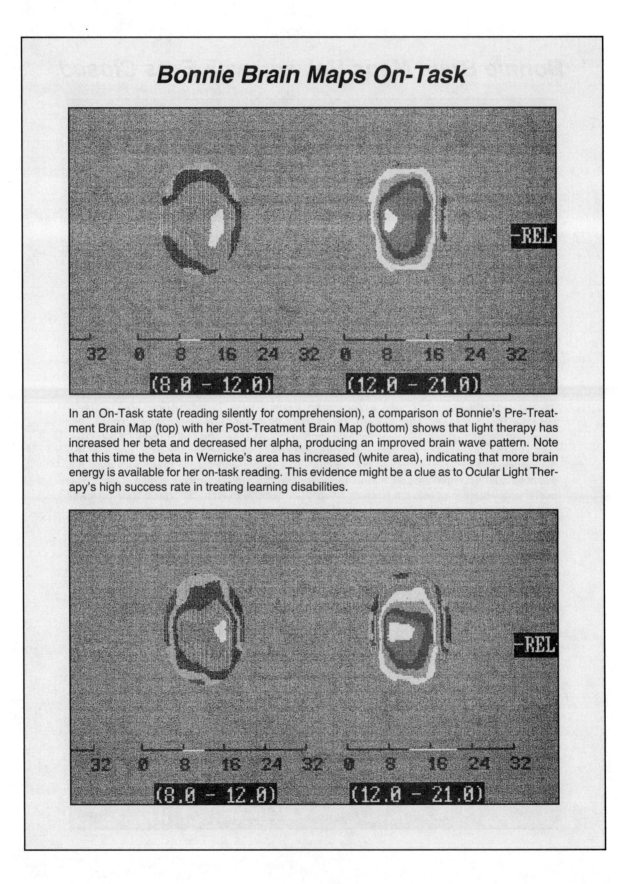

Bonnie Brain Maps On-Task

In an On-Task state (reading silently for comprehension), a comparison of Bonnie's Pre-Treatment Brain Map (top) with her Post-Treatment Brain Map (bottom) shows that light therapy has increased her beta and decreased her alpha, producing an improved brain wave pattern. Note that this time the beta in Wernicke's area has increased (white area), indicating that more brain energy is available for her on-task reading. This evidence might be a clue as to Ocular Light Therapy's high success rate in treating learning disabilities.

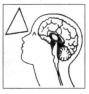

Case – Carol – *Poor Memory, Poor Concentration, Poor Speech Enunciation, Chronic Fatigue, Overly Emotional with Severe PMS Symptoms, Light Sensitivity, Dry Eyes, Repressed Memories*

Carol was the 38-year old daughter of an alcoholic mother who had herself been a *chronic alcoholic* for eighteen years. She had incurred multiple head injuries and tolerated continuous neck pain, resulting from a previous *automobile accident,* many *falls* and numerous *beatings* sustained from her "boyfriend." The primary reason she sought light therapy was to improve her memory, concentration, and speech enunciation. She was also experiencing such low levels of energy that she admitted that she felt herself to be like a "walking zombie." She was overly emotional, with severe PMS symptoms. Her light sensitivity was so severe that she wore sunglasses constantly and her eyes were chronically irritated from dry eye syndrome. In addition, she suffered from memories of childhood physical abuse from her alcoholic mother. Four months prior to seeing me she had fallen on her tailbone, which was now causing a great deal of lower back pain. She was confused, disoriented, and felt angry and inferior; she was sleeping ten hours a night and had lack of motivation. She expressed being very worried because she felt she could never get back to normal.

Upon determining that **Carol was a neurological slow type,** I began Ocular Light Therapy, using **Lumatron™ red light at 15 cps for twenty minutes each session.** In her second session of red light, she felt an increase of anxiety in her chest, which released. After six sessions she noticed more energy, more alertness and better concentration. The pain had begun to go away from her tailbone and she reported that everything in her life was getting better. After twenty-one sessions her PMS symptoms were much less and she wasn't as emotional. The red was making her feel a little on edge with a little tightness in her stomach, but this was minor compared to the benefit she was getting. Now Carol was sleeping two hours less at night, and had more energy. The pain had totally gone from her tailbone area. Her light sensitivity had reduced to the point of seldom needing to wear sunglasses, and her dry eye irritation was completely gone, though she felt she had experienced only a slight improvement in her enunciation. She added that the experience of light therapy felt as if a blanket of security had been placed around her.

Though light therapy had produced a dramatic improvement in Carol after twenty one sessions, I was not convinced that she had gone as far as she could go with it. I, therefore, gave Carol a **supplemental stimulus of yellow for two days, followed by orange for three days.** After the orange stimulation she began to have dreams of being sexually abused. These dreams deeply disturbed her throughout the night, but she would awake in the morning feeling even better than usual. I continued light therapy with alternating orange and yellow. **This triggered a spontaneous memory that had been repressed for 24-years.** The memory was that of being raped at the age of 14 by an adult family friend who had lived across the street from her at that time. At this point of discovery I referred her for psychological counseling to help complete her recovery. **This is a good example of the ability of light therapy to flush out painful, repressed emotional experiences held in the limbic system.**

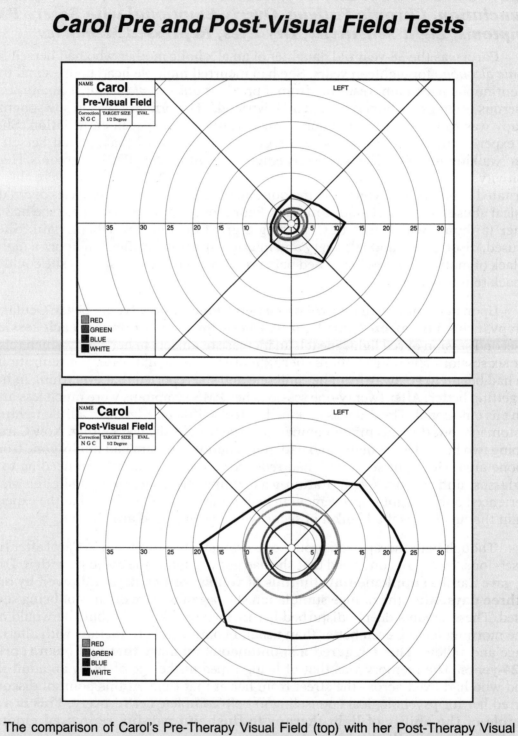

Carol Pre and Post-Visual Field Tests

The comparison of Carol's Pre-Therapy Visual Field (top) with her Post-Therapy Visual Field (bottom), after approximately 30 sessions of Ocular Light Therapy, shows a twelve-fold area enlargement, indicating a significant increase in photocurrent-carried light energy reaching her visual cortex and higher brain centers.

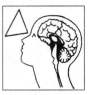

Carol Brain Maps Relaxed with Eyes Closed

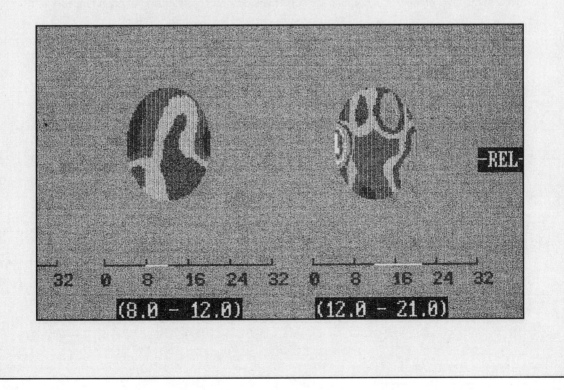

In a relaxed state with eyes closed, a comparison of Carol's Pre-Treatment Brain Map (top) with her Post-Treatment Brain Map (bottom) shows that light therapy has created an improved brain wave pattern of increased alpha and decreased beta.

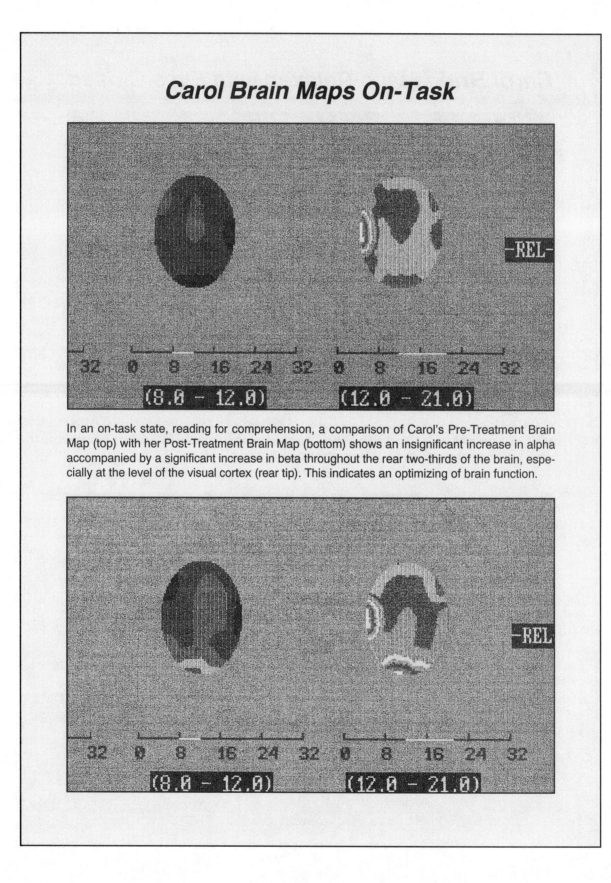

Carol Brain Maps On-Task

In an on-task state, reading for comprehension, a comparison of Carol's Pre-Treatment Brain Map (top) with her Post-Treatment Brain Map (bottom) shows an insignificant increase in alpha accompanied by a significant increase in beta throughout the rear two-thirds of the brain, especially at the level of the visual cortex (rear tip). This indicates an optimizing of brain function.

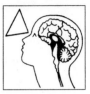

Case – Linda – *Severe Depression, Chronic Pain, Fibromyositis, No Sense of Smell*

Linda was a 30-year-old classical pianist, whose years of sitting tensely at the concert piano in rigidly held positions had resulted in chronic muscle pain in her back. The pain was so severe that she wore a *Transcutaneous electrical nerve stimulator (TENS unit)*, an electrical stimulation instrument used for chronic pain, strapped to her back, and kept it on all the time. Linda said that the TENS unit was the only thing that gave her any relief. Linda had also been severely depressed for about seven years, and the pain made her all the more depressed. Another symptom, which was the most interesting thing about the case for me, was that she had lost her sense of smell about four years previous to seeing me, and she'd never been able to smell the bouquet in wine in her entire life.

I determined Linda to be a **neurologically fast type,** and **Lumatron™ violet light** was determined to be the best stimulant. Astonishingly, after only her first 20-minute session of violet light stimulation, she was standing at the bus stop, waiting for her bus ride back to San Francisco, when she began to smell the fragrance coming from a nearby bush. After that the other scents of her surrounding environment began registering in her brain. **Her sense of smell had returned after four years of absence.** This brought to her a keen sense of wonderment as to whether or not she would be able to smell the always elusive bouquet of wine. As destiny would have it, her destination bus stop put her right in front of a restaurant that was having a wine tasting. She discovered then that her sense of smell had returned more completely than ever before, as she could now smell the bouquets of even the subtlest vintages. **This is another interesting example of ocularly perceived light's stimulating effect on the limbic system, the center of smell perception.**

After nine more sessions of violet light stimulation, the pain from her fibromyositis had not decreased at all. However, her depression had totally disappeared. She told me "It's the weirdest thing, I'm still walking around with intense pain, but I feel happier than I've ever felt before."

I have known light in its purity and I consider it my duty to strive after it.

— *Goethe*

The device used to produce the necessary color stimuli is the ***Lumatron Light Stimulator***™, which I first made available to practitioners in 1986. Acupuncturists use it as a needle of light going directly into the hypothalamus. Chiropractors use it as an adjusting tool for the autonomic nervous system. Optometrists use the Lumatron™ for enlarging visual fields and rehabilitating the neurovisual system. Psychologists and psychiatrists use it for the alleviation of mental and emotional problems, and physicians and naturopaths use it for the full scope of physiological imbalances.

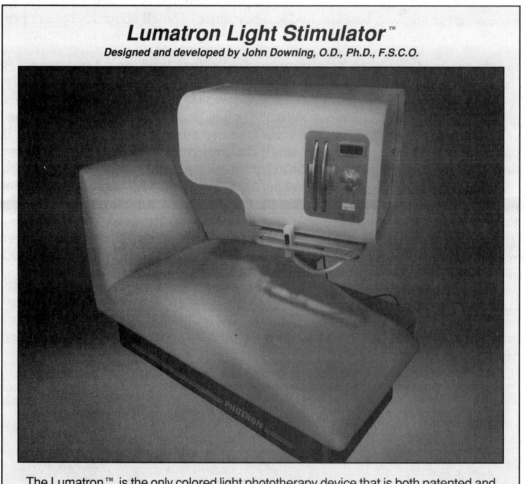

Lumatron Light Stimulator™

Designed and developed by John Downing, O.D., Ph.D., F.S.C.O.

The Lumatron™ is the only colored light phototherapy device that is both patented and has a Class 2 rating by the Food and Drug Administration for non-medical devices.

The Lumatron Light Stimulator™ is the first advancement in Ocular Light Therapy instrumentation since the development of the original instrumentation by **Harry Riley Spitler, M.D.** in the 1930s. It utilizes the highest quality glass filters combined with a full spectrum plasma gas light source, producing pure and precise wavebands of colored light held to a strict tolerance of accuracy. The available flash rate is adjustable in .1 hertz increments from 0 to 60 cycles per second.

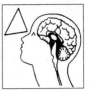

The New Photron® Stimulator

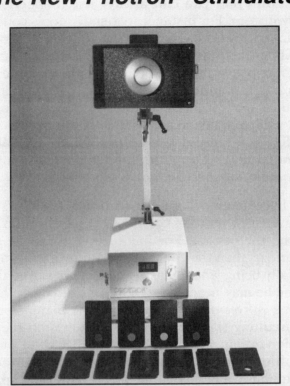

The new Photron® Light Stimulator in the open position (above) and with the case closed (below) for travel and transportation. The Photron® incorporates the colored strobe light technology of the original (and larger) Lumatron™ with an improved design. It is more portable (22lbs) and versatile (in terms of brightness and flash rate adjustments), and less expensive.

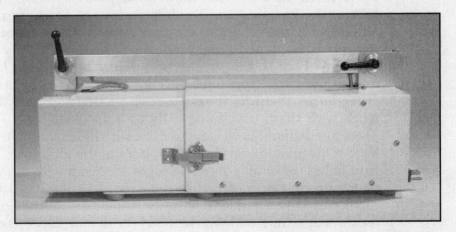

It is currently available from Applied Light Technology, Inc, in San Rafael, California. See *Resource List* for information about this product.

QUESTION: How do you determine the specific colors you use?

DR. DOWNING: I've developed a profile for looking at certain symptoms. However, **I don't feel you can always use a specific color for a specific symptom**. For instance, two individuals could walk into your practice with a headache, and one individual might need a red stimulus, while the other individual might need a blue stimulus. Again, the color books that are out there, the esoteric color books, are very much in conflict with each other, because one says you should use "this color for this symptom," and then you open another book, and it will recommend a different color for the same symptom. **So I feel that you should use colors which are directly related to the individual's *Constitutional Type*. The proper color stimuli are *individual-specific*, not *symptom-specific*.**

I have developed a **Constitutional Profile** (*see following page*) that gives me a starting color, and I give a certain weight to the problem and the person. For instance, if someone comes in with severe *fatigue*, then the client gets a minus four — a high rating for potentially being what I classify a **slow type**. And this is one indication to me he may need a **red light stimulus**. On the other hand, if someone is *hyperactive* or if their mind is racing so fast that it is short-circuiting their mental processing; then they get a plus four or a high rating, on being a **fast type**. This type of individual would need a **blue light stimulus**. I do about an hour-and-a-half case history, similar to a homeopathic physician's workup, in order to determine whether their constitution makes them a fast or slow neurological type. This helps me to choose the color I begin with. I also sit them in front of the Lumatron™ and go through the different colors to see what their individual responses are.

I give them the color that immediately starts making them feel better. Dr. Vazquez and Dr. Liberman use a different, though still quite effective, approach that's more of a psychotherapeutic approach to working with the light, which they will talk about. As I see it, the psychotherapeutic use of light is more of an *antagonistic approach*, giving them the color that most *antagonizes* them, is most reactive to their system. Then you work with them psychologically to help clear their reactions. There are definitely two ways to work with light, and it's the personality of the practitioner that makes a lot of the difference. I feel you have to be a psychologist to do a lot of this work with the antagonistic approach. I personally like the ease of letting the color be the "doctor" and being able to have the patient be on the Lumatron™ for days at a time without the need for doctor supervision. I do a follow-up about once a week to modify their colors and guide them through the Ocular Light Stimulation process. *(Continued on page 157).*

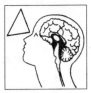

Constitutional Profile

Name_____ Age_____ Date_____

Street_____ Birthdate_____Referred by_____

City_____Zip_____ Sex: M F

Phone (Home)_____ Marital: S M D W SS#_____

Phone (Work)_____ # of Children_____ Payment by: CASH CHECK

Spouse's Name_____ Spouse's Occupation_____

Parents' Name_____
(List if you are a minor)

Your Occupation _____

Activities_____

Please fill out the following portion carefully, as this information has a great bearing on the diagnosis of your case. It will be treated confidentially.

Check the conditions which apply to you:

CONDITION	Present	Past	CONDITION	Present	Past
Allergies			Influenza (frequently)		
Anemia			Measles		
Appendicitis			Menstrual Problems/severe cramps		
Arthritis			Mumps		
Asthma			Nausea		
Blood disorders			Nutritional Deficiencies		
Blood Pressure (High)			Rheumatic Fever		
Blood Pressure (Low)			Pneumonia		
Cancer			Polio		
Car sickness			Pregnancy		
Circulation (Poor)			Scarlet Fever		
Colds			Sinus Trouble		
Dental Problems			Smallpox		
Diabetes			Sore Throat		
Digestion Problems/Gas			Stroke		
Diptheria			Tonsilitis/Removed		
Dizziness			Toxic Condition		
Earaches			Tuberculosis		
Epilepsy			Typhoid		
Fatigue			Varicose Veins		
Genital Problems			Venereal Infection		
Goiter			Whooping Cough		
Hay Fever			Gout		
Headaches			Other		
Hearing Difficulties					
High Fever			Body Injury		
Hypoglycemia			Head Injury		
Infections			Broken Bones		

©1996 John Downing, O.D., Ph.D.

CONDITION	Present	Past	CONDITION	Present	Past
Pain			Whiplash		
Poor Postural Alignment			Other		

Check the problem areas that apply to you:

AREA	Present	Past	AREA	Present	Past
Brain			Pancreas		
Pituitary			Stomach		
Thyroid			Small Intestines		
Thymus			Colon		
Lungs			Bladder		
Heart			Ovaries		
Liver			Uterus		
Spleen			Prostate		
Gall Bladder			Testes		
Adrenals			Other		
Kidneys					

List your surgical operations:

OPERATION	Date	OPERATION	Date
1.		3.	
2.		4.	

General Health—Emotional:

CONDITION	Present	Past	CONDITION	Present	Past
Anger			Lonely		
Irritability			Nervous		
Anxiety			Nervous Stomach		
Fear			Sexual Problems or Concerns		
Cry Frequently			Stress		
Emotionally Dependent/Clinging			Tension		
Feel Inferior			Other		
Feelings Easily Hurt					

General Health—Mental:

CONDITION	Present	Past	CONDITION	Present	Past
Confusion			Lack of Motivation		
Depression			Nervous Breakdown		
Disorientation			Other		
Frightening Thoughts			*Learning Disabilities:*		
Irrational Thoughts			General Poor Learning		
Negative Thoughts			Concentration Poor		
Disturbed Sleep			Dyslexia (Poor Perception Registry)		
Insomnia			Reversing Numbers and Words		
Neurosis			Math Poor		
Psychosis			Memory Poor		
Retardation			Pronunciation Poor		
Suicidal			Reading or Writing Poor		
Worry			Spelling Poor		

©1996 John Downing, O.D., Ph.D.

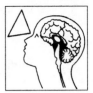

Birth History:

CONDITION	YES	CONDITION	YES
Premature Birth		Instruments Used	
Complications at Birth		Mother Taking Tobacco, Drugs, Etc.	
Anesthesia at Delivery		Other	

Social Development:

CONDITION	YES	CONDITION	YES
Home Unstable/Martial Conflict		Medical Problem in Family	
Parents Separated or Divorced		Emotional Problem in Family	
Poor Child-Mother Relationship		Mental Problem in Family	
Poor Child-Father Relationship		Learning Problem in Family	
Poor Sibling Relationship		Other	
Poor Peer Relationship			

Present Character:

CONDITION	YES	CONDITION	YES
Introvert		Poor Balance	
Extrovert		Difficulty Expressing Self	
Underactive		Behavioral Problems	
Hyperactive		Unhappy	
Sleep over 8 Hours		Other	
Sleep under 6 Hours			

Visual Health:

CONDITION	YES	CONDITION	YES
Blurred Vision		Conscious of Eyes	
Poor Peripheral Vision		Affected by Sunlight, Light, Glare	
Tunnel Vision		Bump into Things	
Decreased Vision at Night		Eye Strain	
Double Vision		Eyes Tired	
Tropia (Turned Eyes)		Eyes Ache or Painful	
Poor Color Recognition		Eyes Water Excessively	
Color Blindness		Eyes Itch	
Poor Eye Movement		Eyes Burn	
Poor Eye Teaming		Eyes Get Red	
Poor Hand/Eye Coordination		Have Floaters in Vision Field	
Get Sleepy When Reading		Have Styes Frequently	
Eyes Feel Heavy		See Haloes or Rainbow Around Light	

List any eye injuries or infections which you've had? _____

_____

_____

_____

_____

List any eye surgery you've had? _____

_____

_____

_____

_____

_____

_____

Which problems are you seeking help for from this office? _____

_____

_____

_____

_____

_____

_____

_____

_____

_____

_____

_____

_____

_____

_____

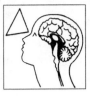

So there is a technique for everyone in this room, and as far as I know, they all work quite well. The final thing about how I use the color is once I do all my determining and start a patient on a particular frequency of light, then their response to the light is going to dictate to me if they stay on it or not. I tell them to call me immediately if they have any negative reaction. **Should they have a negative reaction, then I will change the color, usually going to the opposite side of the spectrum.** If they don't have a negative reaction, but within six days don't start getting any improvement in their symptoms, then I will also change their colors, probably one-hundred and eighty degrees, to the *opposite side of the spectrum,* to see if I can get a clearer fix on what color they require. **The patients are the ultimate determiners to the practitioner as to what color they're going to need**.

QUESTION: Do you reach any aggravation or antagonistic responses with the flicker rates?

DR. DOWNING: I haven't, but I know Dr. Vazquez and Dr. Liberman have, and they talk about that. For me personally, I have generally found a flash rate combination that works with the different colors that for my own type of optometric practice has held up pretty well. **Since the reds are usually entraining a faster brain wave pattern, I set them at a higher flash rate. I set red at fifteen cycles per second, which is slightly into the beta brain wave range and, if I'm giving blue or indigo, the flash rate will be around seven cycles per second, and violet will be around six.** If I've got a really active patient that I want to try to "nail to the wall," to slow them way down, I could go as low as four cycles a second or even to two cycles a second. Sometimes the patient can't tolerate the flash. So again, with the Lumatron™, since you can put it all the way up to sixty cycles a second, I'll turn it up to fifty or sixty cycles a second, which is flashing so fast that it's no longer perceivable as a flash, and that looks to the patient the same as a steady light. **With those individuals who can't tolerate a low flash rate I will do a steady light, which tends to be less evocative.**

QUESTION: I've been working with the Lumatron™ for about two years in Seattle. For choosing the color we use a ***Hand Dynometer,*** which is a muscle-strength procedure that's readily available in every medical clinic and medical supply store. Then you take the Hand Dynometer reading on the person, and it might come out to say ten or whatever it is. They squeeze this with their dominant hand; looking at, for example, red light. I expose the person to red without the flash. I let them squeeze it again. Invariably it'll come up with twelve, or it'll show a strength increase immediately. I'd like someone to tell me how it works with them in our next conference.

DR. DOWNING: How do you use it as a diagnostic tool?

RESPONSE: Diagnostically, what the Hand Dynometer reading means to me is that the light was affecting their whole neuromuscular system, including their entire muscle system, for them to have an increased muscular strength with that color through their hands. Therefore, you can start with that color.

DR. DOWNING: So, sometimes if you showed them red, they wouldn't be as strong, right?

RESPONSE: It's so individual, like you said, it's unbelievable. The next person would be blue or red or violet; and when you did that color, it would increase their strength.

DR. DOWNING: This is interesting, to use a strength test. We can use EEG to validate color selection as well. Dr. Liberman uses a galvanic skin-response (GSR) technique. So there are many different techniques. Thanks, I haven't heard of that one. That's a new one to add to our armamentarium.

QUESTION: Dr. Downing, how do you interpret visual field tests?

DR. DOWNING: I interpret the visual field in a quantitative way. **If you're able to expand the visual field, you're getting more light energy back to the visual cortex**, because that's the part that's "seeing" that visual field. **It's a measure showing that you're grossly increasing the amount of photocurrent stimulation to the brain, and therefore you're feeding the brain with more electrical energy. The brain loves electrical energy; that's what it runs on. You're also stimulating all the cells in the body with this same light generated energy.**

Let me illustrate this with an example. The Lumatron™ is currently being used a great deal in Norway to treat *stroke victims.* One of my Norwegian students in her busiest times is seeing thirty-five patients a day. She has four Lumatrons™ in four booths. The first time she noticed that Ocular Light Therapy had any effect on stroke victims was with a woman who was about 55, which is young for a stroke patient. This patient had a retail business when the stroke occurred and had to close her business. She lost the use of her left hand and she had to drag her left foot behind her. During the woman's tenth session, **Phyllis Nyquist,** the practitioner, heard a scream from the room, and she said, "Oh my God. What did I do now?" So Phyllis ran into the room and the patient was moving her little finger. Within two more weeks she could move her whole hand. Not only had she regained functioning of her hand, but she was no longer dragging her foot behind her! In another twenty sessions she was basically back to normal.

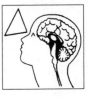

I'm using this case as an example to show that the expansion of the visual field indicates that more photocurrent is not only going to the visual cortex, but continuing beyond it to the cerebral cortex as well. The part of this woman's brain that was affected by her stroke was the part of the cerebral cortex (called the motor cortex), which controls the voluntary movement of muscles. The stroke had debilitated the motor cortex cells controlling her left hand and foot. As her visual field enlarged, increased amounts of photocurrent spread throughout the cortex, including the motor cortex. It is a logical conclusion that the regaining of the movement in her limbs was a result of this increased photo-electric stimulation to the non-functioning motor cortex cells, which re-stimulated them back into action.

Keep in mind these are serious stroke victims. This last lady came in a year-and-a-half after she had her stroke. It's very customary to see improvements within the first six months, they just happen on their own. But after a year or a year-and-a-half, these patients are usually pretty well crystallized into staying where they are, which makes the fact that light therapy still works at this stage very significant.

QUESTION: Dr. Downing, do you have any experience with the use of light in treating *cerebral palsy?*

DR. DOWNING: I haven't personally treated anyone with cerebral palsy. I do know, however, that **Deiter Klinghardt, M.D.,** the director of a Santa Fe pain clinic has had success with this type of condition. One such case that comes to mind is of a woman that was flown in to see him who had been bound to a wheelchair for some time. After several sessions of Ocular Light Therapy she was able to start walking and, to my knowledge, never had to return to the wheelchair.

QUESTION: Has light been used to treat *epilepsy?*

DR. DOWNING: Epilepsy has been affected by light therapy, and I have given two previous examples of this. *There is a caution to working with an epileptic patient, however, and that is the potential of triggering a photoconvulsive seizure.* Some epileptics can be triggered into a seizure by a flashing light or even a flickering television set. If you do have an epileptic patient who wants to do light therapy, you can either do non-flashing therapy or determine that they are non-photo-convulsive so that you can do flashing therapy. I have found that flashing therapy is usually more effective and, therefore, preferable when possible. If the patient does not know whether or not they are photo-convulsive, their neurologist should be consulted.[2]

---

2. See Concerns and Cautions Regarding Phototherapy under Photoconvulsive Seizures and the use of Light Emitting devices in Health Care Practice, *Page xvix.*

What to do if a Patient has a Convulsive Seizure

Convulsive seizures are rare and photoconvulsive seizures are even more rare, occurring in about one in 3000 patients; thus, you will probably never experience one in your office, but if you do, these suggestions will serve as first aid guildelines:

- protect person from nearby hazards
- loosen ties or shirt collars
- place folded jacket or towel under head
- turn on side to keep airway clear
- give support and reassurance when consciousness returns

If a single seizure lasted less than ten minutes, ask if hospital evaluation is wanted.

If multiple seizures, or if one seizure lasts longer than ten minutes, take to emergency room.

This treatment guide was prepared by John Downing in 1987, and has been approved by the Department of Neurology of The Bowman Gray School of Medicine.

Additional information about epilepsy may be obtained from the **Epilepsy Foundation of America,** 4351 Garden City Drive, Landover, MD 20785; and the **Epilepsy Information Service,** Department of Neurology, Bowman Gray School of Medicine, Winston-Salem, NC 27103.

Many times light can significantly strengthen the system to help patients be better able to cope with certain medical problems, even if it doesn't correct that specific problem. **It's far better not to say you're going to cure something, but to just focus on optimizing the patient's ability to take in photocurrent. Let's balance their hypothalamus with light!**

QUESTION: Are you moving toward feeling comfortable with full spectrum light, or are you working towards the specific color that's going to cause a change?

DR. DOWNING: We're all looking for the specific color frequency that's going to cause the change; that's right.

Going back to the epileptic case I mentioned earlier, **I gave him twenty sessions of red light and then followed by twenty sessions of orange light. Immediately the color started neutralizing his condition. The same is true with the cases of *chronic fatigue* and *depression*.** I will pick a color, and then my goal is to immediately start balancing the patient's system and have them get better. The ***antagonistic color approach*** that **Dr. Vazquez** and **Dr. Liberman** use is to pick a color that starts to bring out things that have been buried in their patient's unconscious, and by then working these things out, the patient will start to get better. The final goal

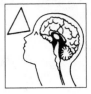

in all of our approaches is to have the patient balanced and not needing any light stimulus[3].

In summary, the great majority of patients undergoing light stimulation have been able to eliminate or significantly reduce physiological imbalances, such as: fatigue, stress, headaches, pain, hormonal imbalances, PMS, insomnia, depression, poor concentration and memory, learning dysfunction, and selected vision problems.[4]

To know God is the most important way to heal all disease - physical, mental, spiritual. As darkness cannot remain where light is, so also the darkness of disease is driven away by the Light of God's perfect presence when it enters the body.

— Paramahansa Yogananda
WHERE THERE IS LIGHT

---

3. For additional information regarding classes, training and treatment in Ocular Light Therapy, Dr. Downing may be contacted directly. See *Resource List: Section One, page 341, Light Years Ahead Authors.*
4. See *Resource List: Section Two, Page 343,* for a list of *Lumatron™ Master Practitioners* who have experimented with this phototherapy instrument within their areas of professional specialization.

This is what patients* have said about their experiences with Lumatron™ Light Stimulation:

> *"I am grateful for being referred for neurosensory stimulation. I have been experiencing problems as a result of chronic fatigue immune dysfunction syndrome for six years. Therapies I had tried prior to your Lumatron™ treatments provided only minor relief.*
>
> *After using the Lumatron™ Stimulator, I noticed a shift right away. Even though it was small at first, the cumulative effect of 20 1/2-hour sessions was that I felt 100% better and had achieved new levels of health, including greater physical strength and endurance, increased ability to concentrate, improved memory, the lifting of depression and a cloud of confusion, the return of a more normal appetite, better communication through increased vocabulary (my memory had returned), more restful sleep (leaving me feeling rested in the mornings), clearing of a scalp problem, and an improved ability to read because of my increased memory and concentration ability.*
>
> *Thank you again, Dr. Downing, for the Lumatron™ and my restored health."*

— N. C., Editor

> *"The effect of my Lumatron™ treatments has been "sensational." I have become more efficient. I am accomplishing more with less stress than I could have imagined. I feel a refreshing relief from the bonds of stress that had always engulfed me. This allows me to perform at a level which not only amazes me, but my wife and associates as well."*

— R. F. B., C.P.A.

> *"This is what happened after my series of light stimulation: the visual fields of both eyes dramatically enlarged; eye tension and resulting eye fatigue were eliminated; insomnia was replaced by a sound night's sleep; dreams became colorful and lively; my erratic pulse abruptly stabilized, as my arrhythmia shifted to a regular, steady beat; my balance has improved and I seldom stumble anymore. I feel my sense of smell is keener, and my depression lifted abruptly from the beginning of the therapy. (**I am tempted to write that the light lightened my life.**) Thank you for making it possible for me to have treatments. I am very grateful and very enthused over the results."*

— V. J., Retired

*Excerpted from Preventive Medical Center of Marin Newsletter, Volume 2, No. 1, Winter 1993.

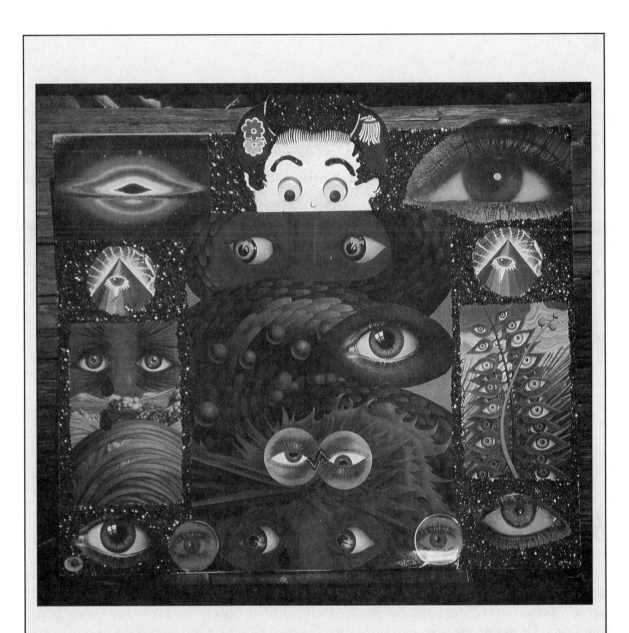

Persistence of imagery, the eye is the canvas of the universe.
Each perceives the same seen/scene differently.

Collage by Bethany ArgIsle

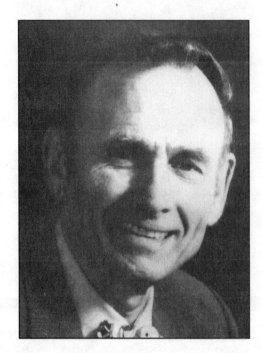

Norman Shealy, M.D., Ph.D.

*D*r. **Norman Shealy is Founder and Director of The Shealy Institute** of Springfield, Missouri, noted for its pioneering use of holistic treatment modalities for chronic pain, depression, and stress-related disorders. Dr. Shealy developed a number of techniques now commonly used in pain and stress management, including *Transcutaneous Electrical Nerve Stimulation (TENS)* and *Biogenics,* an integrated system for reprogramming body functions. He is currently researching the effects of *Ocular Light Stimulation* on neuro-chemical responses in the brain. Dr. Shealy received his medical training at Duke University. He is a co-founder of the American Holistic Medical Association and **President of The HOLOS Institute of Health,** a non-profit clinical, research and educational organization. He is the author of several popular books. His most recent published books include *The Self-Healing Workbook* (Element, 1993), *Aids: Passageway to Transformation* (Stillpoint Press, 1988), *The Pain Game* (Celestial Arts, 1975), *Ninety Days to Self Health* (Ariel Press, 1988), *Third Party Rape* (Galde Press, 1993) and *The Creation of Health* (Stillpoint Press, 1993) with Caroline Myss, and has written over one hundred articles that have appeared in professional journals. His most recent book is *Miracles Do Happen* (Stillpoint Press, 1995).

CHAPTER SEVEN

The Reality of EEG and Neurochemical Responses to Photostimulation – Part I

Norman Shealy, M.D., Ph.D.

*I*t's always a pleasure to speak to people who already agree with what you're going to say. Every once in awhile you get invited to go to a medical school, and everybody just sits there and stares at you in cold silence. I had that opportunity a year and a half ago, and it happens to have been a place which specializes in the management of RSD, reflex sympathetic dystrophy. And it just so happens that one of the men who failed to get well at our place went there. I had a letter from his mother this week, and it was the most disastrous experience of his life to go to this place in Philadelphia, and eventually she believes that he got well, because he finally worked through some of the things that we had taught him. If there's anything that I can most agree with, and I certainly have no disagreement at all with Jacob Liberman, it is that ultimately attitude is the only thing there is. **Attitude is the basic cause, and I believe at this moment in time, the ultimate primary cause of most disease.**

The Shealy Institute is located in Springfield, Missouri. We have six circular pods connected together. It was designed with attention to light and energy as a concept of how a building should be, so that the floors are all either marble or there's crushed quartz crystal under the carpet. And everywhere that there's plaster, there's crushed quartz crystal mixed in the plaster. The building contractor who was hired to build the clinic told me: "Norm, I want you to know that good energy is going into this building," and I knew we had the right elements going into the building.

Jacob Liberman earlier referred to the concept of light coming off of people and artists' rendition of this light. The picture on the cover of a book called *Sacred Mirrors: The Visionary Art of Alex Grey* (Rochester, VT: Inner Traditions International, LTD: 1990) is, I think, one of the more beautiful examples of this work showing the human *aura*. This shows, of course, where it comes from to some extent, and this is the physical manifestation which allows some of the light to be reflected. We have all of these wonderful organ systems inside, and we have both the arterial and venous systems in which we're carrying around electrons and ions and magnetic substances, and we have the nervous system, which he pictured in yellow. This particular picture doesn't show the bones; the bones are actually one of the more interesting electromagnetic generators, because bone is one of the few substances that has something called a *piezo-electric effect*. When you tap on a bone or vibrate a bone, such as with speaking — if you speak in a proper way so that you're not projecting your voice out the top, but are projecting it throughout your body, you actually can feel the vibration all the way down to the tips of your toes and up to the top of your head. And that vibration is translated into an electrical current. If you touch a piece of piezo-electric material with just a tap, it emits an electrical current. Just by speaking you are vibrating your entire skeletal system and adding to the electromagnetic emanations from your body. **There's not only the light around the body, but the thought forms and the myriad connections in the *subtle bodies*.**

Now we get into what people who see optimally see when they look at you. I've always seen energy around people, I just thought that was the way they were. I didn't realize until I was about forty years old that other people didn't see that. That was ninety years ago! Although I've always seen this energy around people, I don't see the *chakras*. I'd love to be able to see those as well. I'm sure they're there because I can feel them, I can sense them, but I don't see the colors of these *individual energy centers of the body*, the chakras, as some people do.

Different folks have different amounts of energy. When a person walks in the room, I can tell you whether they're schizophrenic in an instant; schizophrenics and psychotics have a "tornado" type of energy going on around them, usually on the right side of the body. I will come back to that idea again. Another picture, also by **Alex Grey,** shows the *halo* or energetic pattern around the head. Some people have an energy field that goes out quite far, but not very many; and some people have practically no energy field at all, because they're very depressed. I mean we are the most marvelous creation known on the face of the earth! And when two people get together the energy obviously merges, and sometimes leads to the creation of a new entity.

One of the ways my wife and I support our life energy is by how and where we live. My wife and I have chosen to live in a gorgeous spot in nature for the last twenty-five years, called Brindabella Farms. We believe that this is the nicest way to surround ourselves. We raise Appaloosa horses and try to get out of the "rat race" as much of the time as we can.

For the last twenty-two years I have dealt almost exclusively with chronic pain sufferers, and I soon recognized that what I was actually dealing with was chronic stress. I believe that, basically, all of us who are in the so-called "health professions"— which really are the "disease professions"— are dealing with one illness. **There's only one major illness, and it's called depression.** Sometimes people are angry, and anger is actually good for you, if it doesn't get carried on for too long a period of time, because it's a great antidote for depression. People who go through life with a mixture of anger and depression actually don't do badly. They only die seven years earlier than people who seem to be reasonably well-adjusted, according to Hans Eysenck's research work.

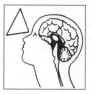

Hans Eysenck is a psychiatrist at Denmark Hill Hospital in London, who with Dr. Grossarth-Matticek in Heidelburg, followed over thirteen thousand individuals for almost twenty years. What they found is that there were:

The Four Basic Types of People

1. Those who are **depressed** all of their lives die on an average of three-to-five years earlier, mostly from cancer.

2. Those who abide with **both anger and depression** — these people usually can't make up their minds whether they're more angry or more depressed and they actually only die seven years earlier, rather than three-to-five years earlier, as the solely depressed people do. So if you've got to be depressed, at least get a lot of anger in there too!

3. Those who are **self-actualized** — these people believe that happiness is an "inside job," not an "outside job."

4. Those people who carry a lot of **anger and blame** all of their lives are the ones who die of heart disease.

Actually there is only one basic emotional problem, and that is fear, that's all there is. There's fear and there's joy, the two primary emotions. There are a very limited number of reactions to fear. **The natural reaction to fear is to be angry; that is normal and healthy and it should lead to action. If it doesn't lead to action, it will lead to depression.** Sometimes it leads to guilt, because people then blame themselves. And occasionally, not infrequently, people don't want to admit fear, so they call it anxiety. That's all there is. **Every other emotional reaction is a synonym of fear.** *Anxiety, guilt, anger, or depression* are also reactions to fear, resulting primarily from either this feeling of abandonment or of abuse or of being wronged. **Pain is then created when we want things to be other than as they are or when we are not accepting of what is perceived as reality.** That pain, which is primarily psychological pain, can also become physical pain, because physical pain can be aggravated by the muscular tension created when one wants something that they feel cannot be changed.

The goal of our work with individuals is to teach them to live the transcendent will, the *will of the soul*, that is, detachment from all that you cannot or choose not to change and have no need to know why. It's non-judgmentalism, being at peace and having a desire to do good to others, which is the only definition of love that fits every situation.

Everything perceived as lacking, which is desire, has nothing to do with love. Now, if one could live from this transcendent will 100% of the time and could do this from early on in life, my suspicion is that there would be almost no illness, and we'd get kind of bored with the world, because everybody would live forever. **The causes of disease occur when we move away from this principle and we know that we are not living our life in harmony with our own basic inner rightness.**

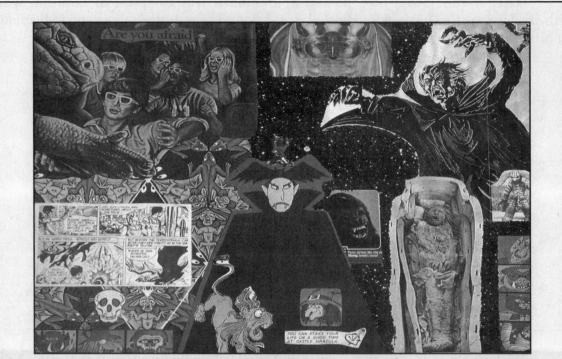

Fear . . . Can You Hold It Near?
Collage by Bethany ArgIsle

Shealy's Five Basic Fears

1. **The Fear of Death.** For some peculiar reason most people, even though they say that they believe in life-after-death and the continuity of the soul, still seem to fear the dying process. Although, as we know, many of those who have gone through it and have sort of "come back at the last moment," often wished they hadn't come back, because they say it's really nice over there! So those of us who really believe in the continuity of the soul should have no reason to fear death.

2. **The Fear of Illness or of being an invalid.** A lot of people fear this, some of them enough to actually make themselves ill.

3. **The Fear of Abandonment.** Abandonment is something that everyone has experienced, probably from the moment of birth. Maybe you were picked up roughly or were beaten on the behind or the chest and then taken away from your mother. Abandonment happens throughout childhood and sometimes people don't get over that; they actually go through life feeling constantly threatened with abandonment. It's a deep fear in the lives of many people.

4. **The Fear of Poverty.** This fear is actually insecurity, it's a feeling of being unable to be sufficient unto oneself and not be supported financially or socially.

5. **The Fear of Abuse** or of being morally or ethically wronged. I would also put it in the same general category as the existential fear that there is no meaning or purpose in life.

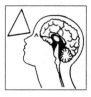

Ten years ago I began to look at a lot of the neurochemical changes in patients. We've looked at all kinds of ratios of these five different neurotransmitters, but it appeared to us that **there are four ratios that may be more important than the actual individual transmitter values themselves, and all of these neurotransmitters are totally interrelated.** First, the ratio of sympathetic to parasympathetic activity as seen in the **ratio of norepinephrine to acetylcholine** is important. We believe the maximum range of acetylcholine one could say is normal would be from 9 to 35 micrograms. The **ratio between norepinephrine and melatonin** is also very important. Melatonin does significantly affect almost all of the other neurochemicals. The **serotonin to beta endorphin ratio** seems to be very important as well. **The serotonin to melatonin ratio** is also important. Again, that would almost have to be true, since these two neurotransmitters are so interrelated in their basic biochemistry.

The Five Most Important Neurotransmitters

1. **Melatonin** is one of the more crucial neurochemicals of the brain. There is an estimated normal range of melatonin in micrograms in the blood. In ten people who were totally normal, by all the standards that we have, we found that some of them had a little higher than average melatonin levels in the morning. This is the early-morning level in the blood, not the late-night level.

2. **Norepinephrine** is basically adrenaline, the primary chemical of stress. Eighty percent of the norepinephrine that runs around in your bloodstream comes from the sympathetic nervous system. To make norepinephrine you've got to have amino acids **tyrosine** and **phenylalanine**.

3. **Beta endorphin** is a natural narcotic and, although the lab we were using said the upper limit was 8 micrograms, I actually believe that the upper limit of normal is probably more likely 10 micrograms; the lower limit of normal is 4 micrograms.

4. **Serotonin** is actually a precursor of melatonin; you can't make melatonin unless you can make serotonin. So if you're deficient in one, you have to be deficient in the other; and you can't make melatonin unless you have an essential amino acid called **tryptophan**, which the FDA recently has forbidden from being on the market. To make serotonin you also have to have vitamin B-6 and lithium. So it becomes more obvious that you've got to have certain basic building blocks to make every one of these.

5. **Acetylcholine** is the transmitter of the parasympathetic nervous system, the opposite of the sympathetic nervous system; and **cholinesterase** is the enzyme that breaks it down.

For a number of years we played primarily with these neurochemicals in looking at people with depression, and what we found is **of all the depressed clients we've tested, 92% were deficient or excessive in one to seven of these neurochemicals. Actually, the average depressed person had about three abnormalities. In fact, 67% of the depressed patients had three to seven abnormalities in just this small profile.** Remember, this is just a tiny piece of a phenomenally complex neurochemical system. So we got interested in treatments that would help bring these neurotransmitters back to normal.

Again, I believe depression is really the only illness there is. When we began looking at other things, like magnesium, we found that **roughly 60% of our patients with depression have a white blood cell magnesium that is well below the lower limit of normal.** But 100% of them have a deficiency which shows up on a test that is probably even more sensitive, called a *magnesium load test*. **Whether or not you can see, whether or not you can function, whether or not you have panic, whether or not you have depression, whether or not you have high blood pressure, or any of a whole bunch of other things, is dependent upon magnesium. Magnesium is one of the most critical chemical regulators of the body.** It is present in much smaller quantities in the tissues than is calcium; but when you don't have the right ratio between calcium and magnesium, you have some real problems. It's the complex of magnesium and calcium together that create the *piezo-electric effect*. The word *magnesium*, in fact, means *magnetic;* and it is a regulator of membrane potential at all cellular levels, including, of course, the nervous system and the muscle tissue. **One-hundred percent of the depressed people who were seen at our clinic were really deficient in magnesium, because they have the cellular need to take up more than a normal person would take up.** At this simple level of the white blood cell system, which is part of the immune function, roughly 60% of them were deficient.

We've now extended this, we're now finding that **well over 90% of depressed people are also deficient in one or more of the essential amino acids. And 86% of them are actually deficient in taurine.**

QUESTION: Are you measuring magnesium intracellularly?

DR. SHEALY: Well, white blood cell is an intracellular measurement. Whole blood, red blood cell and serum tests are useless, as far as I'm concerned. Those tests are a waste of money and time, and they give you a false sense of security, and we've done enough comparisons to find out. We've experimented with all of it, and the only one that is accurate is the *magnesium load test*.

There are many causes for magnesium deficiency. I can't look at light as the only thing there is, even though we know that's what it "all" is. These are manifestations of light, and **I believe that everything ultimately is a manifestation of light**. And if you want to get into understanding that, read the wonderful book written forty-plus years ago, *The Secret of Light* (University Science and Philosophy, 1947) by **Walter Russell**. This book really says that **light is the secret of the universe.**

There have been three major papers done in the last twelve years which demonstrate that if you have a *heart attack* and they give you a shot of magnesium, your chances of surviving are 70% greater than if you don't get a shot of magnesium. Is it routinely done? No. Carry your magnesium ampules with you. If you ever have a heart attack, you will need them.

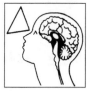
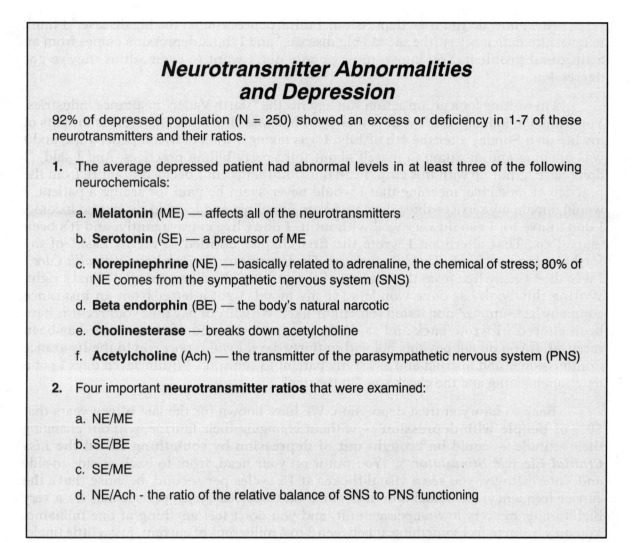

Neurotransmitter Abnormalities and Depression

92% of depressed population (N = 250) showed an excess or deficiency in 1-7 of these neurotransmitters and their ratios.

1. The average depressed patient had abnormal levels in at least three of the following neurochemicals:

    a. **Melatonin** (ME) — affects all of the neurotransmitters

    b. **Serotonin** (SE) — a precursor of ME

    c. **Norepinephrine** (NE) — basically related to adrenaline, the chemical of stress; 80% of NE comes from the sympathetic nervous system (SNS)

    d. **Beta endorphin** (BE) — the body's natural narcotic

    e. **Cholinesterase** — breaks down acetylcholine

    f. **Acetylcholine** (Ach) — the transmitter of the parasympathetic nervous system (PNS)

2. Four important **neurotransmitter ratios** that were examined:

    a. NE/ME

    b. SE/BE

    c. SE/ME

    d. NE/Ach - the ratio of the relative balance of SNS to PNS functioning

So we've got two major illnesses: we've got depression and we've got magnesium deficiency. There are other factors, I'm not saying that these two are all there are. They are just big ones. Can you overdose on magnesium? No, but you can, however, actually over do it to the point that it will make you more deficient. Since magnesium is a natural laxative, if you take too much, you may speed up the transit time through the gut, so you actually will absorb less. It's a very delicate thing; and if you're totally magnesium deficient, that is, if you've got over a 50% retention of a magnesium load, which is equivalent to 60 milligrams per kilogram of given body weight, you probably need about ten shots of it to get your body built up quickly. Then you can take magnesium orotate in order to avoid some of the gut problems and other things.

The foods that have the highest amounts of magnesium are: carrots, beets, sesame seeds, and peanuts. However, you would have to eat seventeen tablespoons of peanut butter a day to get the recommended daily amount of magnesium. All the soils in the world are known to be deficient in magnesium, except those in Egypt; so a lot of our foods are very, very deficient.

Now, how do you treat depression? I think depression is "the big disease." I think magnesium deficiency is "the second big disease," and I think depression comes from an attitudinal problem. You know, most people don't want to even admit they've got depression.

I'm waiting for a group action suit against the "Darth Vadar" insurance industries. You think I'm kidding, don't you? A year ago I had one of the most marvelous insights of my life on a Sunday after the 4th of July. I was taking a walk between paperwork, and I was bitching and moaning to myself about third-party billing practices. And I said, "I don't have to put up with this crap! I can quit." At that point I decided to retire from the practice of medicine, meaning that I would never again be paid for seeing a patient. I would donate my services three days a week to our clinic and I would receive no income. I don't have to; I can do very well without it. I don't live extravagantly, and it's been marvelous. That afternoon I wrote the first chapter entitled, "Free At Last," of my forthcoming new book, *Third Party Rape: The Conspiracy To Rob You Of Health Care*.[1] I was then finally free from the tyranny of the current "third-party mafia!" That's right. Writing this book has done wonders for my mood. I got a letter from an insurance company last summer, and it said something like, "We will not pay this; your records have been altered." I wrote back and said, "Your obnoxious and libelous letter has been received. If you do not pay this bill within thirty days, I will report you to the Insurance Commissioner and instruct and assist my patient to sue you." Within seven days I got a letter apologizing and the check was "in the mail."

Back to how you treat depression. We have known for the last fifteen years that **50% of people with depression** — without changing their taurine, without changing their attitude — **could be brought out of depression by something called the *Liss Cranial Electric Stimulator*** ™.[2] You put it on your head, front-to-back or side-to-side and, interestingly, you see a visual flicker at 15 cycles per second, because that's the carrier frequency; the actual output is going up to 20,000 cycles per second. It's a very high-frequency, very low-amperage unit, and you don't feel anything at one milliamp. You may begin to feel something at between 3 to 4 milliamps of current, just a little tingle, but **it stimulates beta endorphin, melatonin, and serotonin production.** This is very interesting, because it raises both melatonin and serotonin at the same time, as well as beta endorphin, and quite strikingly! **If you use this device every day for two weeks, about 50% of the people will come out of their depression**. And, of course, over a period of a month or two or three afterwards they go back into depression, because all that has been done has been temporary. It's been done electrically and/or through light stimulation; I'm not quite sure which factors are relevant, but it has only temporarily changed their neurochemistry.

---

1. Available from Galde Press Inc., St. Paul, Minnesota: 1993, or Self-Health Systems, Fair Grove, Missouri: (417) 267-2900.
2. For product description and ordering information on the Liss Cranial Electric Stimulator, See *Resource List: Section 8, page 377, Other Instruments Mentioned in this Book.*

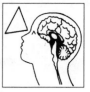

The Causes of Magnesium Deficiency

1. **Inadequate Intake**

2. **Poor Absorption**

3. **Diarrhea**

4. **Renal Wasting.** There are people who just excrete excess magnesium and excess vitamin D. You know, there is a lot of vitamin D in almost everything in our food markets, and there are a lot of multivitamins that have a 1,000 units of D, which is not good for you.

5. **Malabsorption.** If you get your magnesium at the same time that you eat a high protein diet, you don't absorb the magnesium. Today, milk and excess calcium are in cereals with too high a protein level.

6. **Negative Lifestyle Risk Factors.** Other factors that interfere with magnesium absorption are:

    a.   **High Fat Meals**

    b.   **Soda Pop** in our diets. Phosphate of soda interferes with both magnesium and calcium absorption

    c.   **Sugars**

    d.   **Margarine**

    e.   **Alcohol**

    f.   **Smoking**

    g.   **Diuretics**

7. **Stress.** When you are stressed and raise your norepinephrine level, you eat away your magnesium, you lose it; and it's just one of those unfortunate reactions to stress.

8. **Caffeine Abuse and a Sedentary lifestyle** also make you excrete magnesium.

    I really believe that, **second to depression, the most common problem that we have is magnesium deficiency**. For example, 80% of people with high blood pressure can be markedly improved by just giving them magnesium.

Major Diseases Associated with Magnesium Deficiencies

- **Arteriosclerosis**
- **Kidney Stones**
- **Heart Attacks**
- **Eclampsia**
- **Osteoarthritis**
- **Osteoporosis**
- **Cardiac Arrhythmias**
- **Parathyroid Dysfunction (both high and low)**
- **Depression**
- **Miscarriage**
- **Epilepsy**
- **Pain**

Less Serious Diseases Associated with Magnesium Deficiency

- **Premenstrual Syndrome (PMS),** which can often be controlled by taking adequate magnesium with vitamin B-6.

- **Low Birth Weight**

- **Carpal Tunnel Syndrome** (The vast majority of people with carpal tunnel syndrome can be cured within a month by taking huge doses of vitamin B-6 and magnesium, but you must not stay on the vitamin B-6 very long).

- **Hypothyroidism** (especially in infants).

- **Low Apgar Score** (a series of signs of an infant that is weak, sickly, and neurologically damaged at birth).

- **Allergies**

- **All Immune System Dysfunctions**

In other words, **most illness is related to Magnesium Deficiency**.

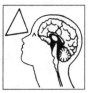

Nutritional and Brainwave Abnormalities and Depression/Review

I. Magnesium Abnormalities and Depression

A. 100% of Shealy's depressed patient sample was deficient in magnesium (Mg load test).

    1. Mg is the most critical chemical regulator in the body.

    2. Mg must be in proper balance with calcium (Ca).

    3. Mg means "magnetic" and gives bone its piezo-electric properties.

B. Dr. Shealy sees Mg deficiency as the second major disease (stress wastes away our Mg supplies.)

C. Mg levels have been implicated in: High Blood Pressure, Arteriosclerosis, Kidney Stones, Heart Attack, Eclampsia, Osteoarthritis, Cardiac Arrhythmia, Parathyroid Dysfunction, Panic Attacks, Depression, Miscarriage, PMS, Low Birth Weight, Carpal Tunnel Syndrome, Hypothyroidism, Allergies, Immune Dysfunction, Epilepsy, Pain (especially myofascial pain).

D. Food sources of Mg: (in addition to intravenous or dietary supplementation) carrots, beets, sesame seeds, peanuts.

    1. All the world's soils are now Mg deficient[1], except Egypt.

II. Amino Acids Abnormalities and Depression

A. 90% of Shealy's depressed sample were deficient in one or more amino acids.

B. 86% were deficient in the amino acid named taurine.

---

1. Read current USA Vice President Al Gore's book *Earth in the Balance, Ecology and the Human Spirit,* (New York: Houghton-Mufflin Co., 1992) for more information about soil and changing weather conditions worldwide.

The Shealy Relax Mate ™ is also something we've used a lot. It is a set of portable goggles with a flashing light instrument — the evolution of fifteen years of work. It's so small you can wear it and, by the way, it's wonderful for *jet lag*. I use it routinely when I travel internationally. The flicker rate goes from 3.1 to 12 cycles per second, which is all within the relaxation and safety range. **This, too, significantly alters neurochemistry.** It helps people sleep if they use it properly. So it's an adjunct we use, but this alone won't be enough for lasting improvement, either.[3]

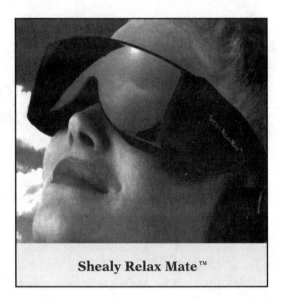

Shealy Relax Mate™

We've used ***music*** now as part of our regimen for the last four years, as well. We not only use music through the ears, but we use it through the bones. We have four different ***Vibrating Music Beds*** at the clinic, and patients are encouraged — coerced sometimes, because they often don't like it at first, as it often brings up repressed emotions.

Patients are instructed in ***autogenic training, biofeedback***, and ***self-regulation skills***, and there's an ***educational component***, as well. Patient education includes all the information about fear and the transcendent will, the chakras, interpersonal relationships, the critical balancing technique and ways of getting rid of your "unfinished business." It's interesting. We've worked with these techniques over the last four years, and **we get more than 70% of patients to *stay out* of depression. In the last two years we have used the Lumatron**™ **as an adjunct, in addition to the Relax Mate**™.

We may soon get to a place where we can get almost everybody out of depression. **We've worked with about 450 chronically depressed people.** In our experimental work they had not previously responded to drugs or psychotherapy. These are "the worst of the worst" of the depressed, the ones who have tried up to seven or more different antidepressants, none of which worked. What we found is that at the end of forty hours of education over 90% of them are out of depression. **In a week 90% of these people *can get out of* depression.** Now I thought, "Wow!" What we've done in the past is have them come back for various things like the Lumatron™ light work, some music and maybe a Relax Mate™ at home. We've given some of them magnesium; we've also given some of them taurine. And this year we decided we would teach a group of people to do their own ***intuitive insight work*** to help them get rid of the root causes, because **ultimately it is their "unfinished business" which causes depression**. The same conflicts of personality and interpersonal relationship that **Jacob Liberman** was talking about earlier are the same basic causes here. So, teach people how to be intuitive, and that can be done. We actually taught these people how to be intuitive, and then we encouraged them to come back to use techniques for enhancing intuition, such as music.

---

3. For ordering information on the Shealy Relax Mate™, See *Resource List: Section Eight, page 377, Other Phototherapy Instruments Mentioned in this Book.*

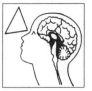
We also put them in front of a **copper wall. Dr. Elmer Green,** at the **Menninger Foundation in Topeka, Kansas has worked with a copper wall for the last eight years to enhance lucidity in normal, non-sick people.** Thus, we decided that we would add the use of the copper walls, an isolated, non-grounded (it's separated from the ground) wall of shiny copper. The person sits on a non-grounded chair, so there's no possibility of electrical connection. And they just sit with a magnetic field over their head, 250 milligaus, and look at the copper wall. Now if you hook up an electrocardiogram to a copper wall ten feet away, you can pick up that person's EKG. If they move a finger, and you have a strain gauge attached to your copper wall, you can pick up the movement. What do you think is happening to me with one hundred people's

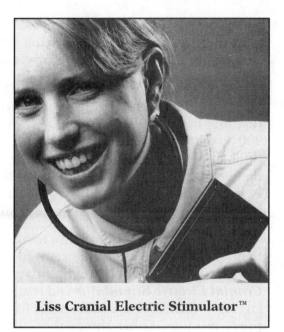

Liss Cranial Electric Stimulator™

EKGs projected up here at the podium? This is what's happening to all of us every day. **What happens when you sit in front of the copper wall with a magnet over your head is that it seems to enhance the release of those things to which you are psychomagnetically attracted — mainly, all of your "crap," your "unfinished business," to give it a nice, scientific term.** What we found was that in the past four years before this treatment only 4 to 5% of patients would drop out of this kind of program; with the wall 22% dropped out. They couldn't take the forced de-magnetization of their "unfinished business." Even though they'd come out and say, "That gives me nightmares,". . . I'd say "That's wonderful, what an opportunity!" So, 22% would not do it. Every year we wind up with about 70 to 72% who will persevere with this treatment. No matter what we do, we can't seem to get that last 30% out of depression and that's okay. I mean I'm comfortable with what we've done, considering that the people we started with were intractable already; that's the best we have been able to do with these most severely depressed people. By this time next year we'll have a package of these techniques, a protocol that any therapist can take and use.[4]

In the next research study we're starting we're going to divide our people into two groups. They're all going to get the same treatment, except that the **educational component** is going to be done live to half of them, and by videotape of the material to the other half. My prediction is that the videotape education will be more effective than the live education. It's a sad commentary on our system, but I believe the people have been so brainwashed that they believe more easily what they see on the tube than what they hear coming out of my mouth. You know, I could give the same lecture on video — I've done it many times and I have videos of some of my lectures — and the patients, no question, believe it more when they see me on the video! Results: Longterm, 80% of the video patients and only 68% of the live lecture patients do well.

---

4. Dr. Shealy's research on the non-pharmaceutical treatment of depression appears in the journal: *Subtle Energies*, Vol. 4:(2), 1993.

So, by the end of next year, I believe we will be able to say this specific combination of treatments is what will work for depression. It includes a combination of both types of light therapy, the Lumatron™ and the Relax Mate™.

With the *Liss Cranial Electric Stimulator,* for instance, **there is an increase in serotonin, beta endorphin, and a little bit of norepinephrine in the bloodstream** *(nothing in the cerebral spinal fluid),* **and melatonin.** Some people will go up 100% to 200%, this actually happens! We have done these transmitter levels on cerebral spinal fluid, and you get about twice as great a beta endorphin response in spinal fluid as you do in blood, and you get a slightly greater serotonin response. You get no norepinephrine in the cerebral spinal fluid. With melatonin you actually get a stronger response in the blood than you do in the cerebral spinal fluid.

About three years ago we thought that beta endorphins were the key. We thought they might be the most important of these chemicals, so we looked at **those things in normal people which might raise beta endorphins** 50% or so. We used the *Liss Cranial Electric Stimulator* and that worked. *The Relax Mate™* worked and so did *slow jogging* — just twelve minute miles for thirty minutes, basically two-and-a-half miles for thirty minutes. Other things that raised endorphin levels were *receiving a total body massage, but not giving one.* This I found quite disappointing, because I thought you ought to get something back out of giving. *Music, guided imagery, laughter* — just doing artificial laughter for five minutes will double your beta endorphin level. We've done it.

What we found did *not* raise beta endorphin levels were: *giving a massage, yoga* for thirty minutes, and *masturbation.* I was quite disappointed in that too. I thought, "My God, it's not worth it if it doesn't raise your beta endorphins!" We got four couples to volunteer to let me come out to their home and draw blood, and I would go away for forty-five minutes, and they would have sex in one of three ways for thirty minutes. Then I would come back and draw the blood again. And they would go have sexual intercourse, or masturbate in separate rooms, or masturbate one another. Then they had to grade what they had experienced on a scale of 0 to 10 how much fun it was and whether it was a stressful experience or not. What we found was, as my secretary — this very lovely, meek person — said in big headlines, "Attitude is more important than sex." We found that masturbation can actually raise beta endorphins among other things, but it depends upon whether you're feeling okay about it or stressed about it when you do it. This was the first time we'd done it at the clinic — in private treatment rooms for God's sake — not out in the lobby!

We also found that with photostimulation — although it didn't raise the beta endorphins as much as some of the other things did — oxytocin, the nurturing hormone, was raised as much by the Lumatron's™ red light as it was by having sex! Now we've got a lot of volunteers lined up wanting to try sex with the photostimulation, and we haven't done that experiment yet!

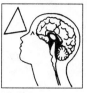

Shealy Center's Depression Treatment Program/Review

I. Results after 20 hours/week for 2 weeks

A. Of 450 chronically depressed people who were previously unresponsive to anti-depressant medication and/or psychotherapy, 72% showed no signs of depression neurochemically or behaviorally at 6 month follow-up.

II. Program Components

A. Education — 40 hours, including information on the transcendent will, the chakras, interpersonal relationships, critical balancing technique, ways of letting go of unfinished emotional business, and intuition development.

B. The Liss Cranial Electric Stimulator™ — 20 minutes daily

    1. Shealy's data indicate a 100-200% increase in levels of BE, ME, NE and SE.

    2. With this treatment alone 50% of his severely depressed sample will remit within 2 weeks time.

C. Light Therapy

    1. **Lumatron**™ increases:
       a) neurotransmitters and neurohormones, such as beta endorphin and oxytocin (the relaxation and nuturing hormone);
       b) EEG symmetry.

    2. **Shealy Relax Mate**™ (portable light goggles) alters neurochemistry, decreases insomnia and jet lag symptoms.

D. Nutritional Intervention — intravenous or oral Mg., amino acids, B-6, etc.

E. Vibratory Music Bed — to increase bone oscillation and emotional catharsis.

F. Self-Regulation and Relaxation Skills Training, Biofeedback, Autogenic Training

G. Copper Wall — self-therapy to facilitate emotional release of repressed unconscious conflicts.

H. Aerobic Exercise — 30 minutes a day; i.e., slow jogging, walking

I. Yoga — 30 minutes a day

J. Massage Therapy

K. Artificial Laughter Therapy — 5 minutes a day

L. Guided Imagery

M. Homework Exercises — journal writing to let go of unresolved conflicts and to gain additional insights

The *Relax Mate™* also has some nice effects. We've also looked at computerized electroencephalograms; and, believe it or not, these *brain maps* actually come from those squiggly little lines, and the computer does all these wonderful things. This is an example of a depressed individual at rest with the eyes closed. Instead of having a nice symmetrical brainwave pattern, he has a right frontal-temporal lobe dominance. It's like there's a broken record going on here on the right side of the brain. It doesn't have to be a frontal-lobe asymmetry, by the way. We could just tell you that **100% of people who are depressed have asymmetry of electroencephalograms**. Sometimes it's back here; sometimes it's over here. Sometimes they have a black spot over here. The left hemisphere is indicating that nothing is happening here in the logical part of the brain. Depressed patients always have EEG asymmetry *(see Brain Maps on following page)*.

We've never seen a depressed person who follows photostimulation appropriately. Now, since the beginning of electroencephalography, we have known that if you flash lights into the eyes of a normal individual three to ten cycles, or at thirty cycles per second, the brain will pick that up in two out of three normal people. One in three so-called normal people actually will have little response, but they never produce the wrong rate. That is, if I shine light into a normal individual they either increase their ten cycle activity — if there are ten cycles being put in — or they don't do anything. With depressed individuals not only do they not follow appropriately (entrain), but many of them follow totally inappropriately. You put in ten cycles and they may produce more than thirty cycles. Or you put in three cycles and they may produce more than twelve; or you put in twelve cycles and they may produce three. It's very erratic and very individualistic.

Two Common Electroencephalographic Abnormalities in the Brains of People with Depression

1. **Asymmetry** — usually right-sided hemispheric dominance, which can be in any frequency from beta to alpha or theta, and are often more in delta and other slow wave activity than you'd like to see.

2. **Inappropriate following of light frequency.**

After they have been exposed to a minimum of five treatments, and preferably ten or more with the Lumatron™ (we chose the color of light according to the test that John Downing devised for it), most of them develop symmetry, but not necessarily the ability to follow frequency. The first thing to improve is symmetry, and then we try to improve the frequency following.

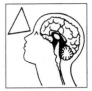

Brain Maps

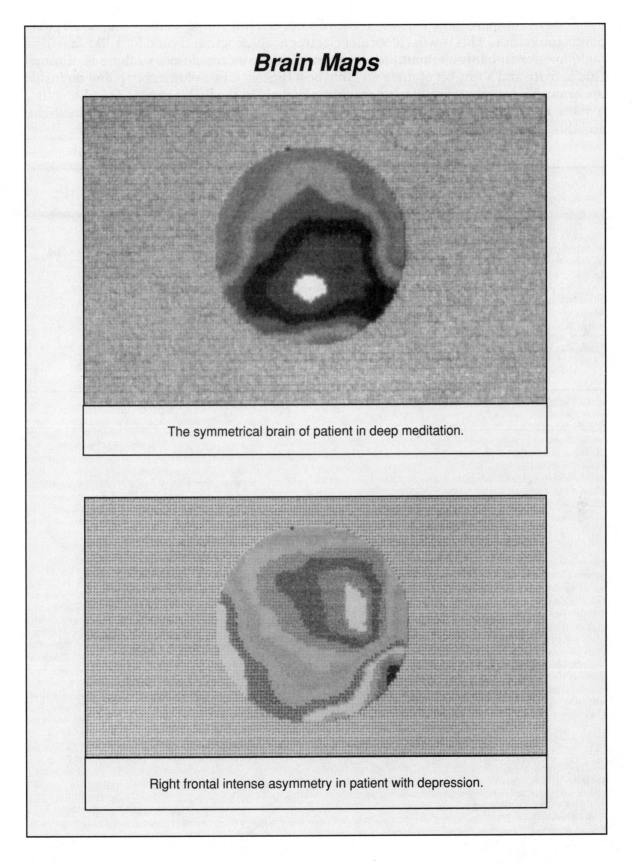

The symmetrical brain of patient in deep meditation.

Right frontal intense asymmetry in patient with depression.

Let's compare these EEGs to those of a normal individual, namely me, undergoing photostimulation. This is what a normal electroencephalogram should look like at rest — high, intense alpha throughout the entire brain. My eyes are closed, so there is minimal beta activity and a tiny bit of theta and maybe a flicker or two of imagery going on inside the brain. This is what should happen when a normal individual is exposed to photostimulation. For example, when 3.1 cycles per second are put into my eyes, I follow the light, and this produces theta.

EEG Abnormalities and Depression

A. Depressed patients exhibit frequent **right hemisphere asymmetry,** a sign of obsessive negative thinking. They also often exhibit:

1. **Decreased left hemisphere activity,** a sign of decreased logical thinking

2. **A preponderance of slow-wave activity,** a sign of withdrawn behavior or reduced external focus, and a tendency to respond to inner stimulation

B. Depressed EEGs do not follow photostimulation.

Progress is directly proportional to controversy.

— Dr. Carl Moyer

All change is heresy.

— Dr. Linus Pauling

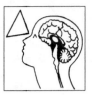

Dr. Norman Shealy's Conceptualizations of Illness and Healing/Review

- The primary cause of disease is attitude.

- There is only one major illness, and that is depression.

- Most people die of depression.

- Magnesium deficiency, also related to depression, is the second major illness.

- All of life's conflicts start at the level of the first, or root, chakra and are **issues related to fear** — sense of safety and security in one's family, how one relates interpersonally, giving and receiving love, etc.

- There are only two primary emotions: fear and joy.

- Fear is the only basic emotional problem (anger, guilt, depression, anxiety and all other negative emotional reactions are synonymous or reactions out of fear).

- Goal of The Shealy Institute's 40-hour In-patient Attitude Education Program

    Learn about the transcendent will, the will of the soul

    Detach from issues that patients cannot or choose not to change

    Develop:

    a. an ability to attune to their transcendent will

    b. an attitude of non-judgment about self and others and about life

    c. an increased sense of peace by accepting more of what is and releasing one's perceived lacks and desires

    d. one's will and intention to do good to others, to love

    e. an expanded sense of self-love

- Physical or psychological pain often stems from chronic stress and wanting things other than how they are, not accepting perceived reality.

- Healing is ultimately triggered when the individual personality allows the light of the soul fully into being.

- Insight is the light of the future.

Dr. Shealy's Hologram of Healing

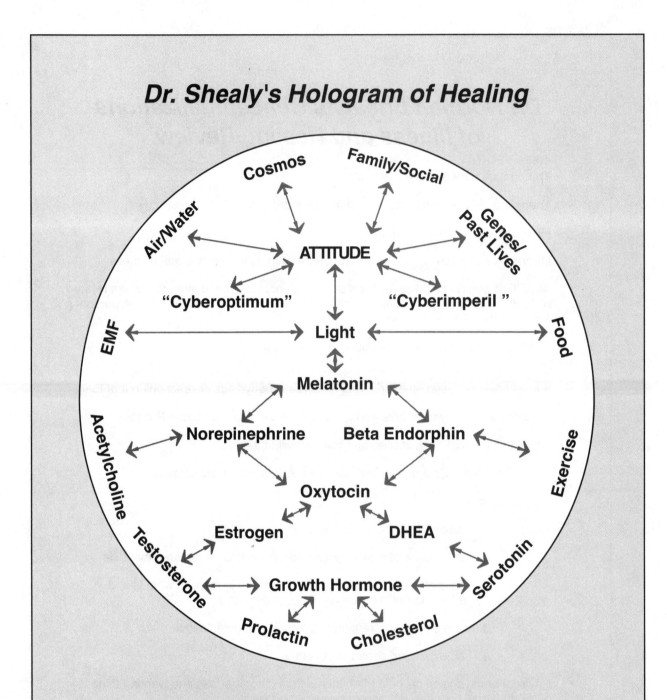

The Hologram of Healing is just a small piece of the phenomenally complex, interactive universe. This is why there are so many therapeutic approaches that all seem to work. You know somebody says, "Well, if I manipulate this, it works." And then somebody else says, "Well, if I do this, it works." And somebody else says, "If I touch them, it works." All you have to do is push the system back toward a state of balance. **For every individual, right down to identical twins, there is a unique pattern of health and a unique pattern of ailments.** Although twins, chemically, seem to be about 65 to 75% identical, even with the same diets and everything else, they do have significant differences. So, I believe everybody is ultimately an individual, and what might be optimal for her might be capable of creating illness in him, or vice-versa. Thus, it's important that we not get too carried away and assume that there is only one way, only one "road to Rome" and to good health.

CHAPTER EIGHT

The Reality of EEG and Neurochemical Responses to Photostimulation – Part II

Norman Shealy, M.D., Ph.D.

As we continue here, I'm just finishing my "basic philosophy of the cosmos" in ten words or less! This is it; this is all you need to know about everything in life . . . everything your mother ever wanted to tell you that you didn't learn. This, **The Hologram of Healing,** is how I understand things. There is no such thing as, "This is the cause and this is the treatment." Everything is influenced by everything else. So basically, if you have too much or too little of anything, you can be in trouble. As I sense it, **the single most important influence, the basis of life is *attitude*,** which is created to a large extent by your *family*, your *social connections*, your *genes*, and your *past lives*. And if you don't happen to believe in past lives, that's your problem, not mine! Ninety-percent of people — even those who don't believe — can, in guided imagery, have spontaneous scenes that appear to be past life experiences, which are often powerful psychotherapeutic tools. *OMNI* magazine (October-November, 1992) has a very nice article on "Past Life Therapy" which is worth reading. And obviously, there's the *cosmos,* your connection through your soul to God.

I have found that attitude is influenced by (and this is the only part which has not yet, to my satisfaction, been scientifically demonstrated) a hypothetical chemical which I call **cyberoptimum.** Cyber means *control*, plus *optimum;* together they mean *optimal control*. It's one of those little *polypeptides* made up of a few amino acids that somehow, when you have it optimally present in your brain, leaves you in a state of perfect lucidity. And perfect lucidity is perfect clairvoyance, *all-knowingness*, optimal intuition, and optimal well-being.

There is also an opposite to that neuropeptide; it may be some distortion of that molecule, or it may be a mirror image of that molecule, I don't know. I would call that polypeptide *cyberimperil.* Because when you've got that present, you feel sick, and you may be crazy. That's when you really become psychotic or have something that feels like the flu that isn't even a virus. I honestly believe that most of the time when you think you've got the flu, what you've got is cyberimperil. You have gotten more "junk," more electromagnetic negativity than your being can tolerate at that point.

All of these things are totally related one to the other. ***Light*, the *amount* of light, the *quality* of light, the *color* of light, or the *frequency* of light, influences everything in your brain and, consequently, everything underneath that**. Food, obviously, is important. Physical exercise and the electromagnetic energy field in which you are submerged, your air and water — all of these are the physical components that determine health. You can be killed with light if it is too intense, it can cook you, you can be killed with food or lack of food. You can be killed with exercise, and you are certainly harmed by a lack of exercise. And so it goes.

In your brain you have (I'm sure there are hundreds of other chemicals that I don't know about) neurotransmitters. Among those which are most critical are: melatonin, serotonin, beta endorphin, norepinephrine, and acetylcholine. There are interrelationships between these, and ultimately it's the ratios between them that are critical.

The next level is getting down to the hormonal system. The neurotransmitters just mentioned are what I would call neurochemicals. This next set of important biochemicals are the hormones: oxytocin, prolactin, growth hormone, estrogen, testosterone, and DHEA.

Oxytocin: When I was in medical school we thought oxytocin was something that a woman produced when she had a baby. Actually, men produce just as much oxytocin as women do (except when the woman is having a baby) and only if the men **feel nurtured**. If they don't feel nurtured, they don't have any; it's that simple.

Prolactin: I was taught in medical school that prolactin was something a woman needed in order to make milk. Yet men produce just as much prolactin as women do when they're not producing milk, yet again, only if they **feel nurtured**. Women who don't feel nurtured don't have any, either, by the way. That's one of the reasons some women don't produce any prolactin after childbirth.

Growth Hormone: We were taught that basically you didn't need growth hormone after you were 18 years of age and it was okay for it to go away. We now know that when growth hormone production stops, you age rapidly. It is thus **a major contributor to aging**. If you give a patient growth hormone, you can reverse many of the effects of human aging. Just from giving growth hormone the skin gets thicker, the subcutaneous fat increases, and the amount of muscle mass increases. Of course, I'd rather not have to take it by injection. I'd prefer to do some of the things that will stimulate it throughout life.

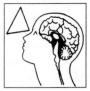

Things that Stimulate Growth Hormone

- **Being outside in natural light**
- **Adequate physical exercise**
- **Adequate sex**

I honestly believe, as did **Wilhelm Reich**,[1] that one of the great regulators, one of the great homeostatic mechanisms, is **sexual orgasm**. And if you don't enjoy it, you haven't had one, so don't bother, you know!

Testosterone and estrogen: After menopause women make more testosterone than they do estrogen — not that they don't make it throughout life. Men throughout life make more testosterone than the average woman makes after menopause. Men throughout life, have a blood level of estrogen higher than the average post-menopausal woman. Now, do you know how you make these chemicals? Out of cholesterol.

DHEA: Dehydroepiandosterone has a linear decrease throughout the lives of those people who are following the usual pattern of aging.

I can't believe that next year I'm suddenly going to stop making all of these things in the same amounts that twenty-year-olds do, but as of this year I still do. And just because I'm going to turn sixty in December, I don't think suddenly my pituitary and hypothalamus are going to atrophy. I believe the reason I'm going to continue this as I have until this point in time is mostly my ***attitude,*** my ***physical exercise,*** and my ***diet.*** **These things all are critically important in maintaining homeostasis, balance, harmony, and good health.**

I want to show you, for instance, what happens when we flash lights of different colors into the eyes of individuals. Now, we've measured not only the neurochemicals but the neurohormones in some of our staff, who are normal, healthy people. We used 7.8 cycles per second as the flicker rate frequency, which is theoretically the human frequency and the Schumann resonance, the frequency of the earth. We used ***red, green,*** and ***violet-colored light from the Lumatron™.*** If you look at the amounts of norepinephrine, serotonin, beta-endorphin, cholinesterase, acetylcholine, melatonin, oxytocin, growth hormone, DHEA hormone, prolactin, progesterone, and so on — we're missing the testosterone and estrogen levels due to a lab error — but looking at all these chemicals, **we found increases in *fourteen* out of forty measurements with *red light,* *twenty* out of forty with *green,* and *fifteen* out of forty with *violet.***

---

1. Wilhelm Reich, M.D., was a psychologist and psychiatrist who studied the relationship between the emotional, physiological and physical functions of biological energy. He saw the orgasm as the key to the body's energy metabolism, discovering that the biological emotions governing the psychic processes are the immediate expression of a physical energy he called "orgone." He is the author of a book; *The Function of the Orgasm,* which is one of the most important books of this century in our understanding of human sexuality.

So in this particular experiment using healthy, normal adults, if you look at all of these neurochemicals, they had about a 50% chance of increasing their concentrations with a green light. Interestingly, also, green was the least favorite of the colors. We did not choose whether the patient or the individual should specifically have that color; we were just trying the same colors on everybody. Remember, these subjects are healthy people who don't smoke and who are not on drugs. They're just volunteers from my staff, and we don't hire anybody who smokes. And that was what we found in just this one situation. We used a different frequency flicker rate on the Lumatron™ with the same three colors, and we found that for each color at least one individual had a totally different response neurochemically and neurohormonally than the others.

I just want to remind you that typically what most researchers are measuring are globulins, antibodies and lymphocytes and "all that jazz;" yet, all of these are ultimately dependent upon the above, higher-echelon things. **Much more important than T-4 cells is attitude, because attitude is what ultimately determines T-4 cells!** Also, much more important than T-4 cells, really, is what is happening in your levels of beta-endorphin and your oxytocin and some of these other neurochemicals. It's a very complex system, and when you look at it and begin to think about it in these terms, it can be so confusing that you wonder what do you do? How do you decide whether to intervene using *acupuncture, light, or food* for a given individual? I think, ultimately, you have to use your intuition coupled with the patient's intuition and their desires.

Now, I want to go into a little more detail about some of the ways in which we have worked with depression to show you the variety of things that can affect it. Four years ago we did our first major experiment on the treatment of depression. I received a letter from a man with whom I had worked and who has been a friend and consultant for a long time. He is a genius who is very, very intuitive; he is about 83 years of age now. He invented hydraulic brakes and hydraulic steering — with no engineering training. He did it all through intuition. He holds 88 patents in the field of hydraulics. And he said, "Norm, if you'll research whether crystals have any effect in healing, I'll give you a research grant to do it."

So we spent seven months trying to figure out how you study whether crystals can be of help in healing. We came up with the idea that we would take two groups of people and do those things that we knew could have an effect upon depression in everybody, and we would do it in a very short period of time, because we already knew that within two weeks we could get 85 to 90% of them out of depression. Then we would send them home with no further contact with us, giving half of those people a *quartz crystal,* and the other half a *placebo, glass crystal.* Nobody would know what anybody had gotten, thus setting up a double-blind research study.

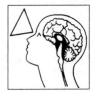

Preliminary Neurochemical/Neurohormonal Data[1] on the Effect of Lumatron ™ Light Stimulation

- Subjects were normal, healthy, nonsmoking, nondrinking staff members at the Shealy Institute.[2]

- The photostimulation effects of 3 colors of light through the eyes were examined at a constant flicker rate of 7.8 Hz (the so-called "Schumann resonance" or the earth's frequency).

- 40 blood measures were examined that looked at individual, combinations, and ratios of the following neurotransmitters and hormones: norepinephrine, beta endorphin, serotonin, melatonin, cholinesterase, oxytocin, prolactin, DHEA, growth hormone, and progesterone. (The lab tests for estrogen and testosterone were spoiled.)

Results of Lumatron ™ Ocular Light Stimulation (7.8 HZ)

COLOR VIEWED	RED	GREEN	VIOLET
Number of blood tests showing increases per 40 measures	14	20	15

---

1. Flicker rate may be an important variable to look at in future research.
   These results are only preliminary and require much further experimentation.

2. Dr. Shealy did not mention how many normal subjects were originally tested.
   All these chemistries were run again with another individual (N = 1) at a different flicker rate (unspecified) which yielded totally different responses (unspecified).

We worked with one hundred forty-one depressed patients the first time. As usual, we put them through forty hours of our various therapies at the clinic — twenty hours a week for two weeks. We gave them ten hours of *lectures*. We gave them ten hours of vibratory music on the *music bed*. We gave them twenty hours of *music therapy* in a large room which has quartz crystal under the carpet and big stereo speakers; so as they were lying on the floor, they could literally feel the music coming through the floor. We also gave them ten hours of *cranial electric stimulation* every day for two weeks, and we did it Monday through Friday for two consecutive weeks. The above treatment helped a lot of people with depression. At the end of two weeks 85% of them were out of their depression. But half of them took home a quartz crystal and half of them took home a glass crystal, and we had them *mentally program the crystal by willing joy into it*, *which they were to redo every day*. We also sent them home with a tape of the music selection that they had chosen. Three months later and then six months later they were to come back for a remeasuring of their neurochemicals and for some basic psychological tests. What we found in the follow-up was that only 28% of those people who had gotten glass were still out of their depression, while 70% of those who had quartz crystals were not depressed. Now, I don't know what that means, all I can tell you is that's what we found. It appeared in that particular experiment that quartz crystal was almost three times as effective as placebo in helping people maintain a normal mood once they had gotten out of depression.

Now remember, we did nothing else. We talked about *nutrition*, but we did not offer any chemical interventions into their lives. We didn't even change their magnesium or their taurine, or any of the other amino acids. We just suggested they might eat a better diet, they might get more exercise, that sort of thing. Most of them probably didn't make these sort of changes. **Again, what we found for this group of depressed people was 70% of those who had quartz were able to stay out of depression, whereas only 28% of those who used a glass crystal were able to stay out of depression**.

So, the next year we decided to research the people who had failed. We had to get a few new ones, because we wanted one hundred people this time. Actually we took fifty people who had failed and fifty people who had done well. We wanted to compare them, and we wanted to see if the people who had done well were that different from the people who had not done well. We measured magnesium levels and amino acid profiles, and interestingly, we found that even those who were no longer depressed — those who had done well — still were deficient in magnesium; yet, somehow they had been able to get back into a state of attitudinal happiness without improving their magnesium level. We also found that there was no difference in the amount of amino acid deficiencies; and so, does that have any meaning?

Then we took those people who were most deficient in magnesium, those who had a white blood cell magnesium test, and we gave them five shots of magnesium intravenously and recommended that they go on to magnesium by mouth. Nothing else, no other changes. Now, this time we gave them five days of *music therapy*, the *patient education* again, five days of *one* hour each on the *Lumatron*™ at the color chosen by the examination method Dr. John Downing uses; and then we sent them home. We had them come back later to see what the results were. We wound up with 70% of those who were depressed at the beginning being free of depression at the end of this time period.

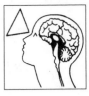

Now we wanted to try something a little different. So, instead of working with magnesium, we worked with taurine and did one or two other slightly different things. This year we had to get about half new patients, because we couldn't find many of our original group who were still depressed — which is a good sign! In the next experiment we took fifty people, all of whom were depressed, and we measured their magnesium and their taurine levels. If they were deficient in taurine, we gave them taurine; **86% of them were deficient in taurine.** We gave them thirteen sessions on the Lumatron™ and thirteen sessions on the music beds and then thirteen hours in front of the copper wall. We'd also given them some other homework, which we asked them to do every day for the whole six-month period, so that they could work through their unfinished business. **Once again we wound up with 70% of them who were improved at the end of this period of time.**

I've already indicated that **those whose depression improved changed their brain maps primarily to become much more symmetrical, and they also began to follow photostimulation better than those who did not improve. But none of them got to a state which is what I would call normal, electrically, or electroencephalographically.** Not one achieved a state which was both symmetrical and followed photostimulation appropriately.

Preliminary Findings on the Positive EEG Responses to Shealy Treatment Programs

Comparisons of those depressed patients who improved versus those who did not improve showed changes in their brain maps suggesting:

- Hemispheric functioning became more **symmetrical**

- An improved ability of the brain to begin to **follow Photostimulation (entrainment)**

- However, of those patients who improved, no one achieved a normal EEG state of both symmetry and appropriate following of photostimulation

---

Now what does all of this mean? Well, again, it means that there are many different "roads to Rome." I've often said to my staff, who really get upset with me sometimes, "It does not matter what we do with our patients; what matters is our attitude while we're doing it." I believe that's more important than any of this stuff. **Our attitude of encouragement, of relating, of getting people back into living, seems to be more important than the individual treatments that we do.**

Does that mean that I don't think light's important? Of course not! It's part of a very critical process. **Light is an adjunct that is cost effective, valuable and useful. But without somehow coaxing the patient into an attitudinal change, it probably won't work, or it won't last. The critical element is finding a way to give people tools that will assist them in rebalancing themselves long-term, so that they can cope with the stress and strain of daily life.**

191

For the last twenty years I have worked with **talented intuitives**, individuals who know medically, physiologically and psychologically what's going on in a person without seeing them. Now, all physicians, and I think almost all practitioners in the healing professions, use their intuition every day of their lives in deciding what tests to do and what therapy to use with a patient. But there are individuals who can be remarkably accurate — 93% to 96% accurate — without seeing the patient. For years, in difficult cases, I would call **Caroline Myss, Bob Leichtman, M.D.,** or **Henry Rucker** and ask them to help me with a particular patient. They almost never told me a diagnosis from a medical perspective that I didn't already know. Perhaps occasionally, but usually, it had something to do with a psychological hang-up that I may or may not have known about. I'm going to give you two examples, because I think these show you what I'm talking about.

Case – *Uterine Bleeding*

One was a woman — this was a very simple one — who came into my office with a problem of intense *uterine bleeding*. She did not want to have a hysterectomy. I took her history; I did her exam; and I didn't know what to offer her. Acupuncture, or that sort of treatment, was probably not going to work. As for light, I didn't yet know how to use light to turn off a menstrual cycle, especially one where the bleeding was rather copious. So I called Caroline Myss. She said, "Well, did she tell you about her two abortions?" I was on the phone, and the woman was sitting there, and I said, "You didn't tell me about your two abortions?" She broke into tears. It became clear that the cause of her excessive bleeding was her unresolved, unfinished business over her abortions. The problem was getting her to deal with it now, and she was unwilling to do so!

Case – *Depression and Cancer of the Colon*

The next case was one I consider a failure. A man had been going down a highway, up over a hill on an interstate, and he ran into a car that had crossed the middle of the road. The car had already hit five cows, and the coroner ruled that the other man driving that car was dead from hitting the five cows. But my patient allowed himself to go into a deep *depression,* blaming himself for the death of the man in the car. He had an awful lot of pain, among other things. I worked with him, but this was some years ago. I don't know whether I could have helped him better today using some of these other tools or not. But at any rate, I wasn't getting anywhere, so I called Caroline in July, and she said, "Well, if he doesn't get out of his depression within a year, he'll have cancer of the bowel." In November he was operated on for *cancer of the colon*. In February he was still in his depression, so I called Caroline again and she said, "Well, if he doesn't get out of his depression, he's going to be dead by August." So I screamed and yelled and shook him, and I told him he was going to leave a widow — and his wife was sitting there. I was trying desperately to get through to this man. August came, he had a pulmonary embolism and went into the hospital. I said, "Well, he's going to die." But he didn't die yet. On August 31st of the following year he died, still depressed. He died of depression, which is what I think most people die of, however it manifests itself in the physical body. I failed to get through to him; and Caroline failed to get through to him, even though we came very close.

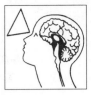

That's why I have decided that without the patient's compliance, it's not useful to call Caroline, or anybody else, and use their intuition, because the patient doesn't pay any more attention to them than they pay to me. I mean, I have had hundreds of patients where we have given them great intuitive insights, like, "Yeah, it's your two abortions that you haven't dealt with." So what! They still have to deal with them; I can't force a person to deal with their unresolved issues.

As I pointed out, we now have some tools that I think can assist people to at least raise from the depths of their souls what has been ignored or buried, but I can't force them to deal with it, even though I offer them support, counseling and everything else. **You cannot force a person to heal. I have come to the conclusion that, ultimately, as healers, we must teach people everything we can about the principles of health and allow them to use their own inner wisdom to solve their own problems, to move inside and deal with the roots.**

Jacob Liberman came up to me at the break, and he said, "All the issues you talked about have to do with the *first chakra.*" And that, indeed, is true! The issues which lead to problems in the second, third, fourth, fifth, sixth, and seventh chakras really start here in the root center, or the first chakra. All these issues start with the original interpersonal conflicts, primarily in your family, in your tribe, in your nation, in your company, in your government. These are the roots — how you relate sexually, your sense of security, how you relate in general to other people, your sense of responsibility, your ability to respond to other people, how you allow yourself to feel, to express and to receive love; how you allow yourself to express your will, your needs and desires; how you allow yourself to use your wisdom and your intuition; how you allow yourself to relate to your soul and to God and to the Divine. All these issues are colored by the root chakra. **The first chakra is the foundation of unfinished business**; there's no unfinished business in life that didn't start at the first chakra. Can you understand what I'm saying? **What I'm saying is that there is no unfinished business in any of your current love relationships that didn't start with basic feelings of safety in the relationships within the family**. There is no problem with will or any other energy system that didn't start here. So, in my opinion, **if you can deal with the root issues, the basic issues, then and only then, can you heal.** Now sometimes *light* will bring that out; sometimes *acupuncture* will bring that out; and sometimes *music* or *massage* will bring that out; and sometimes *postural adjustments* will bring that out. **These are just little tools that assist us in the process of opening ourselves up, of releasing the hooks that are "magnetically attracted" to our unfinished business**.

It is not a question of how much trauma you've had; it is a question of how much you've dealt with. We all know people who have been horrendously abused, and who have thrived. **Victor Frankl**[2] is one of these. He said:

---

2. Victor Frankl, M.D., chronicled his experience surviving incarceration in a Nazi concentration camp: *Man's Search for Meaning,* (New York, NY: Washington Square Press, Inc., 1963); and "Self-Transcendence as a Human Phenomenon," *Journal of Humanistic Psychology,* 6 (1966), 97-106; *The Will to Meaning,* (New York: World, 1969).

You know, much more important than starvation, having typhus and being incarcerated in a concentration camp, is a sense of a feeling of purpose or meaning in life. If you lose that under those kinds of adverse circumstances, you die.

All of us determine our health, our longevity, and our well-being by how well we deal with the unfinished business of our past — whether it is from this life or from a previous life. I have no doubt that many of us have triggered some event in our current life, usually in childhood, that reminds us of a forgotten memory; and sometimes we can unlock that by having guided assistance into a past life.

The light of the future is the light of insight. It is personal insight that allows healing to occur. This may happen with a spiritual healer in the laying-on-of-hands, or it may happen by the exposure to light or to sound. **Ultimately, though, it is the person's individual personality allowing the light of the soul to flow fully into being that is the basic cause of healing**.

QUESTION:	Have you had much experience with healers?
DR. SHEALY:	Yes. I have seen hundreds of patients have their pain disappear instantaneously with the laying-on-of-hands, only to have it return within one to twenty-four hours in most people. **Olga Worrall**,[3] with whom I worked for some years, was a close friend of mine, and I observed her a number of times. I went to her church and I was with her at a number of healings. When Olga died, we had established the **Ambrose and Olga Worrall Institute for Spiritual Healing** at our place in **Springfield, Missouri.** You don't understand what that means in a town that is 42% fundamentalists! But as Olga said, "You know, nobody gets well from a single shot of insulin." Similarly, most people don't get well from a single shot of healing.
	I believe that miraculous, spontaneous healing can sometimes occur instantaneously, but usually it's over a period of weeks. That kind of healing is almost invariably associated with a profound attitudinal healing. So, occasionally it occurs as an act of grace.
DR. LIBERMAN:	The thing I consistently find is more powerful than anything — and all the little gadgetries are merely peripheral to that — is me, or you, or anyone else. As **Tony Robbins**[4] says, "If you want to learn how

---

3. Olga Worrall was one of the most famous American healers, whose healing abilities were widely studied by scientists.

4. Tony Robbins is a national authority in the science of "peak performance" and the "psychology of change." During the past decade, more than a million people have bought his audio tapes, his video tapes and books. He is author of several bestsellers including *Awaken the Giant Within: How to Take Immediate Control of Your Mental, Emotional, Physical and Financial Destiny!* (Fireside, 1992), *Unlimited Power* (Fawcett, 1987) and *Giant Steps* (Fireside, 1994).

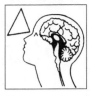

to do something, find someone who does it well." So it is in this matter of life. Find someone who does life well. I think perhaps this is best summed up by the expression, "Healer, heal thyself." I think the auric field or the energy around our body contains our intention, and what I also believe is that a *carrier wave* comes out of that. So, if my intention is to tell you that I really appreciated your presentation, and I really felt like you were right there, then I exude this; I think that's the formula. When someone comes into your presence and feels that kind of relationship with you, then the possibilities for healing open up for any treatment you do.

DR. SHEALY: Let me just summarize, if I may, for those who may not have heard Jacob Liberman. Basically he's paraphrased what I said. **It does not matter what you do. It is your attitude, your intent, the thought field you create around you that helps trigger the healing process in the other individual.**

DR. LIBERMAN: Those of us who are in the healing professions sometimes get caught up in the game of results — "It's my job to fix them. If I could fix things, then I'd be better at my job." One of the things that I realize is — I don't think we know anything about anything! And we certainly don't know when it's the time that someone is supposed to pass on or not. So perhaps the fellow that died of the pulmonary embolism . . . we don't really know whether it's appropriate for us to even violate that process.

DR. SHEALY: Actually, what you've triggered is a talk about the times we are in and whether or not we have a right to try to "force healing" on someone. Obviously I don't think we do, but ultimately as healers we are not healers if we are either *co-dependent*, which means we ourselves are suffering and will do anything to make somebody heal; or we are rescuers, in which case, we go beyond what we should and feel some sense of loss if we don't succeed. **A true healer is only a conduit, not a "forcer of healing" upon the patient.**

A Tibetan Lama said, "You can't interfere with someone else's karma by assisting in the healing process." And basically, I believe that to be true. Only when your intent is right and the patient is willing to cooperate with you is healing allowed to happen.

DR. DOWNING: When you researched the red, green, and violet light stimuli, did you find any set of chemical reactions that showed that one of those specific colors tended to influence the sympathetic versus the parasympathetic nervous system?

DR. SHEALY: Actually, there was relatively less activation, if you will, of either the sympathetic or the parasympathetic systems with these colors. What we'd really have to do to measure whether what we were doing was, in fact, leading to optimal functioning of the autonomic nervous system would be not to measure the instantaneous effects of norepinephrine and cholinesterase, but to measure the 24-hour urine output. **Dr. Herbert Benson demonstrated, for instance, that if you do deep relaxation 30 to 40 minutes a day, you can actually cut in half the total 24-hour production of catecholamines. I think you can take a person and, let's say, use only the Lumatron™ or light photostimulation and accomplish exactly the same relaxation response.** My suspicion is if we were to measure it — not in the blood, which is an instantaneous event, and doesn't tell you what's happening over the whole day — but measure the 24-hour output of catecholamines, we would find that properly done, light therapy would cut down catecholamine production 50% for the whole 24-hour period. We're revving up to do some more research work on urines now, instead of blood, to try to see what's happening over the whole 24-hour period.

If you're interested, the next chapter of my life will be the book that I created entitled *Third Party Rape*. Everybody in the country needs to understand the insurance system.

The Research reported in *Chapters Seven* and *Eight* was supported by research grants from The Charlson Research Foundation.

There is a place in hell for those who in the face of a great moral dilemma, maintain neutrality.

— *Dante*
THE DIVINE COMEDY

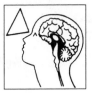

Ten Steps to Total Health

© Norman Shealy, M.D., Ph.D., 1992

Here's to your HEALTH! You can save it, prolong it, enhance and improve it, but money can't buy it. Choose to be healthy!

1. Eat 3 healthy meals every day.
   Eat lots of different foods; avoid caffeine and sugar.

2. Eat breakfast every day.
   Statistics show that those who do, live longer.

3. Do not use tobacco and avoid the environment of those who do.

4. Minimize or avoid alcoholic beverages.

5. Exercise regularly at an enjoyable activity.
   Start slowly and build up to at least 3-4 sessions weekly.
   Double the heart rate for at least 20 minutes each time.

6. Sleep 7 or 8 hours in each 24-hour cycle.

7. Keep your weight within 10% of your ideal.
   Exercise and eat a low fat, high complex carbohydrate diet.

8. Relax and rebalance regularly at least 30 minutes daily.

9. Have a positive attitude and create meaning and purpose in your life.

10. Resolve your anger and fear daily through prayer, counselling, communication or Biogenics (Shealy's patented system of affirmations and autosuggestion).
    Never go to bed with a grudge inside you or beside you.

The Healing Light:
A Guided Imagery Exercise

Close your eyes, take a deep breath and just let it all go. Now pay very close attention to your body. Always start by getting the feedback from your body, and you can do this instantaneously. Pay attention to the sensations in your face . . . neck . . . and throat . . . shoulders . . . arms . . . hands . . . chest . . . breasts . . . abdomen . . . back . . . buttocks . . . pelvis . . . sexual organs . . . thighs . . . calves . . . feet.

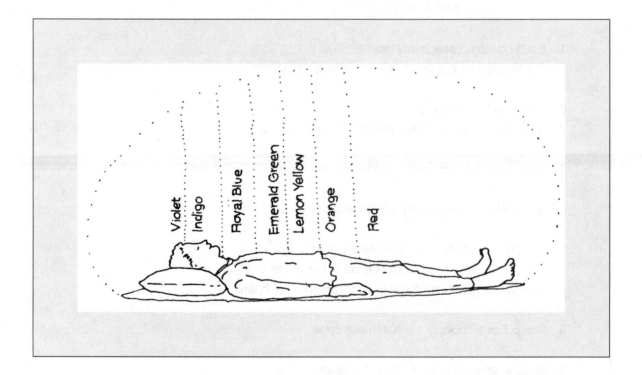

There are only a limited number of feelings, all of which include synonyms for feeling tension and discomfort or those sensations of having no feeling at all or the absence of feeling. Just be aware that anything but an "okay feeling" is actually a lack of communication between your body and your mind, for whatever reason.

Now imagine that you have coming into the top of your head an unlimited amount of energy, and that energy is focused in the form of a marvelous, powerful **Violet** light, connecting you with your soul and God. In the center of your brain, in the region of your pineal organ, this light is now being transformed into a deep, **Purple-Indigo** color, a color that sustains your wisdom and intuition. And as the Indigo moves down through your mouth . . . and neck . . . and throat . . . and arms . . . and hands . . . it becomes a **Deep Royal Blue** that feeds and nurtures your personal will, your needs and desires, and your ability to communicate them. And as this Deep Blue moves into the center and throughout

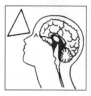

your chest, it becomes a beautiful, rich **Emerald Green**, allowing optimal flowering of your ability to love yourself and other people. And as this beautiful Emerald Green moves down and fills your entire solar plexus, it becomes a **Lemon Yellow** color, sustaining your interpersonal relationships, your sense of responsibility and self-esteem. And the Yellow now swirls throughout your pelvis and becomes a **Pure Orange** color, nurturing your sense of security, your sense of sensuality, and sexuality. And as this Orange flows down through your legs, it becomes an **Earthen Red** color, and it flows out the tips of your toes and the soles of your feet. The Red is now purifying all of your relationships with your family, with your tribe, and all of your past experiences.

Be aware now that you have this **Unlimited Rainbow of Energy** available to you, to flow into you from the top of your head through the pores of your skin and through your eyes, anytime you choose and at any frequency you need, balancing you, harmonizing you, and healing every cell in your body. And all you have to do is have an attitude of joy and love and openness, and your Rainbow of Energy will be perfect.

And with that knowledge take another deep breath and slowly and pleasantly open your eyes and stretch, feeling and seeing your Rainbow of Energy in perfect attunement.

You are a system of light, as are all beings. The frequency of your light depends upon your consciousness. When you shift the level of your consciousness, you shift the frequency of your light.

— Gary Zukav

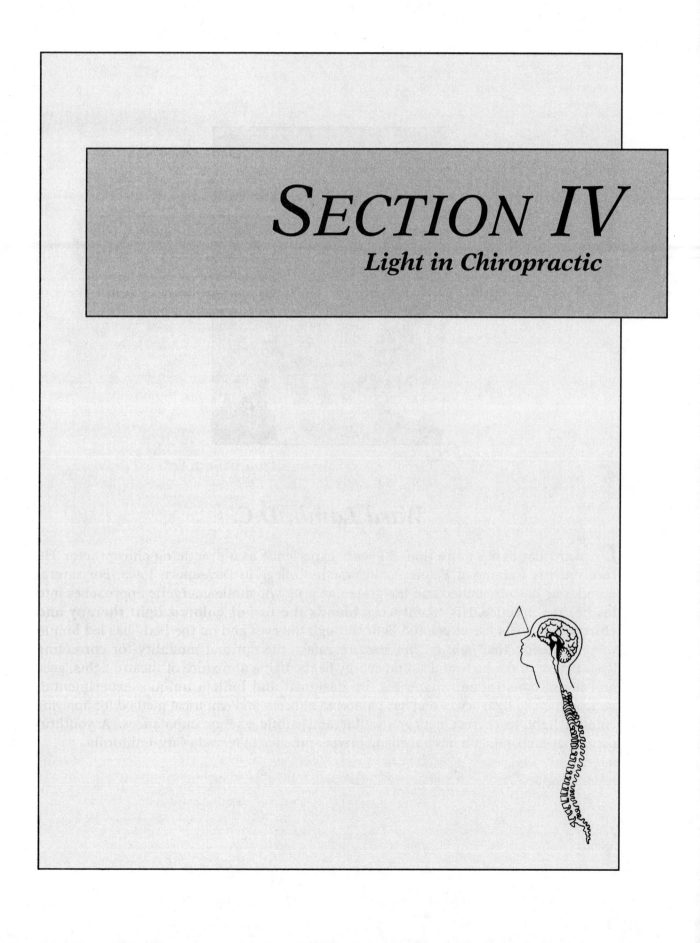

SECTION IV
Light in Chiropractic

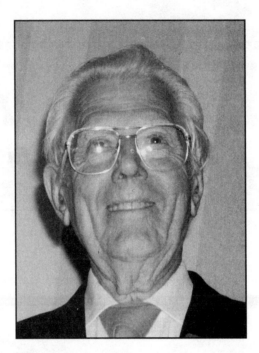

Ward Lamb, D.C.

Dr. Ward Lamb has more than 50 years experience as a practicing chiropractor. He received his training at Palmer Chiropractic College in Davenport, Iowa. For several decades he has researched and integrated a variety of subtle energetic approaches into his healing practice. His recent work **blends the use of colored light therapy and chiropractic.** His use of colored light through the eyes and on the body has led him to the conclusion that *light is "the great revealer,"* the optimal modality for correcting dysfunction in the body and subtle energy fields. Using a mixture of theatre lights, gels, and home construction materials, he designed and built a unique, experimental, noncommercial light device and has pioneered a theory and empirical method for applying colored light to correct neuromuscular and subtle energy imbalances. A youthful octogenarian, Dr. Lamb has a thriving private practice in Nevada City, California.

CHAPTER NINE

One Man's Journey Into Light:
The Use of Colored Light in Chiropractic

Ward Lamb, D.C.

What a joy it is to be here today. Fantastic conference! And did you know that all of you are making history? This is the first time that there has been a conference of this nature on light-based therapies in the whole world. Give yourself a hand!

The book *Light: Medicine of the Future* **by Jacob Liberman** virtually fell off the shelf into my hand. I read it voraciously from cover to cover a couple of times, and it built a "fire" under me like nothing has for a good many years. So intense, it's still burning! I just had to know about this energy called light and how to use this energy. Another thing occurred to me. Why are we, and why have we *been,* so inattentive to light? How has light escaped us for so many years that it could only now be of therapeutic use? I thought about it for awhile, and I decided it's probably because it's free!

I'm not here as an expert on light therapy. I'm one of you seeking, searching, wanting to know how to use this ubiquitous stuff that's all around us as part of the electromagnetic spectrum, termed light. How do we use light therapeutically? Any of you who are interested in exploring colored light, the book *Let There Be Light* by **Darius Dinshah** would be very helpful to you, because it gives you all the color gel formulas to make the color-specific frequencies that you need to apply to the body or through the eyes for phototherapy. When I became interested in color therapy, I realized there had to be some way to introduce light to the systems of the body. In my initial experimentation I combined two systems of light therapy that I knew about. One was **Syntonics,** fostered by the optometric profession, and Dinshah's **Spectrochrome.** My experience led me to work with light through the eyes and on the body. I began making my own light instruments using a combination of inexpensive and easily available equipment. Using the **Roscalene gels** and holders, I made up color filters according to Dinshah's original Spectrochrome formulas.

Dinshah mentions Roscalene filters. That was a brand new word for me. I said, "What the heck is that?" I thought, "Boy, I'd probably have to call New York to get that." But, as it turned out, one local phone call, and I had them in my hands. So while I was there at the theatrical supply, I was looking around, because I didn't know what kind of lights to use to transport the light to where I wanted it to go. By that time I had learned a little bit about Syntonic Optometric Principles (see *Chapter Two* for description of Principles). I knew

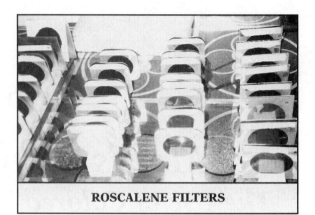

ROSCALENE FILTERS

I had to get light into the eyes. I didn't know how I was going to do that, so I looked around a bit and found an old strobe light that I had gotten from Radio Shack, and I said, "Well, that will flicker; that will give us a beat." And, with a little tinkering around at Home Depot's plumbing department, this apparatus is what I came up with.

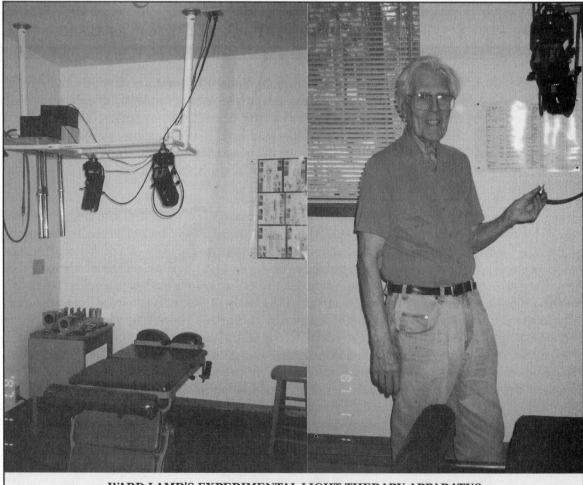

WARD LAMB'S EXPERIMENTAL LIGHT THERAPY APPARATUS

Today the media has gotten a lot more interested in the brain, as we can see from the covers of three recent magazines. These two are from the covers of *Discover: The Magazine of Science* in May 1984, and in December 1988. There is also a special issue of *Scientific American* on "Mind and Brain" in September 1992, in which the whole issue was dedicated to the brain and how it works in learning, memory, sex, vision, and language. **There's all this interest in the brain, and here we have light, with direct access via the retina!**

This is the first light instrument I made, right here *(see photo on previous page)*. So now I was ready to treat myself. I've always done anything that was "new" on myself first. If I survived, then I figured my patients would probably survive as well!

By way of a little personal history, in the late 1930s and early 1940s I lived in San Francisco. I grew up walking around the flatlands of Santa Clara Valley, and when I hit the hills of San Francisco, something went wrong with my right knee. It got pretty bad. It kind of crippled me, and I didn't know much to do about it. But I was a country boy, so I used hot and cold compresses, Ben-Gay, and an Ace bandage. And in about ten days it got better, or so I thought. In the early 1940s, I was a "guest of Uncle Sam." I was in San Francisco and, as luck would have it, I was still living in my apartment when I had another episode with the right knee. I saw the military doctor, and he was very honest. He said, "I don't know too much about that; here's some pills; see me next week." I thought, "Well, if it worked the first time, I'll try it again." So, I tried hot compresses, an Ace bandage, and Ben-Gay again, and I got well. That was 1940, folks. Remember, 1940! I haven't had another real serious episode with that knee until it resurfaced and I began my experimentation with light.

If we have a pain or bodily discomfort that hangs around, pretty soon we say, "Oh, that's normal for me." Many times conditions will go on for months without our attention. The body goes through *denial;* and by the operation of denial, we disconnect our awareness from the area of symptomology. And once that's done, although the pain and discomfort may disappear, the body is simply in a state of *adaptation* and shuts down. **Light seems to be able to reach in behind the denial and allow the reconnection of the various energy systems in these symptomatic areas to make a fresh beginning as far as healing is concerned.** The renewal that occurs as a result of the impact of light frequencies penetrates deep into the body. We're not exactly sure how this occurs, but we are sure that the outcome of using light through the eyes creates the re-emergence of old denial patterns and symptoms as a person moves towards healing. As in my case, this state of denial and adaptation where the symptoms are no longer evident, can go on for fifty years or more. During a *healing crisis* a mindbody reconnection occurs and we temporarily re-experience old physical and emotional symptoms. **Getting well is going beyond denial, and this is what light therapy is about.** So after my initial *light tonation,* I got a brand new knee and haven't had any problem since. If anything is a kicker, it's what happens to yourself. If I needed any further convincing about light's powerful effect, I had it right there, for sure.

One reason I moved beyond crystal research was because I was frustrated. In working with crystals, there was only one frequency available. You could do a certain amount of healing with that frequency, but then you were all through. **My gut told me**

when I looked at the light, here was an ideal modality to approach the chakra system once again, but now with the potential to have an even greater effect than we'd ever been able to accomplish with the crystals alone. In my view, the chakra system not only receives energy, but transmits it as well — it's dual in its function.

When I started talking about light therapy and describing a few of the details about how it is done through the eyes, I had heard remarks from several people in a row, and I have to tell you I think all of us have an instinctive feeling that there is something good and right about the therapeutic use of light. After having read the book *Let There Be Light*, which talks about using light directly on the body, and after I had been a little bit informed about *Syntonic Optometry's* use of light through the eyes, I said, "Wouldn't it be interesting to combine these two approaches? Wouldn't that have an interesting effect? At least, **why not simultaneously shine light through the eyes and on the body and see what happens?"**

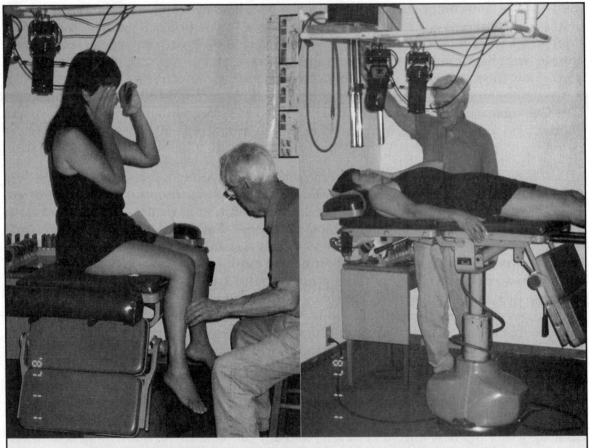

DR. LAMB ASSESSING AND UTILIZING LIGHT THROUGH THE EYES —
Demonstrating with a patient, doing a Kinesiological test — long leg, short leg.

So I had this piece of gear, and I decided I would also need to have something to apply color to the body. A theatrical spotlight came to mind. I had to brainstorm how to get light onto the body and how to handle my patients so that they were at least reasonably comfortable. Now you're seeing a photo of my table in my office; the plastic PVC plumbing pipe frame you see, the one that's holding the lights, is a result of a Sunday afternoon's work. Now I was able to begin to Spectrochrome (Dinshah's term for light therapy) the subtle energy of the body and the eyes simultaneously. **I particularly found that colored light placed on the body over the chakra locations was very effective in balancing the** *core energy system.* **Later, I observed that colored light stimulation directly to the brain via the eyes and retina was perhaps even more effective than going to the chakra areas on the body.** It was a step-by-step learning process, moving from one concept to another and learning through experience on myself and others.

Now a little past history. I worked closely with the late **Dr. Marcel Vogel.**[1] We did a lot of pioneering research on the subject of subtle energies, including the early work with quartz crystals. At that time we were particularly interested in how we could affect the core energy system of the body. **When I say core energy of the body, I'm talking about the chakra system. The core energy seemed to be very important to what goes on in the well-being and wellness of individuals. If the chakra system is "out of sync," then the whole mindbody system is out of sync.**

I must tell you I ran a group of patients through my "dining room table laboratory." Well, it works, folks! It's been about a year-and-a-half now, and I've run a clinic on my day off, because I had to know and establish some treatment protocols. How did I know what was going to happen to people when I gave them light through the subtle energy of the body and through the eyes at the same time? I had to have some guidelines when I talked to people, and I had to be able to say, "Well, this might happen or that might happen."[2]

After reading Jacob Liberman's book, I understood that you could have some pretty weird reactions. And, believe me, you can. I can tell you about a few of those, but I won't right now, because I have a couple of people here whom I call my *Courageous Recruits.* They're courageous recruits because they were willing to start with me, to teach me how to do light therapy. So, with your permission, I'd like to have them come up here one at a time. It's not for me; it's for color, for light, to give you a little overview of what they experienced while working with light, okay?

I'd like to introduce you to Gwen.

Case History – Chronic Fatigue: Courageous Recruit #1

GWEN: I'm a little more formal than you are, so I'm going to read. And I have to say, as I'm standing here before you as an "intimate stranger," it kind of dawned on me that this really isn't exactly how I had

---

1. The late Dr. Marcel Vogel was a renowned research physicist who patented the technique to make liquid crystal while working at IBM for over twenty years; he was also a passionate explorer, with his friend Dr. Lamb, of the nature and therapeutic application of subtle energies. These two men co-founded the Psychic Research Institute in San Jose, California.
2. To date, nearly four years later, Dr. Lamb has successfully used colored light through the eyes with chiropractic adjustments (which he terms Chromotherapy) with more than 300 "courageous recruits."

planned my "Andy Warholesque" fifteen minutes of fame — to point out to you how sick I was — but we'll just go with it.

My name is Gwen, and I have been a very willing and very satisfied guinea pig for Dr. Lamb's light therapy experimental treatments for about the past eight months. As a point of reference, I'd like to give you just a little bit of background on myself. I had been working in Washington, D.C., in a very stressful position for about twelve hours a day, weekends included. That was pretty much the norm. I had been told a time or two that I have a Type A personality. Combined with my personality, I was constantly travelling and seemed not to have the time for exercise, nor the ability to eat properly. I had absolutely no balance in my life. I was a professed *workaholic,* but I didn't seem to give my frantic lifestyle much thought, because I believed that my health was truly dispensable. I'd been keeping up this pace for about three to four years when I finally decided that I should, and maybe deserved to, take a vacation to visit the Mayan temples that I had wanted to see for many years. Ironically, that was where my problem began. Toward the end of my stay, in the wee hours of the morning, I suddenly awoke. I was salivating as one usually does before vomiting. The pain in my stomach was excruciating, but I just dismissed it, because I thought I had become just another victim of *"Monteczuma's Revenge."* Once home, that *"old Mexico feeling"* stayed with me for a good two weeks; yet, I assumed that my system would simply work it out.

I returned to work at my same old pace and tried to put my *stomach pain* and my *nausea* out of my mind, but my symptoms began to increase. It seemed like clockwork that every month a new ailment appeared. In addition to my constant abdominal pain, I became increasingly *constipated.* The next month my knees began to ache. The following month I began to feel *feverish* a good percentage of the time, followed by constant *sore throats.* In addition to the *ringing in my ears,* there were bouts with *nightmares;* I felt like I was "going mental." Having a host of other ailments as well, I finally acknowledged that there was, indeed, something wrong when my *eyesight began to blur.* At one point in time I felt so miserable I was unable to drag myself out of bed to make it to work. At that point I decided I would take a leave of absence from my job in Washington and return home to California to get what I thought at the time would be a quick diagnosis, take whatever vitamins, herbs, and treatments were necessary, and return to work in a few months. That was two years ago. I bounced around for the first six months or so in search of a specific name for all of my ailments, and I baffled specialist after specialist. I really, honestly, did not know what to do. **It was at one of those rare moments when I wasn't looking for an answer that I found Dr. Lamb. And I'm convinced that, though**

not yet completed, it was here that my odyssey back to good health began. I first began to see Dr. Lamb as a chiropractic patient. I heard he had a very good success rate in treating obscure cases such as mine. At this time Dr. Lamb was not yet practicing light therapy.

I continued with my treatments faithfully; yet, progress was slow. One day about eight months into my treatment Dr. Lamb pulled out this blue piece of cellulose material, shoved it against my chest, told me to hold it, and measured the length of my legs.[3] Then he took away the *blue gel* and muttered, "Wow, we could really be onto something, but we're not ready for this yet." In the next month or so Dr. Lamb formally approached me and asked me if I would be a willing participant in his experimental light therapy treatments. Even with the consistent chiropractic care that I had been under for the last eight months or so, my first four to five visits to Dr. Lamb for light therapy revealed the need for light tonation in all seven of the chakras. I had a limited response to the initial treatments, and nothing terribly dramatic happened to me. But then slowly the importance of the treatments began to emerge.

What we found in my particular case was that the **light therapy began to reveal certain muscle and neurological disorders which Dr. Lamb was unable to identify during my chiropractic sessions. Quickly we discovered one of the most important rules of light therapy, that light is the great revealer. It became very apparent that my chiropractic treatment was greatly enhanced by my weekly light tonations, and my progress began to move along at a much quicker pace.** This is not to say that after every light and chiropractic treatment that I felt, or feel, great. Sometimes it is just the opposite. A number of times the treatments would release energies within my body that had been blocked for a very long time. The release of this energy has the potential of creating what Dr. Lamb affectionately terms *"whoop-ti-do,"* a healing crisis. While temporarily painful and uncomfortable, healing crises are beneficial, because they bring forth hidden dysfunctional energy that needs to be incorporated in order to restore the proper energy flow in the body. Just as the combination of light and chiropractic treatment created the healing crises, the combination is also responsible for incorporating this new-found energy back into my total body energy.

This became known as my "one-step-forward, two-step-back period," which, I will honestly say, I am still experiencing from time to time. **In the beginning of my light treatments there were certain**

---

3. A kinesiological testing method (muscle testing) that measures the body's response to a particular healing stimulus.

colors that I didn't like. Ironically, they were the colors I needed the most. In my particular case it happened to be green and yellow. There was simply something about these two colors that I just didn't like or trust. Other colors such as blue and indigo, in my case, I took to immediately. **My treatments in the beginning consisted of treating the seven chakra areas only. Then, as I continued to improve and my chakras began to stabilize, Dr. Lamb expanded my treatment by introducing other colors to induce healing, but also to try to reveal potentially hidden disorders — disorders not demonstrated simply through chiropractic care.** The expansion of these light treatments was fascinating and we have discovered many things.

It was during this experiment that I had my most dramatic reaction to light therapy. In analyzing all of my symptoms, Dr. Lamb was led and found a need to reverse the energy flow of what he believed to be one of the most important nerves in the body, the *vagus nerve*. Within less than twenty-four hours of treating my vagus with what appeared to be a "little innocent" *red and green light*, I was experiencing my biggest "healing crises" to date. My whole system completely shut down, and I was bedridden for at least three to four days. As I laid in bed, trying not to think about how miserable I felt, I felt different from all the other times that I went through "whoop-ti-dos." Underneath all the pain there was for the first time a stirring sense, a sense of "core energy" that was trying to emerge.

Usually, my temporary setbacks created not only an onslaught of physical pain, but mental pain as well. They would dredge up the recurring thought that I was never going to get better or the feeling that I've been completely abandoned by my body. But this time I really felt different. While I was in a lot of physical pain, I was overcome with a *sense of hope*, a feeling that I had desperately tried to experience throughout my treatment with Dr. Lamb, but never truly captured until then.

That was after about three months. I'm currently continuing my light treatments on a weekly basis, as I am with chiropractic. **We have found that spacing light and chiropractic treatments about three days apart allows the light therapy to reveal conditions that can be treated chiropractically, and vice-versa.** Meanwhile, admittedly, I'm still experiencing "healing crises" from time to time, but I feel that my progress has truly been enhanced by Dr. Lamb's light therapy treatments. We just simply have more work to do.

At this point in my treatment I've begun to establish a rather deep personal relationship with each color. While I'm still not a huge *yellow* or *green* fan, I have found that the more tolerant I became of them, the less my body demonstrated a need for them, particularly green. I fought with this color for a very long time, but I think with my personality type, that's probably easy to understand. Usually about five to ten minutes after I've been exposed to **green,** **my entire system calms down,** and I experience a sort of humming sensation and a feeling of inner peace. And you don't know me, but for me, that's saying something!

For me there's one color, *blue,* that I can actually feel working while I'm being exposed to it. I've been susceptible to *sore throats* for a long time, and while I've been going through this health crisis, it seems I can get a sore throat at a moment's notice. While Dr. Lamb is treating me with blue, I can feel the energy moving almost in a clockwise direction near my tonsils, and the swirling motion moves toward the side of my neck and dissipates slowly, allowing me to swallow once more, very easily.

Indigo is my favorite color. I know that when I've been exposed to *indigo,* I'm going to feel better almost immediately. Dr. Lamb has used indigo light throughout my entire abdominal cavity where my problems began. It really seems to **quiet down the inflamed tissue** in that area, and it's a color in which I have confidence. Also, with my *vision problems,* at times I feel congested in the forehead area, and by exposing this area to indigo, it seems to **release that energy blockage,** allowing my vision to improve and ridding me of my headaches.

At times between treatments, if some of the symptoms start to flare up, I have found it helpful to imagine a particular color shining on the area of pain; for me it's usually indigo. By visualizing this, I am able to relieve the pain for a few minutes at a time. Actually, I'm becoming quite good at knowing what colors I'm going to need for a tonation. Then there are times when I think I'm feeling pretty good and I go in for a tonation in which I don't think I'm going to need any colors, only to find that I need some fine-tuning. All I have to say about working with Dr. Lamb is that while we do have more work to do, there has been a significant change that has been taking place inside of me. I truly believe that I would not have gotten this far without Dr. Lamb or his light therapy treatments.[4]

---

4. Courageous recruit #1, Gwen, two years post-light treatment, is back at work full-time and experiencing lots of energy.

Case History – Chronic Fatigue: Courageous Recruit #2

JAN: Well, like Gwen, my claim to fame is that I've been ill for over four years and finally have found something that is helping me to get well. I'm totally convinced, and I'm very happy to be here, because, as professional people in many healing fields, you're working with light, and I'm here to tell you that light works! Four years ago — I had a very balanced life, or so I thought. I worked at Tandem Computers as a training specialist. I haven't worked for two years now. I took a class at John F. Kennedy University; I hiked with the Sierra Club; I did aerobics; my social life was good. I went to the opera, the symphony, and the theater. You know, I thought I had it all. And one day I could not get out of bed, so I went to my internist; and she said, "I don't know what you've got; go home and rest." So, I did — for a couple of weeks; and friends would call me and say, "Did you take an Epstein-Barr test?" And I'd say, "No." So, I went back, and she diagnosed me as having *mononucleosis*. So, I stayed home for two-and-a-half months, went back for a couple of weeks part-time, thought I was well, and started working again. A few months later I collapsed. This time my internist couldn't find anything wrong. I went to a new internist for a second opinion, and he said *chronic fatigue and immune deficiency syndrome*, which is kind of a lightweight title . . . *fatigue* . . . for a very heavyweight illness. It's devastating; it's depressing. You lose everything. At the time I came to Dr. Lamb I was getting up one hour a day, max. You can't do too much in one hour a day. And I had a house to run and whatever.

I want to speak a little bit about chronic fatigue, because there are more people with chronic fatigue than there are people who have AIDS. It's a little-known illness, because we're all too tired to do anything about it! There are support meetings, but we're too tired to go! There is research going on, but it's limited. There's a lot of help out there, but you have to get to the right people. What chronic fatigue does is it affects the immune system and affects the endocrine system. They think it's a retrovirus called aspumivirus or human foamivirus. They haven't really said this yet, because other clinics or laboratories have to come up with the same findings before they will really say, "Well, this is what it is." So, right now we don't know what starts it. And all you know if you have it is that you feel like you're dead!

The Center For Disease Control has to research the criteria before your doctor is supposed to diagnose it. You have to have eight out of eleven symptoms, and your activity level has to decrease by 50% for at least six months. At the time I was diagnosed, I had nine out of the eleven symptoms. There are an additional thirty symptoms, but they didn't count. Some of the symptoms I had were: *sore throat, swollen lymph glands, severe headaches, muscle pains, like fibromyalgia*

— so painful that I couldn't lift my arms or hold a telephone — *fevers, a flu feeling* — *nausea* — where you wake up in the morning and you just know you have the flu — *rashes, heart palpitations, thyroid dysfunction, and cognitive problems.* All of a sudden *I couldn't concentrate*, and while I was still trying to work at that time, I had to put my head down on the desk. When I finally found that I was lying on the floor in my office, I thought, "Okay, Jan, get it together, find somebody who can help you."

The most debilitating part was the fatigue. It was a little discouraging, because I'd have friends call and say, "God, I had such a hard day. I'm tired, too." I'm not talking about being tired; I'm talking about just being "dead." And I'm not a "California cornflake." So I want you to know that I'm a responsible person, and I was not in a depression.

A lot of people want to say, "Well, you're depressed." I have not been depressed through this whole illness. I'm a real upbeat person. I've got a good sense of humor. And because of my background, I feel this illness holds for me a lesson to be learned. I don't know what the lesson is, and I don't know how I'm going to get out of this, but I'm going to learn something, and I'm going to be a better person for it.

So, at first, when I'd go to the American Medical Association (AMA), they didn't really have a whole lot to tell me. They'd say, "Rest," and they'd try to give me some help with the pain, because there's a lot of pain with chronic fatigue syndrome. That's why I was in bed a lot. When you're lying in bed, you don't have the pain. There are no painkillers that can help any of the pain that you're feeling. And then they'd say, "We want to put you on high doses of Prozac." Well, I knew I wasn't depressed, and I wasn't about to take Prozac. I decided that if I was going to have this illness, I should go and get some counseling, because I've always believed that there's a strong tie between body, mind, and spirit. And I found somebody who was very helpful. She had other people with chronic fatigue, and she found me a doctor through one of the other clients. She sent me to Dr. Shamlin here in the San Jose area, who was the first doctor who could talk to me about chronic fatigue.

I did a whole lot of different therapies. I did visualizations. I did absolutely everything that would help my body, my mind, and my spirit. I had church practitioners coming to me. Absolutely *everything* that's out there I've tried! I've tried to get well. A lot of things helped; Dr. Shamlin helped me a whole lot. But nothing really stayed; I still couldn't get out of bed! I got very interested in angels, and I was reading a book that said you could ask for what you want; be very direct with them; angels don't like you to be subtle. So, I sent out a "mental prayer-fax," and I said, "Look, I've been ill. I've been a good sport about it; I haven't gotten depressed. I've tried everything. Would you please send me someone." Suddenly, Dr. Lamb appears, and he says, "I'd like to do light therapy with you. You're my most challenging client. I want to know why you haven't gotten well." The book that I was reading was called *Messenger of Light.* I went home and thought, here's my "messenger of light," my angel.

And he has been, because I started over a year ago. And in the first six months absolutely nothing happened. I'd go. I'd need all the colors. I'd need them a long time. I didn't feel anything, and I'd go home to bed. Six months this lasted. And, of course, he had some other people he was working with that he had pulled out of his practice, and I'd keep saying, "How are those other people doing? Are they gone?" Everybody was leaving and getting well, and nothing was happening to me. It's like, "God, when is it my turn?" **Finally, something started happening. Then, when I would go in, I was still very fatigued and in pain, but I didn't need all the colors anymore. Some of the chakras, I guess, were finally holding; and I just needed some colors of different varieties.** Each week it was different, so there wasn't a pattern yet.

But finally, about two months ago the lower three chakras were holding, and I only needed some of the upper ones. And I could leave his office and feel some energy in my body. I mean I hadn't felt any energy in two years! When I would wake up in the morning, there was no restoration. I felt just as tired as I had the night before without doing anything. Nothing was coming to me. But finally it started happening; and about six weeks ago I needed only one or two colors, and I started waking up in the morning restored.

Now it's like I have energy. I can be up six to eight hours now. I mean it's finally happening. It's taken well over a year, but it's working. And last Tuesday when I went in, I just needed *magenta* for the spleen. That's the only color I needed, and he needed to lessen the dosage at that point. So something is really happening. I had a very spiritual experience at the end of February; it lasted three days. I was just lying in bed, and I had this great, great, surge of energy, unlike anything I've ever had before. And I always knew there was a reason. When I first went to see Dr. Shamlin, she said, "Chronic fatigue is a spiritual transformation." So I had my spiritual experience, and the one thing I knew for sure was that my spirit was healed. I didn't know if I was going to have a miraculous healing right then and just get up and move. I didn't, but I knew the physical body comes along a little slower, and I knew that I was going to get well now. I still don't know why it took so long, but I'm a very stubborn person.

I just can't tell you enough about how well this works. I know what my next career is going to be. I'm not going back to high tech; I'm continuing my journey to wellness with Dr. Lamb. If you know of people with chronic fatigue, I would like to help them. I can give them support; I can give them practical help; I can give them inspiration; and most of all, I can give them hope, because I've always had hope. I knew I was going to get well. And people get very depressed and even commit suicide, because at a certain point you just can't believe you're ill that long when you've always been healthy. So what I would like to say to all of you who are in the healing field, I hope you'll be "messengers of light." There are a lot of people like me who need more "earth angels." Thank you. God bless.

DR. LAMB: Okay, folks, that says it all. I don't have to say anything more. Isn't that neat!

Radiologist Dr. Bjorn Nordenstrom of Sweden, internationally renowned for his research on biologically closed electric circuits in cancer treatment,[5] postulates that the arterial and venous system are dual in function. First, they transport venous and arterial blood; and second, they create a pathway for the streaming of energy through the body. Dr. Nordenstrom's techniques capture and stimulate the body's subtle energies to promote healing.

We know that energy streams through the body in the manner stated in acupuncture theory; that is, *life energy* or *chi* streams through the meridian systems. Dr. Nordenstrom also suggests that this energy may travel through the arterial system as well.

I'd like to explain about the ***parasympathetic and sympathetic nervous systems*** as they relate to nerve flow and the possible transmission of life energy *(see following illustrations)*.

The sun shines
Not on us
But in us

—John Muir

---

5. Dr. Bjorn Nordenstrom, Radiologist at the Karolinska Institute in Sweden, published his theories in a book entitled: *Biologically Closed Electrical Circuits*, (Stockholm: Nordic Medical Publications, 1983).

Parasympathetic Division of the Autonomic Nervous System

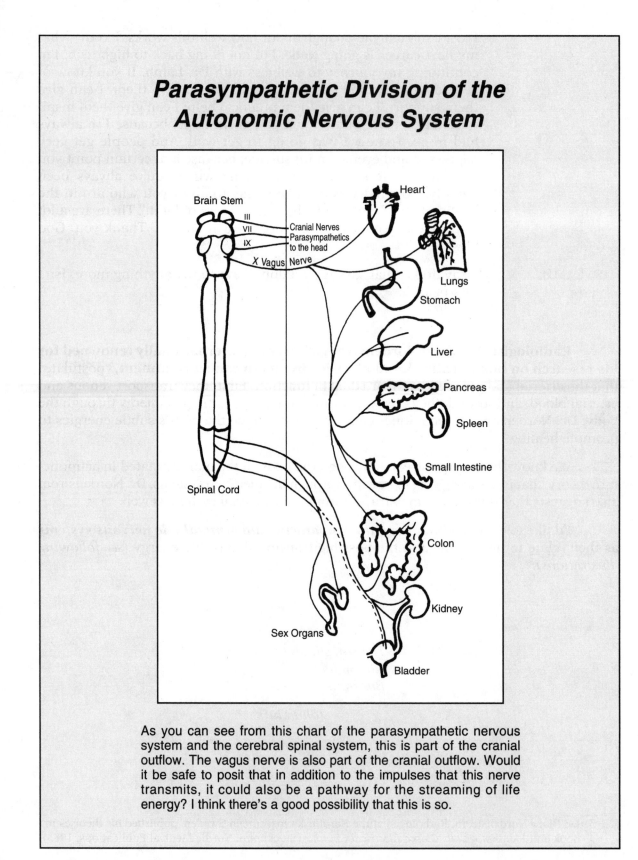

As you can see from this chart of the parasympathetic nervous system and the cerebral spinal system, this is part of the cranial outflow. The vagus nerve is also part of the cranial outflow. Would it be safe to posit that in addition to the impulses that this nerve transmits, it could also be a pathway for the streaming of life energy? I think there's a good possibility that this is so.

Sympathetic Division of the Autonomic Nervous System

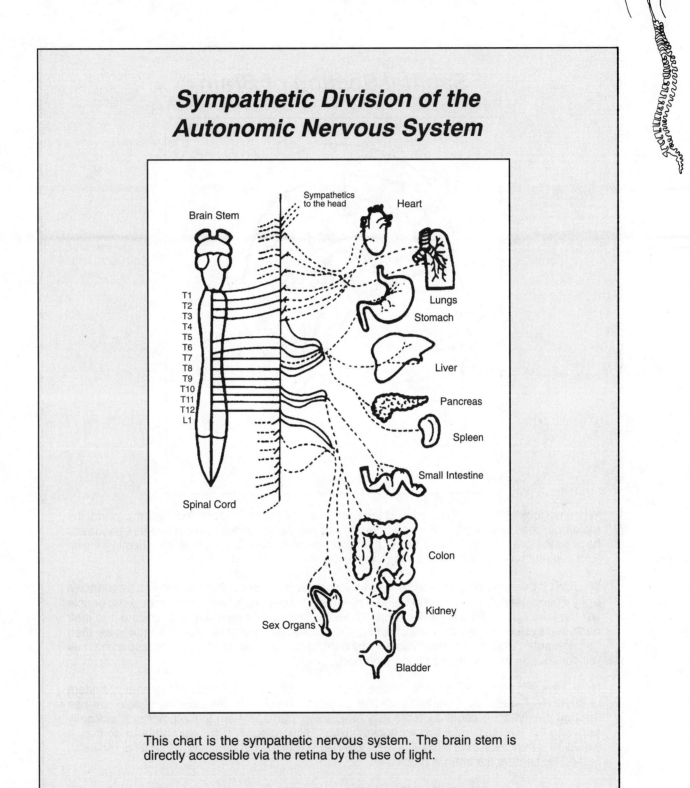

This chart is the sympathetic nervous system. The brain stem is directly accessible via the retina by the use of light.

Sagittal Section of Brain

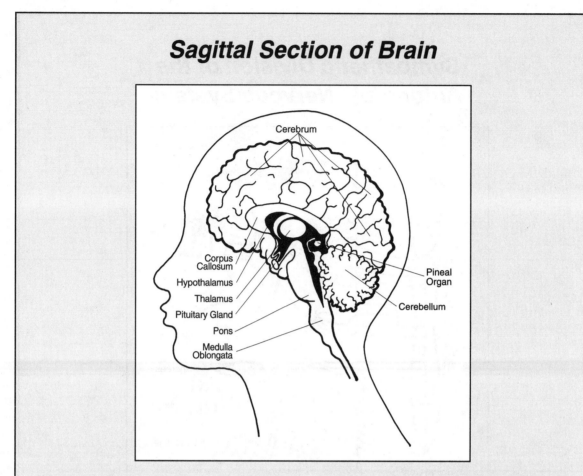

When we look at the sagittal section of the brain, we see the brain stem, the hypothalamus, the thalamus, the optic chiasm, the optic nerve, and the visual cortex, which, incidentally, feeds back to the brain stem. What a target that brain stem is! I think we are really affecting it with light stimulation — and not so haphazardly, either!

Wouldn't it be something if we were able to somehow or other control the specific frequencies of light people need. And I have to preface by saying that I already have found that some people will not take light "full bore," light even at 75 watts. I have to bring it down, attenuate it to their particular system, before they will accept it. Once they have accepted these frequencies, their "big computer," the brain, says, "Okay, it's all right." Then you can gradually increase it and they will continue to metabolize it through their body.

Now, if the "big computer" is that sensitive to what's coming into the milieu of the energy system of the body, I speculate if we had very fine control of the specific frequencies of color we use through the eyes, we could do some very fine tuning, perhaps even to the point of specifically targeting the hypothalamus and its nuclei inside. Think about it; if we were able to do that, it would be a truly awesome thing! Because after all, it is in the hypothalamus that all of the information that enters the brain is processed.

If a patient is suffering from depression or they have some kind of physical problem that can be affected by an acupuncture needle in the arm to stimulate a particular meridian system, what would happen if we were able to specifically target those areas in the brain that had to do with specific cranial outflow that was needed to either tonify or sedate that meridian?

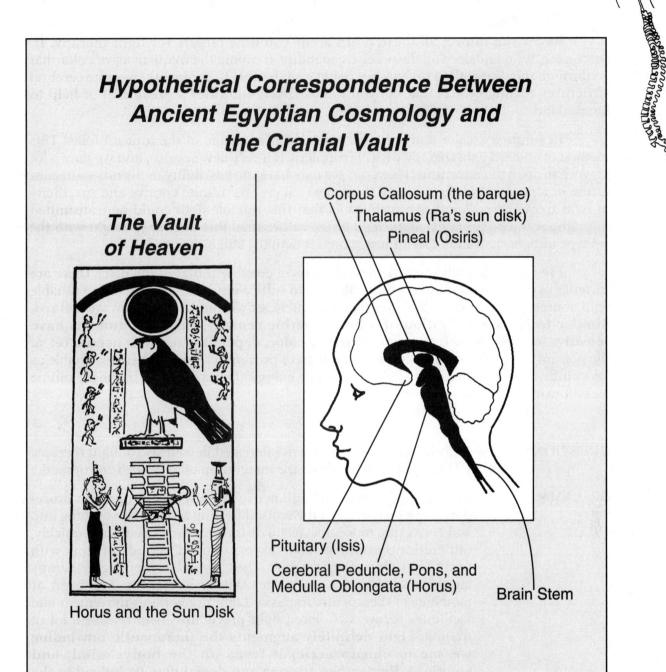

Hypothetical Correspondence Between Ancient Egyptian Cosmology and the Cranial Vault

The Vault of Heaven

Horus and the Sun Disk

Corpus Callosum (the barque)
Thalamus (Ra's sun disk)
Pineal (Osiris)

Pituitary (Isis)

Cerebral Peduncle, Pons, and Medulla Oblongata (Horus)

Brain Stem

Color Therapy is a very ancient science, so ancient that because we are now rediscovering it, it's new! I'd like to show you something I discovered in Egypt a few years ago, a representation found on a bas relief. The Egyptians thought so much of the brain stem that they made a symbol for it. They called it Horus, and Ra was the Sun God. They called this entire symbol "The Vault of Heaven." When we look at this bird and the sun, it has some very interesting correlations. The bird appears to correspond to the brain stem, while the "Vault of Heaven" (barque) appears to correspond to the corpus callosum and the Sun Disk, to the thalamus.

As for the future, all these brain areas could be targets for light therapy. If, perchance, we could develop the precise capability of tuning the frequencies of color that go through the retina, then perhaps we could even be able to contact these same cerebral structures through the retina. As you know, this could offer a great deal of help to humankind.

In summary, color and light are indeed the "medicine of the future," folks! This method of colored light therapy with chiropractic is a very new science, and we have a lot of work to do in the meantime. However, we may have the possibility in the not-so-distant future of a new *tunable light source* that may well give us infinite control and specificity of light frequencies. Another possibility is that this tunable light could be transmitted throughout the body via *fiberoptic light pipes*, rather than this theater spotlight with the gel type of light instrument that I use, which is actually still quite crude.

I've experimentally created combinations of color formulas of my own. There are varieties of color filter hybrids, which will have to suffice until we come up with a tunable light source. For example, there are many frequencies within the spectrum we call red. **Similar to the right dilution of a homeopathic remedy, I believe humans have sensitivities to specific frequency ranges of color, depending on their needs.** Yet, at the present time the colors we have available have proven to be more than acceptable as far as influencing the neuromuscular and subtle energy chakra systems. In the meantime we will work with what we have and enjoy it.

QUESTION: As a chiropractor myself, I'm interested in your use of light therapy. I'd like to hear more about the integration of light with chiropractic.

DR. LAMB: Light is a very valuable adjunctive therapy to chiropractic procedures. I've seen it speed the natural healing process by reaching into and correcting musculoskeletal distortions fairly easily and quickly, difficulties that might have taken extended periods of time with traditional chiropractic approaches. I've also seen light therapy augment chiropractic at times when the person has been at moments of therapeutic impasse. Light precipitates movement and facilitates recovery. Colored light procedures help release a lot of trauma. **Light definitely augments the therapeutic unwinding we see in chiropractic; it frees up the body, mind, and emotions. Remember, trauma and denial may be lodged in the body or organ system, not just the brain.**

Colored light through the retina appears to precipitate profound states of relaxation and mindbody release more easily than if you were to tell your patients to simply relax. Light through the eyes facilitates the process of release which can be reinforced by chiropractic manipulation and by encouraging the patient to verbalize or mentally attend to the emerging memories such that their energy can flow and stream, and as a result, healing can begin. People, like my *"courageous recruits,"* who have had considerable experience with these light treatments, actually sense the effects of different light frequencies and can feel the energy streaming through the body.

Dysfunctional tissue and symptomology can be encouraged to become functional by stimulating the streaming of life energy. And light is a very effective modality whereby dysfunctional tissue or symptoms can be encouraged to operate more functionally. Light complements chiropractic in a very spectacular way. When standard chiropractic procedures are used to restore the subluxations and remove skeletal and muscular distortions, they do a very good job. However, many times disturbances in the energy fields and systems of the body are not reached directly via chiropractic approaches. This is where light becomes useful to reach the subtler energies in and behind some of the problems I see in my chiropractic office. **Light appears to help restore the connection of the energy systems in the body, where, if there are subtle blockages, light helps augment the streaming of energy through the various bodily systems that have been blocked by subluxations and musculoskeletal distortions.**

In chiropractic we depend upon the subtle energies being released by adjustments. In my opinion, it's the streaming of released subtle energies that actually does the healing. So, healing takes place by anything that helps release the blockages and holding patterns, be they physical, mental, or emotional in nature. Light seems to be effective in helping to release these mindbody and subtle energy blockages.

QUESTION: Please describe more with regard to the anatomy of the subtle energy systems and how they fit into Eastern and Western models.

DR. LAMB: This is a very exciting time where Eastern and Western models of healing are being bridged by quantum physics. For example, a **German research physicist, Dr. Fritz Albert Popp,** has discovered that low levels of light frequencies may actually be the way cells communicate. Dr. Nordenstrom's model leads me to expect that our nervous system, like the vascular system, may also be dual in function. That is, it not only puts out and receives nerve impulses, but also may be a channel for the streaming of subtle energy. An Eastern model I'm comfortable with is derived from *yoga theory*. The anatomy of the core energy system consists of three interpenetrating vertical energy channels that go up the midline of the body that are called the *ida*, the *pingala*, and the *sushumna*. If there's a lack of core energy, it is because ida, pingala, or sushumna have shut down. When this happens, denial occurs and dysfunction begins at the energy level which later manifests at a cellular level, and then still later to inflammatory states at the level of tissues, and

221

finally to the gross physiological disturbances we see in a variety of disease patterns. Increasing this core energy is, in my view, the key to getting rid of denial. As I said before, when subtle energies stream through the body, this leads to healing. I believe that energy system disturbances are primary and if not corrected will later create disturbances in physiology and at the level of tissue and organ anatomy. At the most basic level everything we address in sickness and health relates to energy. If something shifts in our consciousness or in our body, it interrupts the flow of this energy; and when energy flow becomes aberrant, it will eventually lead to physical aberration. Many people are walking around dead and not knowing it. They've locked their energy systems in a closet. They're walking around in a daze and are largely operating on the level of unconscious reflexes. These energy level imbalances often start years earlier, and it is only much later that people become aware of pain and physical symptoms.

QUESTION: Can you say more about your experimental light apparatus and technique?

DR. LAMB: Very briefly, the spotlight and or strobe light sources are turned on and used with the set of Roscalene color filters that correspond to the colors of the chakra regions. The patient holds them over the chakra area on the body or over one eye while I do a kinesiological, or muscle testing technique called "the long leg, short leg phenomena." By observing their physical responses to the particular color frequencies, the body indicates the color it needs to rebalance itself. Muscle testing is not only valuable to point out where there are functional difficulties, but by using muscle testing before and after interventions, it allows the patient to be more fully involved with their healing process and helps them understand changes that have been made.

The theatrical spots with various gels are aimed on the appropriate body area or organ system to help change or restore the energy field in an area that is dysfunctional. The strobe light in combination with the colored gels is used through the eyes and is the most frequently used modality.

Switch on your light in all lives. Feel that you are the One Life that shines in all creation.

— Paramahansa Yogananda

Dr. Lamb's 5-R's Healing Affirmation

RELAX

RELEASE

RECONNECT

RESTORE

RENEW

This is the healing affirmation Dr. Lamb's patients recite while receiving Colored Light Therapy through the eyes and on the body. Dr. Lamb monitors his patients' neurophysical responses to light stimulation so they receive the optimum frequencies and quantities of light and color.

As memories emerge from the denial state during sessions, patients who are in a deeply relaxed state are encouraged to address these memories rather than repress them, thereby encouraging the mindbody system to enter a state of *reconnection, restoration, and renewal.*

QUESTION: Are there conditions you've seen respond particularly well to your colored light treatments and are there contraindications or hazards?

DR. LAMB: Light, as an adjunct to chiropractic, appears to work very well with those who have been diagnosed by a medical doctor as having *chronic fatigue* and a variety of metabolic and endocrine disorders. I've also seen it work quite well with *stress-related conditions* that have been previously unresponsive to normal types of medical and chiropractic interventions. It also appears to work very nicely with *chronic pain syndromes* and children and adults who suffer from *hyperactivity* and *difficulties with attention.* Let me say **I've witnessed profound changes in long-standing physical conditions and**

what I've often seen is a dramatic increase in vitality, stamina, and the ability to concentrate.

There are indeed some **cautions and contraindications** to the use of colored light, as Dr. Downing mentioned. You definitely need to be careful with the use of flickered light with the patients who had a history of *seizure activity*. Beyond this, patients need to be aware that they may go into periods of temporary, yet profound, psycho-physical catharsis. During the moments of what has been termed "healing crisis," they might experience *exacerbations of old emotional conflicts* or physical difficulties in the process of releasing old traumas.

Home of Light

Out of mind into body

I've made up my heart

all color is the keyboard our life plays us

do not be clogged with ideas

do not think so much, listen

so full of promise o'child

wear your body all lit up

the joy of giving, of breathing, of living

lie down beneath healer's hands of fire

and let go of all pain of held back desire

you are now free and you are the home of light

— Bethany ArgIsle

Let's leave it to the scientists to figure out at what "atomic or submolecular" level this stuff works. I really don't care. I'm a chiropractor; my main focus in practice and in business is to get that person back to full function, whatever it takes. To break it down to the finest little point of science and the finest little hormone kicking in over here, that's not my focus. How many people here could go into a biochemical laboratory and make a tuna fish sandwich into adrenaline? How many people could go into a biochemical laboratory and make white bread into testosterone? Yet, I want you to know that everyone of you in this room does that when you eat tuna fish and white bread; you do that every day without thinking about it, from the time you wake up to the time you go to sleep, and from the time you're born until the time you die. A lot of these processes cannot be repeated in the laboratory, and they never will be repeated in the laboratory, because there is something other than a strictly physical phenomenon that takes place, which has to do with what chiropractors call "Innate Intelligence" — what the acupuncturists call "chi energy" — what the holistic practitioners call "life force." I don't care what you call it. If you're religious, you'll call it God. That's okay. It exists within us, this force makes things happen, and that cannot be replicated in the laboratory.

Robert Dubin, D.C.

CHAPTER TEN

Downing Technique, Ocular Light Therapy™ and Cranial Sacral Therapy™ in a Chiropractic Setting

Robert Dubin, D.C.

When the eyes and the brain are disconnected from one another — which is the main focus of **Lumatron Ocular Light Therapy™; it reconnects the brain and the eyes so that the eyes can once again become a more effective conduit to get information into the brain** — when this disconnection happens, the brain and the body shut down to some extent. And when this happens, all of the systems shut down simultaneously. So, when you open up the eyes again, all kinds of things that weren't previously metabolized in the mindbody system could very possibly be remobilized and brought into consciousness. Then these thoughts and feelings can be detoxified or abreacted, because now the body is able to do it, whereas before it wasn't. This is just my theory of what takes place.

I use the specific *flicker rates*[1] I learned when I took the workshops from **Dr. John Downing**, and I really haven't varied those. The blue light flicker rate is lower, while the red light flicker rate is higher. I've never gone below 8 hz with violet light for anybody, because as a chiropractor, I believe it's too evocative.

---

1. The flicker rate on the Lumatron Ocular Light Stimulator™ consists of the light source turning on and off at adjustable rates from 1 to 60 flashes per second.

QUESTION: In your treatment protocol when you use the Lumatron™, do you do the chiropractic adjustments on the *cranial sacral level*[2] first, then work with the Lumatron™?

DR. DUBIN: No. Now that's a very good question and it's something that I really wanted to touch more upon today. I don't really propose Lumatron Ocular Light Therapy™ to anybody unless they're not responding well to chiropractic treatment in the clinic. Either that, or patients come in and ask for it, because the word's gotten around now in the area and people know that I have the device, and patients know other people who have benefitted from it. So, from time to time I do get calls specifically for the Lumatron™. I really like to have the patients under both therapies, but I don't push it that hard. I never push very hard in the clinic; I try to give people what they want.

QUESTION: What sequence do you usually use if they are on chiropractic, cranial sacral and Lumatron Ocular Light Therapy™?

DR. DUBIN: I never mix the cranial sacral and chiropractic in the same office visit. I think it's just too much input for the individual, and I basically operate from comfort. I focus on what's bothering the patient today and we go from there. Over the years I've been practicing, I guess I've developed the intuition to know where to go and what to do next. If you're in this business for any length of time, you have a sense of what happens and what needs to be done next. It's a difficult thing to explain; I don't think it can be cataloged, because it's different for everybody.

When a patient comes in to see me with complaints of *musculoskeletal pain*, that's typical. In any chiropractic practice the overriding majority of patients who come in have some type of musculoskeletal pain that's not being addressed properly. When I can't relieve the dysfunction or the discomfort in a couple of office visits, it's rare. Only if treatment doesn't work do I start looking around for other impediments that may be happening. The first thing that comes up, of course, because I have the device and I have the training, is the Lumatron Ocular Light Therapy™.

The Lumatron™ testing procedure to determine the specific color treatment takes only ten to fifteen minutes: that's not a big deal. The Ocular Light Therapy is marvelous, because the patient goes in a darkened room and puts on headphones, and I can't even hear the damn music! They listen to the music; they watch the light; and then

2. Cranial sacral balancing was created by osteopathic physician Dr. John Upledger. It aims to re-establish freedom of movement in the cranio-sacral system which consists of the bones, fluid, and membranes of the skull and spine. Cranial sacral work is often helpful in cases of: chronic neck and back pain or tension, recurrent headaches, insomnia and stress, sciatica, birth trauma, depression and emotional disturbance, temporomandibular joint (TMJ) problems, and recurring discomfort from old injuries.

they go out a "happy camper!" I don't even have to talk to them! The Vietnam veterans that I've treated with this have been on a strictly "research-project basis," if you will. I don't ask them for money if they can't afford to pay me. And I've had no problems, absolutely zero problems with the insurance industry with this therapy. Once I explain it to the insurance people, it's not really a problem.

QUESTION: Clear up one thing for me on cranial sacral manipulation. Does that usually or always involve the temporomandibular joint (TMJ) as well?

DR. DUBIN: You cannot separate the cranial sacral from the TMJ. **The TMJ is the center of the vestibular network.** It's the reference point to the entire proprioceptive system, and you cannot separate the balance of the body and the gross function of the skull as it relates to the rest of the body, without involving the jaw. It's not possible. Unfortunately, a lot of people have had orthodontic work, and that can create cranial distortion, and to reverse this problem is sometimes a "real trick."

Darkness may reign in a cave for thousands of years, but bring in the light, and the darkness vanishes as though it had never been. Similarly, no matter what your defects, they are yours no longer when you bring in the light of goodness. So great is the light of the soul!

— *Paramahansa Yogananda*
AFFIRMATIONS FOR HEALING

Cranial sacral therapy and chiropractic can give people tremendous relief from almost anything that they present with if the problem is mechanically, musculo-skeletally based. If it's psychologically overridden, then you need another avenue or another modality to use to try to break the hold that the psychological problem is having on the system. That's really what happens when a person gets traumatized, at least this is how I perceive it, and I've been traumatized enough to understand. When a person gets hit, the first thing that happens is a recoil. This is not only an outward manifestation, but it's an internal manifestation as well. The internal body cringes from trauma and disconnects. It kind of "folds in" upon itself — I visualize it as the individual being in a fetal position.

Back in the body, it doesn't want to "come out" because something bad is out there that might hurt it again. **It's up to us as health practitioners to unwind that trauma reaction, to bring it out, and to have the person's psyche fill up their body again, to**

have the mind, the body, the brain, and the eyes all be simultaneously in touch with reality. That's really our function as health providers, and until that happens, that person doesn't really regain their health. So, this is what we must do. Now, you can do it psychologically by encouraging people to talk; you can also do it through massage and touch therapy; you can do it through chiropractic adjustments or cranial sacral therapy; or you can do it through Lumatron Ocular Light Therapy™ as well. The bottom line, even with acupuncture, is to get the internal body fully functional and reintegrated into the system. That's really what healing is all about.

The Lumatron™ is probably the most powerful tool you'll ever see for opening up the connection between the eyes and the brain! That's where healing starts, because the eyes bring 85 to 90% of the information from the environment into the body. Unless this channel is open and functioning properly, you will not see a complete healing or complete remission of whatever problems patients may have.

SECTION V
Light in Acupuncture

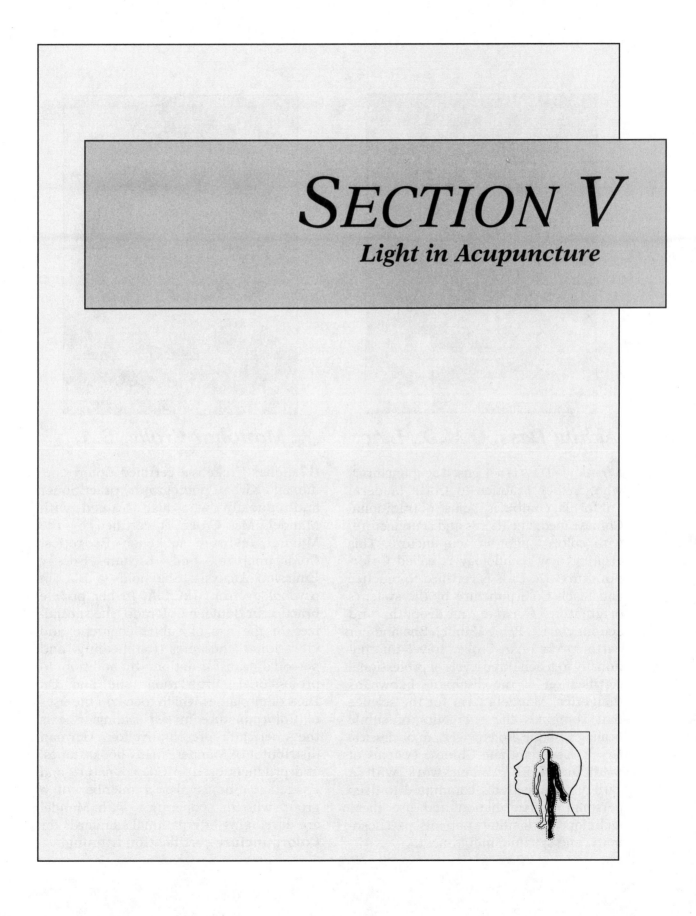

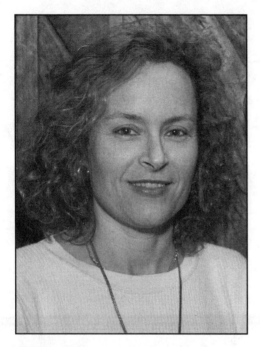

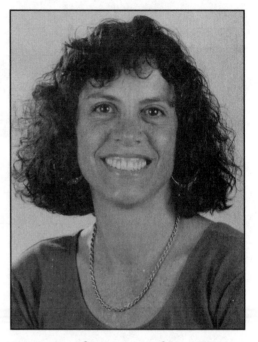

Akhila Dass, O.M.D., L.Ac.

Manohar Croke, B.A.

Dr. Akhila Dass is a licensed acupuncturist, who, in her practice in Corte Madera, California, combines the use of traditional Chinese medicine (herbs and acupuncture) with colored light in acupuncture. This exciting new technology is called **Colorpuncture.** Dr. Dass is certified to practice and teach Colorpuncture by the system's originator, German naturopath and acupuncturist, Peter Mandel. She and her partner, Manohar Croke, travel internationally to teach three levels of professional certification of the discipline known as **Esogetics,** Mandel's term for the science that combines the energetics of subtle healing with the esoteric wisdom of classical Greek, Egyptian, and Chinese systems of medicine. Both women work with a variety of individuals committed to deep personal transformation and use these techniques to facilitate patients' psychosomatic and spiritual unfoldment.

Manohar Croke is a certified Colorpuncture and **Kirlian photography practitioner** and educator who also trained with Mandel. Ms. Croke is certified by the Mandel Institute to teach Esogetics, Colorpuncture, and Kirlian Energy Emission Analysis. She holds a B.A. in psychology from U.C.L.A. In her private practice in Boulder, Colorado, she specializes in the use of subtle energetic and vibrational therapies for healing and personal transformation. In addition to professional certification, she and Dr. Dass offer classes which focus on the uses of Colorpuncture in self-healing. She is the American representative for a German distributor of Mandel's many books, tapes, and products used in Colorpuncture and Esogetics. She is also a member of a group who in cooperation with Mandel are developing international standards for **Colorpuncture certification training.**

CHAPTER ELEVEN

Colorpuncture and Esogetic Healing:
The Use of Colored Light in Acupuncture

Akhila Dass, O.M.D., L.Ac., and Manohar Croke, B.A.

*I*t is our pleasure to introduce you to **Colorpuncture** and the work of **Peter Mandel.** Imagine **a healing system that relies solely on colored light** — not coherent light or laser quality — but of flashlight quality — a gentle, painless system which simultaneously imparts healing information to the body, mind and psyche, by placing different colored glass (silicon) tips of an ***Acu-light Pen***[1] on the skin at selected acupoints. Imagine further that this system would not only support your physical well being, but also become an invaluable tool for expanding your awareness and understanding of who you are and why you are here. Colorpuncture helps people move more easily toward the blossoming of their potential, while gently unwinding and releasing the traumas, emotional scars, and negative beliefs that stand in their way.

What is Colorpuncture?

Colorpuncture is a system of colored light therapy largely based on the concepts of acupuncture.[2] While other methods of phototherapy use the eyes and large areas of the skin as entry points for light into the system, **Colorpuncture uses acupuncture points from Chinese medicine to transmit light through the meridian system.** Similar to acupuncture, Colorpuncture presupposes that the balanced flow of energy through the meridian system will support good health. Whereas acupuncture treatments use needles to move the life force (chi) to create homeostasis, Colorpuncture accomplishes a similar

---

1. See diagram and photo of ***Acu-light Pen*** on *page 256.*
2. Although acupuncture in this country is considered a form of alternative healing, it is the oldest known system of medicine, having been practiced for approximately 5,000 years. Justifiably it could be conceived as traditional medicine.

goal by adding new information to the system via the use of different frequencies of colored light, thereby offering a new and unique dimension of healing.

Many Colorpuncture points are derived from traditional acupuncture points and from other holographic grid systems such as reflexology and applied kinesiology, as well as new points Mandel discovered in his clinical practice.[3] Each color of light is a different wavelength or frequency and sends a different vibration into the energy system. It is thought that when colored light meets the skin, it is translated into vibrational impulses at the molecular level, which travel along the meridian system to the brain at the speed of light. These informational patterns help clear and balance the entire energy system, which includes the meridians and life energy fields around the body.

The History of Colorpuncture

Colorpuncture was originally founded and is still being developed by **Peter Mandel,** a German naturopathic and chiropractic physician and acupuncturist. **Mandel's Institute for Esogetic Medicine** (Mandel Institut Für Esogetische Medizin) is located in **Bruchsal, Germany,** where he maintains an extensive practice and engages in ongoing research and international training activities.

Mandel is the founder of the *Energy Emission Analysis (EEA)* diagnostic system and of Colorpuncture. He is a well-known figure in German medicine. Many of his articles have appeared in scientific periodicals. The books he has authored include: *Energy Emission Analysis, Acu-Impulse Therapy, A Practical Compendium of Colorpuncture (Volumes 1 & 2), and Esogetics: The Sense and Nonsense of Sickness and Pain.* He studied acupuncture in Hong Kong and India. In 1987, with the discovery of the ***transmitter relays,*** an important building block was added to his development of *Esogetic Medicine.*

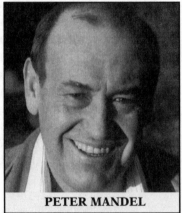

PETER MANDEL

---

3. Reflexology is a system of bodywork based on the premise that there are areas on both the hands and feet that correspond to every part of the body. Reflexes on the hands and feet are stimulated by manual pressure to effect changes in the corresponding glands and organs. Reflexology is the leading form of complementary healing in Denmark and has been demonstrated to be effective in the management of PMS, anxiety, hypertension, and pain.

Applied Kinesiology is a system of assessing (and alleviating) glandular and organ imbalances by the demonstration of weaknesses in certain muscle groups. Kinesiology is often used to augment other diagnostic methods and has been widely adopted by chiropractors in the treatment of musculoskeletal imbalances, and with pain, endocrine, immune, and digestive problems.

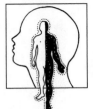

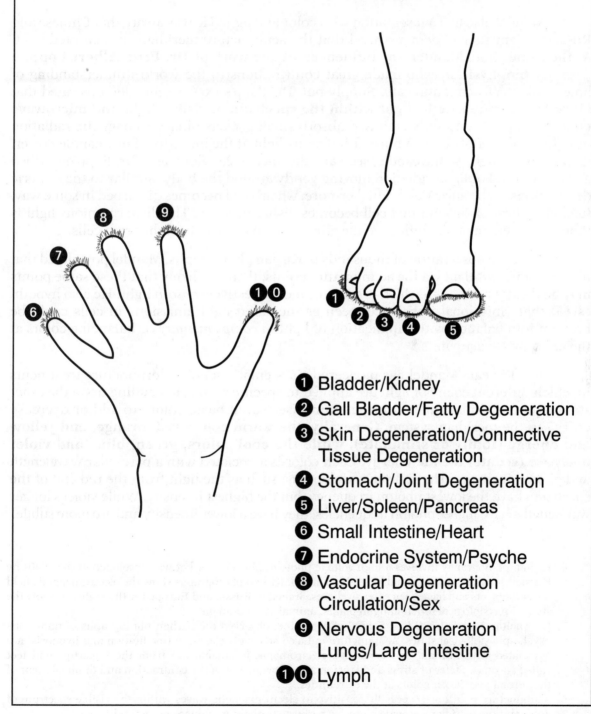

Energy Emission Analysis
Organ/Meridian Correspondences

1 Bladder/Kidney

2 Gall Bladder/Fatty Degeneration

3 Skin Degeneration/Connective Tissue Degeneration

4 Stomach/Joint Degeneration

5 Liver/Spleen/Pancreas

6 Small Intestine/Heart

7 Endocrine System/Psyche

8 Vascular Degeneration Circulation/Sex

9 Nervous Degeneration Lungs/Large Intestine

10 Lymph

Mandel's initial step in the development of Colorpuncture began when he acquired a **Kirlian Camera**[4] in the early 1970s. He began taking black and white photos of the energetic patterns of the fingers and toes, and wondered if the rays of life energy that emanated from the skin in the photos might have something to do with the acupuncture meridians. After extensive observations with hundreds of patients, Mandel confirmed his hypothesis and developed a method of reading specific energy imbalances with Kirlian photography.[5]

Mandel also had a fascination with color and light. He was aware that Chinese and Russian scientists had demonstrated that the acupuncture meridians transmitted light. At the same time, Mandel was influenced by the work of **Dr. Fritz Albert Popp, a German biophysicist,** who made great contributions to the world's understanding of how human cells communicate. Simply put, Dr. Popp's experiments demonstrated that **all cells communicate by light within the spectrum of visible light and microwave energy.** All cells constantly emit and absorb small packets of electromagnetic radiation or light, called *biophotons*. A normal cell emits light at the intensity of one candle power, defined as the light of one candle, seen at a distance of 25 kilometers. Dr. Popp described a constant level of light radiation moving gently around the body (similar to the esoteric descriptions of the auric field). Furthermore, when a cell becomes disturbed in some way, the light vibration around that cell becomes disharmonious. The disharmonious light is thought to detrimentally influence the vibrational patterns of neighboring cells.

After the observation of thousands of Kirlian photographs, Mandel postulated that if organisms *emit* light via the acupuncture points, then it is likely that these same points may be the doors through which organisms most effectively *absorb* light. He also hypothesized that vibrational imbalances seen as increased light emissions in cells could be brought into balance by the application of light in *complementary* or balancing colors at the appropriate acupoints.[6]

For 15 years Mandel has pioneered a systematic set of Colorpuncture treatments in which different colors of light are applied to specific points, depending upon the exact state of energy imbalance. Colorpuncture uses seven basic colors to add or decrease energy to the meridian system. **Generally, the warm colors red, orange, and yellow add energy (tonify or stimulate), while the cool colors, green, blue, and violet decrease (sedate) the life energy.** Each color is associated with a particular wavelength and photon intensity. The shorter wavelengths, such as the light from the red end of the spectrum, have the lowest photon frequency, but the highest intensity. While violet's longer wavelengths have higher photon frequencies, they have a lower intensity and are more subtle.

---

4. Kirlian photography involves a high voltage photographic device that was developed in the 1940s by Russian scientists Semyon and Valentina Kirlian. Kirlian photographs show the electromagnetic field around objects and have been extensively researched in Russia and Europe for the ability to show the state of physiological functioning in plants, animals, and humans.

5. Dr. Thelma Moss, at U.C.L.A. School of Medicine, observed the Kirlian photographs of numerous psycho-physiological states. Acupuncture induced states of relaxation (meditation and hypnosis) are associated with brilliant and expansive electromagnetic emanations from the fingertips and feet called coronas. States of stress and tension are associated with the contraction and diminishment of the corona and darker colors at the extremities.

6. Acupuncture points are especially sensitive to electromagnetic waves within the visible spectrum of light, and the meridians provide a precise pathway for light to induce energetic shifts.

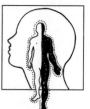

Therapeutic Applications of Color in Colorpuncture

According to Mandel's experience these colors have the following physical and psychological effects when applied on the skin by the methods of Colorpuncture.

RED is the most yang, warm or stimulating color.

• *Physically* it tonifys and produces heat. The most penetrating color, it stimulates vital energy, aids circulation of the blood, and decreases anemia, asthma, diseases of the larynx, certain skin diseases (such as eczema), and chronic coughs. It stimulates the sensory nervous system and energizes sight, smell, hearing, and touch. It stimulates healing of wounds without pus and is used in treatment of chronic infections and insufficiency diseases.

• *Psychologically* Red (caution) is associated with choleric temperament (easily angered, bad-tempered), and too much Red can lead to anger or to becoming more hyperactive and talkative.

ORANGE is a mixture of Red and Yellow and is a gentler, tonifying yang color, less intense than Red.

• *Physically* it stimulates appetite and milk production, relieves cramps and spasms, increases blood pressure, induces vomiting, relieves gas, and builds bones.

In combination with Blue it regulates the endocrine system. Used in the treatment of arteriosclerosis, sclerencephaly, cardiosclerosis, anemia, and anorexia.

• *Psychologically* it can stimulate joy, optimism, and enthusiasm.

This color is used to treat certain conditions of mental illness, as it relieves pessimism, helps lift depression, and warms the heart.

YELLOW is also a yang color, the brightest of all colors.

• *Physically* stimulates and strengthens the motor nervous system, metabolism, and the glandular, lymphatic, and digestive systems; increases gastric secretions and bowel movements and general energy levels. It is indicated for conditions of the liver, bladder, kidneys, and the stomach.

• *Psychologically* stimulates intellectual functioning, such as learning and comprehension in adults and children with learning disabilities. It is associated with more sanguine temperaments (such as with cheerfulness, confidence, detachment, optimism, and sweetness).

(continued on next page)

GREEN is the most neutral of the yin colors and is only slightly cooling.

• *Physically* it is used in the treatment of conditions of lungs, eyes (styes and cysts), diabetes, musculoskeletal and inflammatory joint problems, and ulcers.

It is antibacterial, disinfectant, and aids in the detoxification and cleansing of the body.

• *Psychologically* it calms, soothes, relaxes and balances. It is associated with the phlegmatic temperament, which is slow-moving, unemotional and apathetic.

BLUE is a yin or cool color.

• *Physically* it produces profound relaxation of the body and mind; reduces fever, congestion, itching, irritation, and pain (headaches, migraines); arrests discharges, hemorrhages, and oozing wounds; used to treat high blood pressure, burns, inflammations with pus and all diseases involving heat.[1]

It also contracts tissues, muscles (spasms), hemorrhoids, and hyperthyroid conditions.

• *Psychologically* it is calming and tranquilizing when used on the pituitary and pineal acupoints. It is used in the treatment of attention deficit hyperactivity disorder (ADHD). post-traumatic stress disorder (PTSD), insomnia, phobias, and endocrine imbalances (such as menopausal difficulties).

Should not be used for the treatment of all types of depression, as it is a melancholy (depressing) color.

VIOLET, the most yin color.

• *Physically* it works on the spleen and is used in combination with Yellow to increase lymph production, control hunger, and balance the nervous system.

• *Psychologically* it reduces irritability and balances the right brain.

Violet acts on the unconscious and amplifies the effects of meditation.

---

1. See *Chapter Two:* Light History: An Historical Overview, page 46, for Dr. Baldwin's comments. In the early 1920s, American surgeon, Dr. Kate Baldwin wrote of her successful experience using blue light (Dinshah's color projection methods directly on the body) to aid in pain management and to promote the healing of burns and wounds.

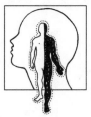

The Soul-Spirit Colors

The *Soul-Spirit Colors* are said to facilitate the awareness of the deeper layers of the psyche and spirit. Working with the four special colors in the context of Colorpuncture Therapy as propounded by Mandel assumes extensive knowledge and experience in treatment using the seven basic colors, particularly because the therapeutic effects of the four special colors can be many times more intense. A special glass color set is used in *mental therapy*, which goes even deeper into the various levels of consciousness. The soul-spirit colors include: **turquoise, crimson, light green,** and **rose.** Treatments with these colors may precipitate sudden strong psychosomatic reactions that generally soon give way to insights and feelings of well-being.

Colorpuncture's Use of Complementary Colors

The use of different colors in Colorpuncture is based on **Goethe's original theory of complementary (*warm and cool*) colors.** Warm and cool colors are used to balance yin and yang energy flows in the meridians. Each color has its own complementary color (yellow-violet, orange-blue, red-green) which is used to create different effects on different meridians or zones on the physical body and subtle body.

Mandel discovered **you can also tonify or sedate the acupuncture meridians by using complementary pairs of colors. Generally, red, orange, and yellow *stimulate*, while green, blue, and violet *sedate*. There are complementary pairs of sedating and stimulating colors assigned to each meridian; and these are used bilaterally to treat the same acupuncture meridian.** First you treat the more painful points (a sign of energy excess) with the cooler color, then you balance with the warmer color. On any given point the energy is balanced by treating the excess with the cooler color first and balancing the energy with the warmer color.

We reserve the right to marvel at color's occurrences and meanings, to admire, and, if possible, uncover color's secrets.
— Goethe

Any kind of disease should be considered as an alarm signal for disharmonies in spirit and soul . . .We have to turn away from our suffering and sickness, because they are the hindrances on our path towards the inner. We have to bid farewell to those frustrations and fears which prevent us from progressing and from coming into contact with our higher selves.
— Peter Mandel

Primary and Complementary Colors Used in Colorpuncture

Color	Action	Indications	Organs	Qualities
RED &	Hot color, color with the greatest penetration, strongly stimulates the flow of blood	Poor circulation, inflammation, chronic cough, asthma, anemia, eczema	Heart, lungs, muscles	Love, anger, wrath, joy
GREEN	Neutral color, treats chronic problems, sedative, soothing, relaxing	Whooping cough, inflammation of the joints, tumors, ulcers, cysts, eye diseases, diabetes	Lungs	Contentment, tranquility
BLUE &	Cold color, has a relaxing effect, used for all diseases involving heat	Pain, congestion, hemorrhoids, warts, sleeplessness, impotence, frigidity, menopausal difficulties	Pituitary gland, endocrine system, contraction of muscles, ligaments and tissues	Quietness, reserve
ORANGE	Gives energy, makes joyful, color of the sun	Pessimism, psychosis, depression, fear, arteriosclerosis, emaciation, anemia, tiredness	Heart	Joy, happiness
YELLOW &	Fortifies the endocrine system, makes chronic processes acute	Diseases of digestive tract, strengthens the nervous system	Liver, bladder, kidneys, stomach	Intelligence, comprehension, cheerfulness
VIOLET	Acts on consciousness, promotes awareness, prepares for meditation	Lymphatic system disorders	Spleen	Meditation

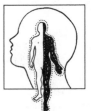

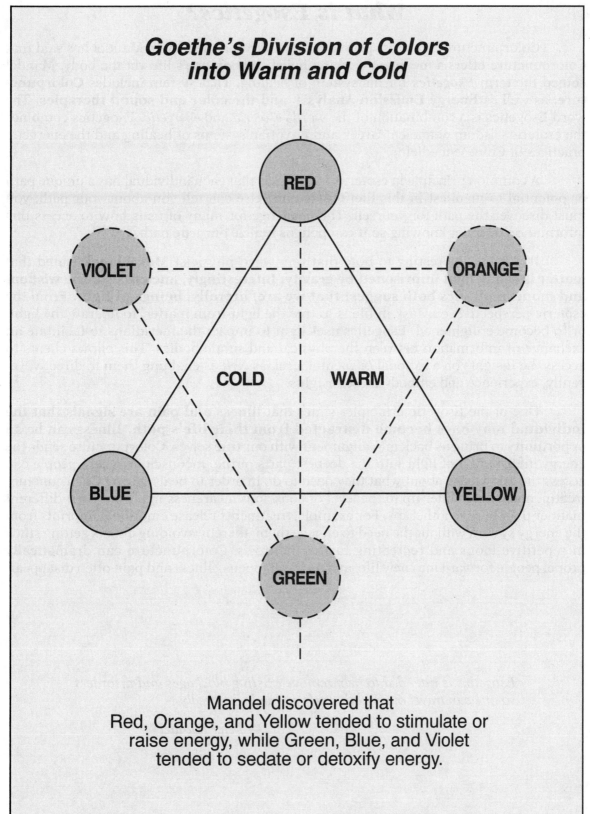

Goethe's Division of Colors into Warm and Cold

RED

VIOLET

ORANGE

COLD   WARM

BLUE

YELLOW

GREEN

Mandel discovered that
Red, Orange, and Yellow tended to stimulate or
raise energy, while Green, Blue, and Violet
tended to sedate or detoxify energy.

What is Esogetics?

Colorpuncture can assist people in transforming their lives. Mandel has said that Colorpuncture offers a means of working holistically on one's life via the body. Mandel coined the term **Esogetics** for his system of healing. That system includes **Colorpuncture**, as well as **Energy Emission Analysis, and the color and sound therapies.** The word Esogetics is a combination of the words *esoteric* and *energetic*. Esogetics combines the esoteric wisdom of ancient Greek and Egyptian systems of healing and the energetic practices of Chinese medicine.

A common principle in esoteric doctrines is that each individual has a unique path or potential to manifest in this lifetime. No one else can tell you about your path; you must discover the path for yourself. The challenge for many of us is how to access this information or inner knowing so it can help us realize our true path.

It is quite interesting to note that renowned physicist **Max Planck** stated that **matter is really light imprisoned by gravity. Interestingly, ancient esoteric wisdom and modern physics both suggest that we are, literally, beings of light.** From the esoteric perspective, our task in life is to free the light from matter, to liberate the light, or to become enlightened. Esogetics uses light to impact the meridians to facilitate an exchange of information between the physical and subtle bodies. This allows clients to access the insights on a rational or mental level, as well as enabling them to directly, yet gently, experience and embody these insights.

One of the Esogetic principles states that **illness and pain are signals that the individual may have become distracted from their life's path.** Illness can be an opportunity to bring us back into alignment with our true selves. Colorpuncture sends the energy/information of light into the deepest parts of the unconscious where people can access the knowledge about what they need to do in order to heal. During Colorpuncture treatments insights filter up to the level of conscious awareness in a somewhat different manner than in psychotherapy. For example, treatments release emotional imprints from the energy system without the need to engage them, thereby avoiding clients getting stuck in repetitive loops and recreating further neurosis. Colorpuncture can dramatically propel people forward into new life, and as this happens, illness and pain often disappear.

Esogetics is intended to help remove existing blockages and disorders so one can travel one's path freely and light-heartedly.

— Peter Mandel

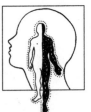

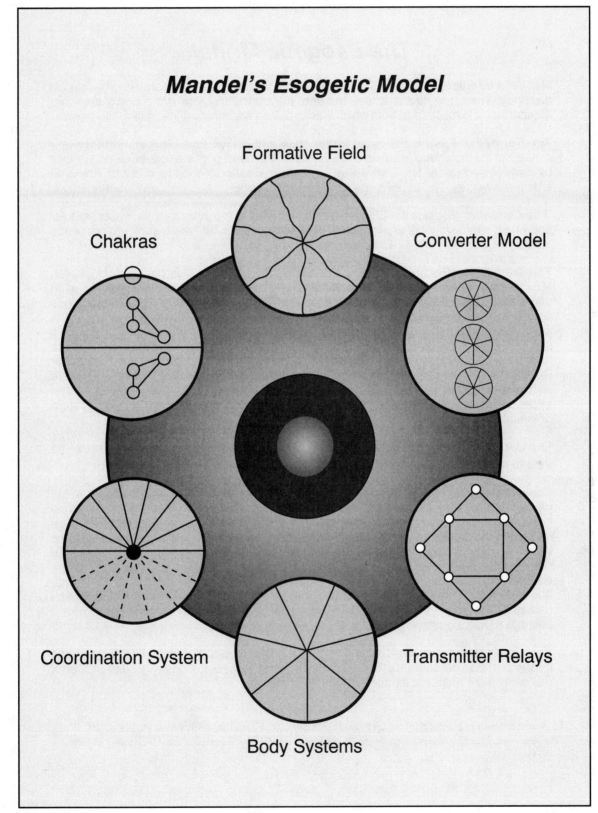

Mandel's Esogetic Model

Formative Field

Chakras

Converter Model

Coordination System

Body Systems

Transmitter Relays

The Esogetic Model

Mandel's Esogetic Model is a holographic representation of how energy is generated in the body. The three circles above the line, from ten o'clock to two o'clock, are what Mandel calls the *subtle level* from which human beings are constantly receiving information.

The Formative Field is the circle at the apex and is likened to **Rupert Sheldrake's** concept of the morphogenetic field and is similar to the concept of the *collective unconscious* by Swiss psychiatrist **Dr. Carl Jung,** or the *superconscious or void* out of which all creation emerges. The upper three spheres represent what Mandel calls "pure energy."

The Converter Model is the Chinese medicine model of the three heaters, upper, middle, and lower; it is the highest expression of pure energy. Out of the three suns you get seven points that evolve into the 147 acupuncture points, our seven subtle energy centers.

The Transmitter Relays are the molecules on the lower right side (four o'clock), which Mandel says are comparable to an executive who sits in a very high managerial position and does nothing but filter out what is good and what is bad for life. This system brings us the information that man as he comes to earth incarnates with a plan or, rather, a partial plan that contains a particular way of proceeding on a particular stretch of one's life. This means that everyone must not only go their own way, understand it, find it, but that there is also someone inside us watching that we do so. Practically, the Transmitter Relays are a series of eight concentric circles around the top of the head, which are treated with light to remove blockages of past trauma. They contain stored memories of all past experiences, including past lives, time in the womb, birth, early childhood, and future potentialities.

The Body Systems are the central lower molecule, representing the organs, and can be treated directly using Colorpuncture.[1]

The Coordination System is the molecule at the lower left side of the model (eight o'clock) that represents parts of the brain: the medulla oblongata, limbic system, pineal gland, thalamus, hypothalamus, pituitary, and corpus callosum. Life has built for us a certain hardware: the central nervous system and the hormonal system and its related structures within our brains. These are what Mandel calls the *coordination organs*. He likens the Coordination System to the puppet operator . . ."It is just the operator. It didn't make the doll; it also has no idea how to direct the play and of course cannot create such a drama. It is a specialist: the one who makes the doll dance." Treating the coordination organs relates to the concept of moving to a higher level of control when confronted with a plethora of mindbody symptoms.

The Chakras are pure light, and it is these subtle levels that contain the energetic imprints of our personal history. The three lower molecules of the Esogetic Model represent the *material* or embodied aspects of energy.

---

1. A more in-depth description of Mandel's Esogetic Model is contained in his latest book, *Esogetics: The Sense and Nonsense of Sickness and Pain* (Hasselbrun, Germany: Energetik Verlag, 1993).

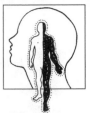

What Happens in a Colorpuncture Treatment?

Colorpuncture offers a tremendous number and variety of treatment possibilities. Typically, sessions begin with the Colorpuncture practitioner talking with the client about any mindbody issues that they would like addressed. Mandel uses a variety of testing methods, but his chief tool in his practice is the Kirlian photograph. A photograph of the client's fingers and toes is taken; and an assessment is made, based on Mandel's Energy Emission Analysis, of the quantity and quality of the movement of the client's life energy. A particular light treatment is then selected and administered to suit the client's needs. At the end of the Colorpuncture treatment another Kirlian photograph is taken so the practitioner and client can see the treatment's effect on the energy system.

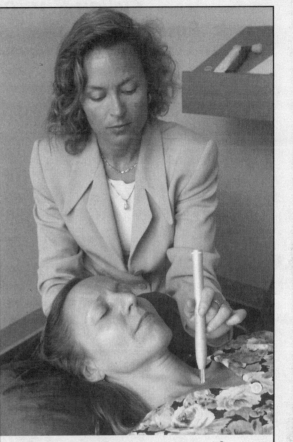

Dr. Dass demonstrating use of Perlux® Colorpuncture Instrument

Kirlian Photographs Before and After a Single Colorpuncture Session

Colorpuncture treatments are hierarchical in their focus and intensity. Treatments usually begin with the focus on the body and balancing the flow of energy. There are a variety of Colorpuncture treatment options that include: treatments to release stress and promote relaxation, energetic detoxification treatments that stimulate the release of stored toxins, or to rebuild energy in degenerative conditions. These foundation treatments help prepare the energy system for higher level treatments so that the energy body can adapt to the inflow of higher level information. Later, more advanced treatments may address clearing out old energetic blockages from prenatal, childhood, or past life traumas, and accessing information regarding the individual's life program.

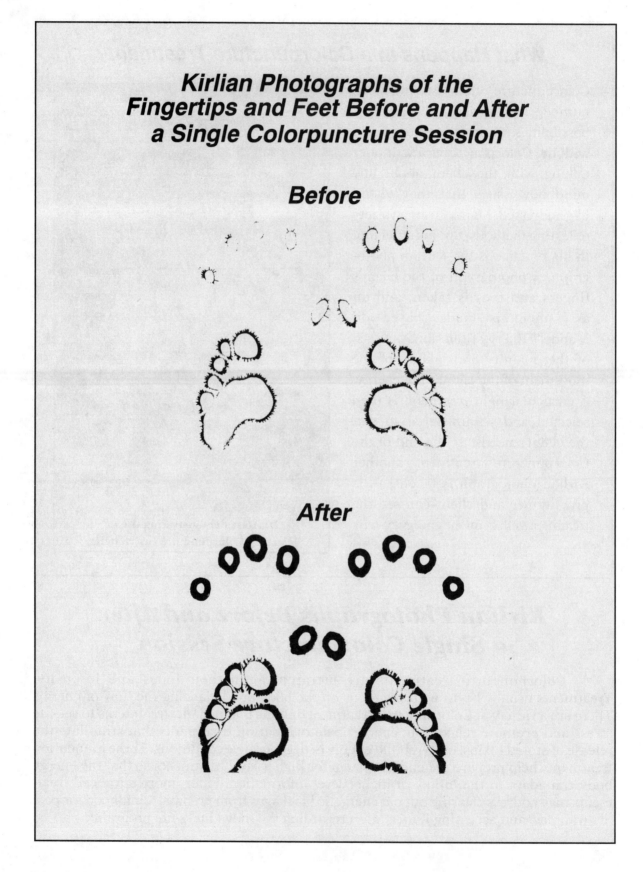

Kirlian Photographs of the Fingertips and Feet Before and After a Single Colorpuncture Session

Before

After

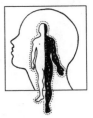

Types of Colorpuncture Treatments

To give you an idea of a few of the main types of Colorpuncture treatments, we want to share a few case histories.

Case History – Dream Zones Treatments

Mandel identified areas of skin on the surface of the body which he calls **Dream Zones.** These zones are the doorways to accessing the information from the subconscious and higher states of consciousness. The Colorpuncturist stimulates these zones with colored light, with the color varying according to the zone. He also developed a particular herbal oil, **Esogetic Dream Oil**, which when rubbed on these zones, causes the person to dream more actively and powerfully. These dreams often allow the person to more easily release a backlog of subconscious material and open this material to more conscious understanding. Mandel recommends daily self-treatments of these areas to facilitate patients' access to their inner wisdom.

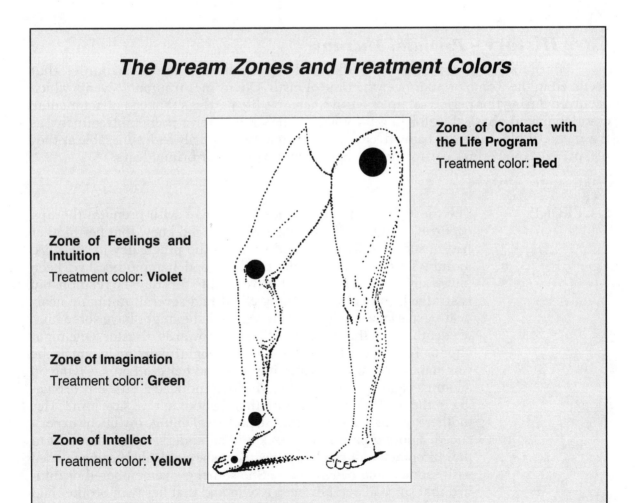

The Dream Zones and Treatment Colors

Zone of Contact with the Life Program

Treatment color: **Red**

Zone of Feelings and Intuition

Treatment color: **Violet**

Zone of Imagination

Treatment color: **Green**

Zone of Intellect

Treatment color: **Yellow**

Ms. CROKE: One of my client's dream experiences clearly demonstrates the value of Colorpuncture treatment of the Dream Zones. The first Dream Zone, located at the hip, is called the *Zone of Contact with the Life Program.* This zone is where people hold unconscious blockages that keep them from moving toward their personal program. A female client presented with a great many physical problems and a lot of uncertainty about how to use her creative potential. I gave her the assignment to treat this zone at home. That night she had a powerful dream. She dreamed she was in her attic boxing up a lot of old junk. One box was labeled, "Too old;" another said "Too fat;" and another said, "Not educated enough." She then took all the boxes down to her backyard and burned them in an incinerator. When she returned to her house, she discovered it had been beautifully decorated. This is a clear example of how the Dream Zones can assist in clearing the subconscious beliefs that prevent us from moving forward on our path. This dream was the beginning of an important healing for this client.

Case History – *Prenatal Therapy*

Prenatal treatments gently evoke and release energetic disharmonies that occurred in the womb or at or near the time of birth. Oftentimes traumatic events which occurred during this period set up repetitive negative life patterns that can affect mental, emotional, and physical well-being throughout one's life. After a prenatal treatment, as the energetic blockages are being released, clients may temporarily feel vulnerable as they reexperience powerful early memories, basic belief patterns or primal fears.

Ms. CROKE: The most dramatic experience I have had with prenatal therapy occurred when I was treating a woman who knew that her mother had unsuccessfully attempted to abort the pregnancy in the third month. Throughout my client's childhood her mother had been physically and emotionally abusive, and to this day the relationship is strained. In her adult life my client had several traumatic near-death experiences. She actually worried she might have some kind of "death wish" that kept impelling her towards disaster. One night after a prenatal treatment, she had an insightful dream in which she was standing beside a swimming pool and her mother was lying on a lounge chair beside the pool. My client noticed a little boy drowning in the pool and asked her mother, "Shouldn't we save him?" Her mother told her not to bother. Upon awakening, my client experienced shooting pain in her neck and shoulders. When she went to the chiropractor, during the adjustment she suddenly became flooded with sadness and began to cry. She somehow remembered or intuited that she had actually been a twin and that her twin brother had died at the time of the attempted abortion. Although she had never

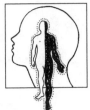

been told this and, in fact, her mother emphatically denied it, my client was sure this was true. To confirm her belief, she went to the hospital where she had been born. Surprisingly, the medical records for her birth indicated that a nonviable and undeveloped male fetus had been born with her! Although this discovery was shocking, my client was very grateful. It helped her to understand many previously unexplained feelings that she had as a child, as well as her conflicted feelings about being alive. This experience opened the door for a new level of healing and completion in her life.

Case History – Function Circle Treatments

There is a set of Colorpuncture treatments which balance the energetic flow in different meridian-organ systems of the body. In Colorpuncture we refer to these systems as *Function Circles,* and we are especially concerned with helping the client understand the emotional qualities and life issues associated with each Function Circle. According to Mandel's *Function Circle Model of Development,* we are born into the *Kidney-Bladder Function Circle.* Kidney-Bladder is associated with *fear,* and the life issues have to do with developing the courage to take our next steps in life. Fear is the first emotion we encounter when we move from one plane of existence to another, as in birth. If, as often happens, we are unable to experience or express this fear consciously, then it becomes an unconscious or repressed energetic burden which we carry with us as we move into the *Liver-Gall Bladder Function Circle.* In Liver-Gall Bladder the emotional quality becomes anger. Our repressed fear is now hidden behind a wall of *anger.* To deal with this anger we must learn about expressing this energy openly, which can lead to the potential for creative self-expression. For most of us the honest expression of anger is not currently or culturally accepted. Anger becomes a part of the repressed emotional baggage which we carry with us as we move on to the *Lung-Large Intestine Function Circle.* Lung-Large Intestine is associated with the emotion of *melancholy* or *sadness.* Here we must learn about loss, letting go and accepting or allowing our grief. As we experience the depth of our sadness we can discover the hidden potential for sensitivity, intuition, and inspiration. If, as typically happens, we are unable to consciously experience the pain of our grief, it too becomes repressed. Now, the accumulation of these repressed emotions begins to turn into stress as we move into the *Function Circle of Stomach-Spleen-Pancreas.* Here our minds begin to express stress in the form of *excessive worry* and *compulsive thinking.* If we are unable to release this stress — for example, by moving the obsessive mind into states of no-mind or meditation and by learning to make life choices for ourselves which are truly nourishing — the stress accumulates and becomes chronic.

Normally, we circle around these four Function Circles many times throughout our lives, moving through fear, anger, sadness, worry, and stress; and the burden of unlived emotions weighs upon us and more. Eventually this energetic burden becomes so great that it begins to weigh upon the last *Function Circle, the Heart-Small Intestine.* The heart-small intestine is seen as higher than the other four Function Circles, as it is symbolized *(see chart on page 251)* as the center or the upper tip of the pyramid. In the heart we normally find the qualities of pure *joy, compassion, humility,* and *love,* as well as the potential for illumination. **Mandel sees the heart as the central meridian and love as an important quality to develop on our journey towards self-realization.**

No stress or problem actually originates in the heart. Instead, the unresolved issues of the other four Function Circles eventually begin to put a stress on the heart and affect it's proper functioning. When we treat the Function Circles, we seek to clear the accumulated energetic blockages affecting these meridians. **Thus, the goal in Color-puncture is to treat the client to bring energetic balance to these meridian systems.** As treatments progress, the client may experience the release of long repressed and strong emotions. As these feelings are released and the client's life understanding deepens, physical symptoms may improve or disappear altogether.

DR. DASS: One of my earliest experiences with Colorpuncture was very simple, yet, life-altering. I had a cold, and I treated the psychological aspects of the cold by applying light to points for the lungs and the colon. As I mentioned previously, the lungs have to do with letting go. Mandel taught us a treatment that involves a set of complementary colors, red-green, that facilitate the bereavement process by targeting points around the lungs. At that point in my life I needed to let go of some feelings and issues around my mother. As the energy was moving through my body, I profoundly understood the deeper message of the cold; and after these feelings were released, the cold was literally gone in a matter of minutes! Even though this was a relatively minor illness, the experience gave me a deeper and clearer insight into the synchronous functioning of the mindbody.

The quality of the sound's energetic structure, frequency, modulation and so on, is such that the same areas of response are reached via the ear as through color, via the acu-sound therapies, which are extremely well suited to prophylaxis and regular self-treatment.

— Peter Mandel

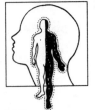

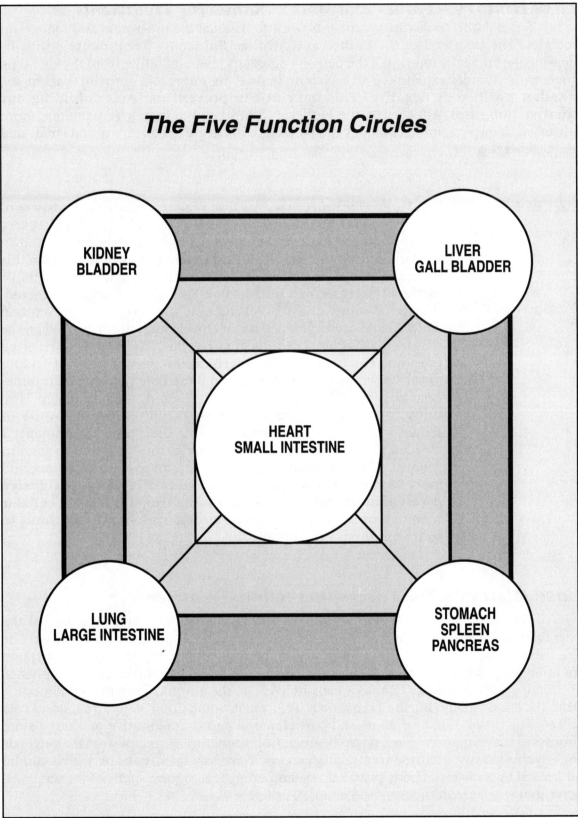

251

Case History – Father and Mother Balancing Treatments

Several Colorpuncture treatments work to balance the male *yang* and female *yin* energies. The first level of the **Father and Mother Balancing Treatments** begins by clearing the energetic imprint of the person's actual mother and father from the energetic system. As Mandel explains, **every parent leaves an energetic imprint within us, whether positive or negative. This imprint can prevent us from unfolding our creative potential.** After using the Father and Mother Balancing Treatments, more advanced Colorpuncture techniques can be used to integrate the client's unique male and female energies.

Ms. CROKE: The Father Treatment was my first real experience of the power of Colorpuncture. My mother and father divorced when I was very young and I had experienced great pain about never having known my father. Even though I had done psychotherapeutic work on this issue and was feeling relatively clear and resolved about it, within a matter of thirty seconds into the first Father Treatment I felt incredible terror in my body. I realized that somehow, as a very young child, I had been frightened for my life around my father. When the treatment was completed, the fear receded. The next day I received the same treatment and I experienced a deeper layer of feeling toward my father. I experienced an incredible rage and determination to protect myself, which later receded after treatment. The third day I experienced the release of an unbearable sense of sadness, loss, and abandonment. After the Father Treatments I noticed a subtle improvement in my ability to relate to men in general. Also, my relationship with my lover became deeper and more satisfying. **I realized that even after doing extensive psychotherapy on an issue, a trauma can still leave a cellular memory or an energetic impression which can continue to subconsciously effect one's life.**

Case History – The Transmitter Relays Treatments

Mandel describes the ***Transmitter Relays*** as the "watchman at the gate of the energy body." These areas contain stored memories from all our past experiences. The Transmitters also contain information about the individual's *life program* or purpose. Treating the points in this area usually consists of a series of ten Colorpuncture treatments. By treating the Transmitter Points we can often release the trauma of negative conditioning from the energy body. During Transmitter Treatment, some Colorpuncturists ask clients to keep a journal of their dreams and participate in certain meditative or altered state processes that support the energetic healing. Colorpuncturists may also make referrals for psychotherapy, as these treatments can elicit archetypal situations which can be addressed by a variety of body-oriented psychotherapy techniques, such as bioenergetics, voice dialogue, gestalt therapy, and breath work.

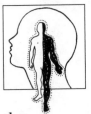

During the Transmitter Treatments, as these blockages begin to dissolve and the energy begins to move, people may temporarily experience a variety of strong feelings and sensations as old memories surface and are released. **After treatment, people report feeling increased physical energy, enhanced creativity, greater clarity of mind, and a reduction in addictive habit patterns.**

DR. DASS: I'd like to give you an example of working with the Transmitter Relays. I had a client who was working in the sex industry, who had extremely deficient kidney and heart pulses. Emotionally, this meant that there was a lack of love in her life and that she had lost her will to live. Her kidney pulse reflected a very deep sense of unworthiness. I treated her Transmitter Relays over the course of a year, and during that time she stopped working in the sex industry, began her first deep relationship with a man, and entered psychotherapy to examine issues around her sexuality and family of origin. After a year of Transmitter treatments her kidney and heart pulses completely normalized, which is quite unusual given the seriousness of her problems. Also, during that time I augmented her Colorpuncture treatments with Chinese herbs and acupuncture. Subsequent to treatment this client also entered sex therapy and recovered sensations in her previously numb pelvic and genital regions. At that point she also began to develop and market her unique skills as a gifted porcelain doll maker.

Everything that flows can be considered as healthy. Strain is only experienced if congestion and blockages hinder the flow, regardless of the cause of these blockages . . . Disease is a reflection of the inner; it is the opposite of health. Health is usually associated with joy, happiness, and a pain-free life; with having ideas and being able to live them out; with being active and being able to laugh; with being able to perceive and recognize things others cannot or choose not to see. Disease means frustration, pain, the paralysis of life . . . Disease is walking on a wrong path, or one that has been taken only because the right path could not be recognized . . . There is only one simple road to well-being: one's own path.

— *Peter Mandel*

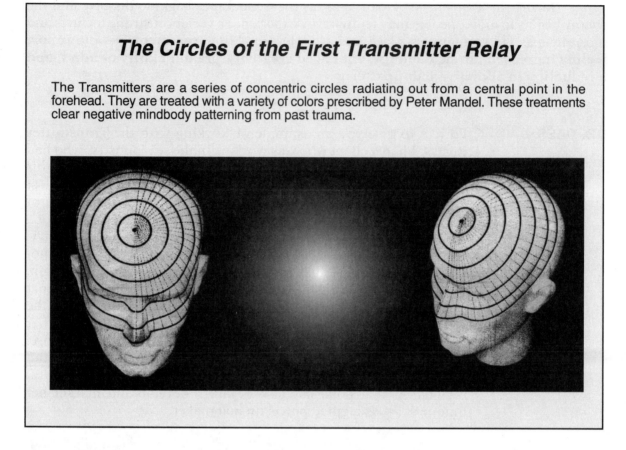

The Circles of the First Transmitter Relay

The Transmitters are a series of concentric circles radiating out from a central point in the forehead. They are treated with a variety of colors prescribed by Peter Mandel. These treatments clear negative mindbody patterning from past trauma.

Case History – Conflict Resolution Therapy

     Conflict Resolution Therapy is a series of Colorpuncture treatments aimed at bringing up an individual's primary conflicts stored as memories in the deeper portions of the brain. During the course of these treatments, deeply conflicting issues and out-moded beliefs surface and are unwound and released, which in turn, dramatically support the person's healing. In Germany Mandel has people come to his clinic from all over the world, and it is reported that he has successfully used these treatments for a variety of acutely and chronically ill patients, such as those suffering from cancer and multiple sclerosis.

DR. DASS: A Chinese-American woman I recently treated was severely sexually abused as a child by her father. Physically, she presented with a complete lack of physical sensation from her waist to her knees. At that point she was facing a major life decision: whether to go back to an abusive husband, whom she had previously left, or to create a new life with a new lover, who was a woman. As a result of her inability to make this decision, she was suffering from extreme nervous tension. After two weeks of Conflict Resolution Therapy, she entered my office, saying that she realized that her conflict was not about whether she should be sexually active with a man or a woman, rather it reflected even deeper issues about her own identity.

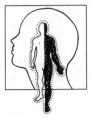

Color/Sound Therapies and Esogetic Sound Patterns

Having explored the therapeutic uses of colored light, Mandel became interested in whether it might be possible to influence energy flow in the meridians with sound and music. Working with a team of composers and music educators, Mandel developed his *color/sound therapies.* These involve audiotaped sound patterns that contain frequencies that are equivalent to the vibrational patterns of the various Colorpuncture treatments. For example, a particular sound treatment might deal with strengthening the immune system, relieving insomnia, stress, or headaches. Mandel's research, in collaboration with **composers and music educators Kay Korten and Ludovika Helm,** led to the discovery of certain frequencies, patterns, and modulations associated with certain brain centers, such as the thalamus, pituitary, and so on. Since improper functionting of these "coordination organs" is associated with psychosomatic illness, the aim of these tapes is to release psychological pressures such as fear and stress, thereby improving the functioning of these centers. By the use of these sounds brainwave activity between the left and right cerebral hemispheres becomes synchronized and gently guided to states of profound relaxation. The Color/Sound Tapes provide an extremely pleasant, comfortable, and mood-elevating experience for the listener.

Next, Mandel developed the *Esogetic Sound Pattern Tapes.* These tapes also translate the vibrations of color into equivalent vibrations of sound to affect the energy system. The Esogetic Sound Pattern Tapes are designed to stimulate different aspects of Mandel's Esogetic Model. Rather than focusing on particular symptoms, these tapes work to expand and deepen the awareness and perception of one's felt experience. These tapes are especially powerful when used in conjunction with the Dream Zone Therapy and Esogetic Oils on the Dream Zones.

Self-Treatments

While many Colorpuncture treatments need to be done by a trained therapist, there are several things that can be done by the client at home, under supervision of a therapist. If the client has an *Acu-light Pen,* he or she can do particular treatments at home between visits to the Colorpuncture practitioner. Mandel also created aromatic *Esogetic Dream Oils* that can be used on the body's Dream Zones to enhance dream activity and recall. Clients can also simultaneously use the Color/Sound Therapy tapes or Esogetic Sound Pattern tapes to enhance the treatment process.

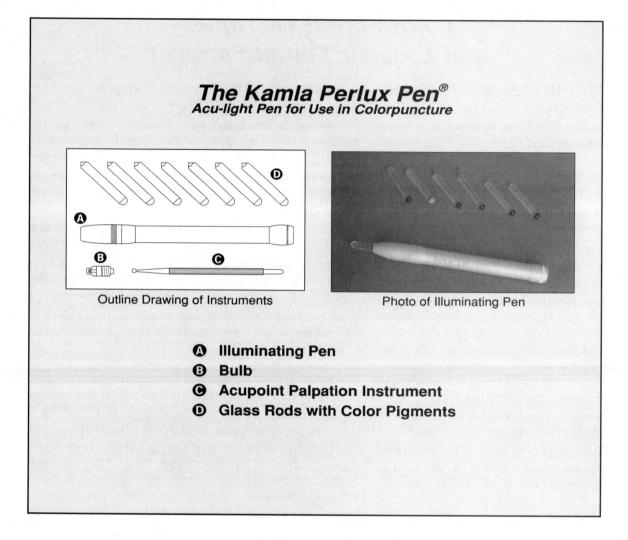

Before we close, we would like to share a quote by Mandel that captures the essence of Colorpuncture:

We who are imprisoned in matter have to bring our "I" out of matter and darkness and into the light. On the level of the spiritual world we humans, in our wholeness are light beings. We must and always will develop toward the Absolute Light which we call God. In this process we are accompanied by light on the outside, and if we allow it, by the light on the inside.

— Peter Mandel

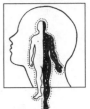

This is a brief sample of the work that is so powerfully supported by Colorpuncture. Colored light is an empowering, direct, yet gentle vehicle to assist us in our journey to the realization of our true selves.

QUESTION: How were you introduced to Colorpuncture?

DR. DASS: In June of 1989, I was living in India where I was one of five acupuncturists who attended a one week seminar on Colorpuncture taught by an Italian medical doctor. This seminar met with such success that Peter Mandel returned six months later to teach a class of over 150 people.

Ms. CROKE: It was also in 1989 that I first met Mandel, when he was invited to the **Osho Multiversity in Pune, India,** to teach Colorpuncture. **My spiritual teacher, Osho, was excited about the potential of Colorpuncture, which he believed was a helpful method for clearing the energy body so that meditation could occur more easily.**

QUESTION: How has Colorpuncture been received in Germany and Europe?

Ms. CROKE: It has been received quite well. We are excited to report that the German government has recently adopted Mandel's System of Colorpuncture as part of the educational requirements for the licensing of naturopathic practitioners known as Heilpraktiker.

Colorpuncture Training

For the last six years we have continued to train with Mandel and are both certified by the Mandel Institute to teach the first three levels of Colorpuncture certification courses, as well as Kirlian Energy Emission Analysis. We also teach a two-day, introductory, self-healing workshop which shows people how to use some of the simpler Colorpuncture treatments, such as the Dream Zones, for their own education and healing. We currently offer a longer, twelve-day, level one Colorpuncture certification course; and in the future we will offer more advanced levels of training.[7] Until recently, Colopuncture training was only available in Europe, and Mandel conducted all of his trainings in German. Today Colorpuncture is being taught worldwide. Mandel has instituted a formal certification process for his instructors. We have both been certified by Mandel to teach Colorpuncture and conduct trainings in English.[8] Students who complete the training receive Certification from the Mandel Institute.

---

7. For information on Treatments and Colorpuncture trainings in the United States, see listings for Dr. Akhila Dass, Manohar Croke and Dr. Helge Prosak in the *Resource List: Section Five, page 371, Colorpuncture Practitioners and Trainers.*

8. Mandel's Colorpuncture and Esogetic Medicine texts are listed in the *Bibliography* under "Light in Homeopathy and Acupuncture" (Colorpuncture and Kirlian Photography).

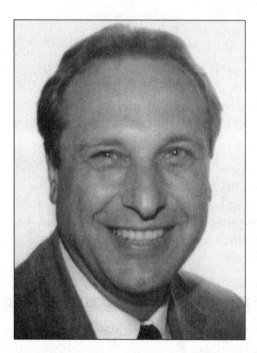

David Olszewski, E.E., I.E.

*D*avid Olszewski is both an electrical and industrial engineer with over 30 years of experience in the fields of electronics, light, and computers. He is the Director of Computer Information Systems for a West Coast petroleum company and the **President of the Light Energy Company in Seattle, Washington,** which markets most of the phototherapy products discussed in this book. As an **inventor and product developer,** Mr. Olszewski, together with his wife **Pamela Baker-Olszewski,** a registered nurse, hold patents in several countries for light emitting diode (LED) devices (an alternative for low power lasers), such as **The Light Shaker**™ and **Tri-Light**™, which are used in acupuncture, pain management, and wound healing. As a popular speaker in the field of holistic health, he lectures and consults across the country on the deleterious effects of artificial lighting and electromagnetic radiation, and the healing potential of sunlight, full spectrum lighting and monochromatic single frequency lights applied through the eyes, directly on the skin and through the acupuncture meridian system. His rich background in electronics, computer science, engineering, and health offers a pragmatic approach to the understanding and application of light in our daily lives.

CHAPTER TWELVE

Getting Into Light:
The Use of Phototherapy in Everyday Life

David Olszewski, E.E., I.E.,
and Brian Breiling, Psy.D.

The purpose of this chapter is to provide you with a review of the key concepts of light and phototherapy to enable you to make informed decisions regarding professional and self-care applications. Phototherapy can be an important supplement and complement to your normal medical treatment and personal health regimen.

Sunlight is a Cornerstone of Mindbody Wellness

Sunlight consists not only of light within the visible spectrum, but also components within the ultraviolet and infrared spectra as well. Infrared light is associated with heating, while ultraviolet is associated with tanning. Each of the visible colors is not just a single wavelength, but is comprised of a broad range of wavelengths that appear to us as bands of color. The sun's rays consist of a rainbow of colors within and beyond the visible spectrum, broken into approximately 700 band widths (or wavelengths) within the visible spectrum, ranging primarily from 290 nanometers to 990 nanometers (nm). For example, green is comprised of 70 different wavelengths within the range of 490-560 nm.

The entire spectrum of natural sunlight is essential for optimal functioning of all living cells in plants, animals, and humans. For example, plant growth is stimulated by infrared light, while the blue end of the spectrum encourages blossoming. Similarly, **Dr. Richard Wurtman, Professor of Endocrinology at Massachusetts Institute of Technology,** states that wavelengths of light are similar to vitamins and minerals since humans also appear to require a broad spectrum of frequencies for physical, emotional, and mental well-being. As it enters the eye each wavelength may have a specific role to play in our mindbody functioning. Our bodies require food, oxygen, and sunlight to live. **Light is the second most important environmental input, after food, in controlling bodily functions.** Thus, a lack of sunlight can lead to disease, just as a lack of food, air, and water does.

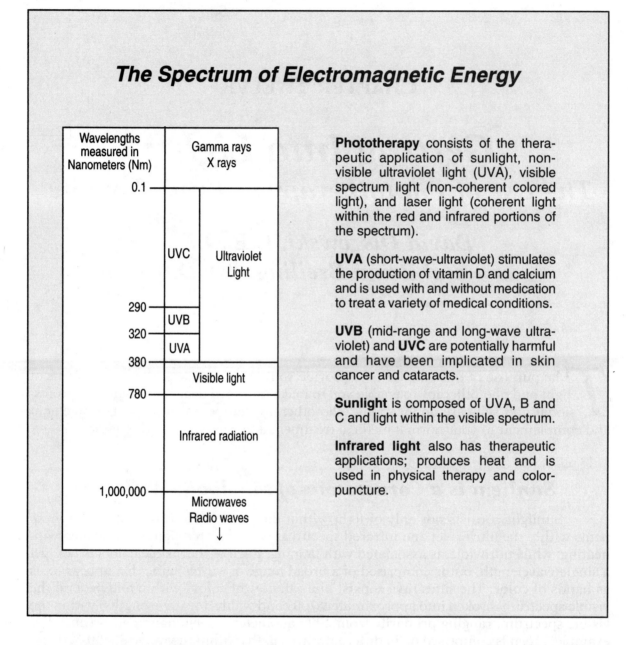

The Spectrum of Electromagnetic Energy

Wavelengths measured in Nanometers (Nm)		
	Gamma rays X rays	
0.1		
	UVC	Ultraviolet Light
290		
	UVB	
320		
	UVA	
380		
	Visible light	
780		
	Infrared radiation	
1,000,000		
	Microwaves Radio waves ↓	

Phototherapy consists of the therapeutic application of sunlight, non-visible ultraviolet light (UVA), visible spectrum light (non-coherent colored light), and laser light (coherent light within the red and infrared portions of the spectrum).

UVA (short-wave-ultraviolet) stimulates the production of vitamin D and calcium and is used with and without medication to treat a variety of medical conditions.

UVB (mid-range and long-wave ultraviolet) and **UVC** are potentially harmful and have been implicated in skin cancer and cataracts.

Sunlight is composed of UVA, B and C and light within the visible spectrum.

Infrared light also has therapeutic applications; produces heat and is used in physical therapy and color-puncture.

Wurtman states that light ignites the cellular metabolism. If we restrict or alter our light exposure, it is akin to fowling the sparkplug of a car — the body won't run properly. Ninety-eight percent of sunlight enters through the eyes, while 2% is absorbed through the skin. Sunlight produces vitamin D and catalyzes other crucial metabolic processes such as the absorption of calcium. Calcium plays a vital role in the transmission of messages in the brain and in the competence of the immune system.

Sunlight plays an important role in the prevention of disease. **Zane Kime, M.D.,** in his book *Sunlight* (Pengrove, CA: World Health Publications, 1980), lists the health promoting benefits of appropriate sunlight exposure as similar to those produced by

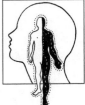

physical exercise. Dr. Kime cites research that suggests that after sunbathing[1] there is a pressure, and blood sugar, while there is an increase in cellular oxygen, muscle strength, endurance vitality, and mental stability.

Historically, sunlight has played an important role in the cure of disease. **Until the advent of antibiotics in the late 1930s, the use of sunbathing (Solar Therapy, Sunlight Therapy) and ultraviolet light (Actinotherapy, from the Greek for "ray healing") were internationally accepted and commonly utilized medical treatments for a variety of acute bacterial and viral infectious conditions,** such as: tuberculosis, viral pneumonia, bronchial asthma, wounds, sores, ulcerations, jaundice, gout, psoriasis, acne, and mumps.

A lack of sunlight impairs the natural defense mechanisms of the body to all forms of stress, both physical and emotional. Generally, the competence of the immune system is lowered in the winter; fertility is lower; fatigue increases; and overall levels of health decline. Winter's darker and shorter daylight hours alter the body's natural internal rhythms, such as the production of hormones and neurotransmitters. With this lack of light many women experience an upsurge in PMS symptoms, while other individuals complain about feeling somehow "out of phase," noticing an increased sense of irritability, moodiness, and difficulties performing intellectual tasks. People often attempt to "self medicate" during the winter months by increasing their consumption of carbohydrates, alcohol, caffeine, and sugary desserts.

Phototherapy pioneer John Ott theorizes that human and animal cells have a process similar to plant photosynthesis, which he calls *biological combustion*, the process that converts light energy into chemical energy. Light enters the eye and goes to the body's power distribution center, the hypothalamus, where it is converted into electrochemical impulses that are sent to important endocrine glands, such as the pituitary and the pineal. These glands, in turn, distribute the hormonal messages via the body's nervous system to virtually every cell in the body. The hypothalamus is the site of the body's pacemaker and *biological clock,* and is thought to regulate a number of bodily functions such as: reproduction, thirst, hunger, satiation, temperature, the regulation of emotions, and sleep patterns. The pineal gland is also a neurohormonal transducer which transforms retinally perceived light waves into neuronal impulses and hormonal regulatory messages that are distributed throughout the body. The so-called "master gland," the pituitary, is itself controlled by the hypothalamus. The pituitary controls the activities of other endocrine glands by the secretion of growth hormone, thyroid stimulating hormone (TSH), adrenocorticotropic hormone (ACTH), prolactin, luteinizing and follicle stimulating hormones (LH) and (FSH), oxytocin, melanocyte stimulating hormone (MSH), and anti-diuretic hormone. Light is thus, one of the most fundamental components of our health and well being.

---

1. Please consult your physician regarding appropriate sunbathing methods for your constitutional skin type, geographical location, time of year and sun sensitizing side-effects of medications. In general, darker-skinned individuals tend to develop less skin cancer than those with lighter skin. It is imperative to avoid burning the skin, as evidenced by the early warning sign of skin reddening. The benefits of sunlight do not require prolonged sun exposure or burning which can place an individual at risk for skin cancer.

Are You Making the Light Choice For Your Health?

Most of us get sun in the summer and very little in the winter. However, the body needs light everyday. We need sunlight to live. Approximately one-and-a-half to two hours a day is a *Recommended Daily Requirement*. A decrease in mental efficiency and depression are two hallmarks of seasonal affective disorder, or winter depression (SAD). Two theories regarding the cause of SAD are that it is related to the ebb and flow of a pineal hormone called melatonin and a hypothalamic neurotransmitter known as serotonin. The levels of both these chemicals vary directly with the amount of light entering the eyes.

Minimum Daily Requirement of Sunlight
1/2 to 2 hours a day of the range of frequencies that comprise sunlight

Or you may experience:

1. Decreases in energy levels
2. Cravings for carbohydrates, sugar, and caffeine
3. Difficulty in getting up and the need for more sleep
4. Decreased desire for sex and other pleasurable activities
5. Decreased efficiency in cognitive abilities such as attention and concentration
6. Mood disturbances from being *"mildly out-of-it"* to severe disorders

---

You don't have to sit in the direct sun to receive the benefits of sunlight, as indirect sunlight and artificial indoor light enters your eyes as well. **While artificial lighting enables us to read and to work without the benefit of sunlight, it can also profoundly affect our body's immune and nervous systems.** Such modern realities as spending too much time indoors, the use of tinted lenses in reading glasses, sunglasses, and contacts, as well as tinted glass and plastic windows, and even smog restricts the quantity and quality of light that enters our eyes. Because of these lifestyle factors, many people suffer from *"Malillumination"* or *Light Starvation* and miss some of the health benefits of light within the red, blue, and purple ranges, as well as parts of the ultraviolet spectrum that may be salutary. **Just as the wrong frequencies of light can cause plants to wilt, the wrong spectral qualities of light can cause stress symptoms in people.** Ott goes as far as saying that malillumination may not only cause fatigue, depression, hostility, immune problems, but it may also be a factor in strokes, Alzheimer's disease, and cancer.

Since sunlight is the only type of light that is optimal or *normal*, all artificial lighting is *abnormal* or second best. We can actually receive a harmful dosage of incandescent, fluorescent and halogen lights of the wrong or improper spectral distribution different from that necessary for health. For example, an overexposure to yellow light can overstimulate an individual's nervous system, causing them to experience increased nervousness, tension, and eye strain. In our daily lives we need to avoid altered light and insufficient quantities of light coming into our eyes. Hospital patients, prisoners, older

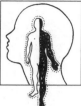

folks, city dwellers and office workers who spend too much time indoors do not get sufficient sunlight and have been observed to have deficiencies of the sunlight vitamin, vitamin D, as well as calcium.

The health promoting benefits of artificial lighting are thought to increase as it more closely approximates the frequency (color) distribution and multiple bandwidths of natural sunlight. Full spectrum fluorescent lighting is the closest approximation to these qualities of natural sunlight and has been found to balance hormones and neuroendocrine functioning. Experiences both within the classroom and the business community demonstrate that full spectrum lighting improves the ability to attend and concentrate. A research study showed that by simply switching the classroom lighting to full spectrum radiation-shielded fluorescents, it decreased the hyperactive behavior of students compared to a control group. Similarly, when Control Data Corporation installed full spectrum fluorescent tubes in their work stations, the data input error rate dropped to the point of saving the company more than $235,000 per year. For many companies lighting has become an important component of office design. The companies that use full spectrum lighting report employee morale has improved, while complaints of headaches and eyestrain while working at video display terminals have greatly decreased.

The physical nature of all "yellowish" light (incandescent, normal fluorescent, and halogen) results in a reflection or glare when applied to white paper (e.g., newspapers and books), causing squinting of the eyes and resultant eyestrain very quickly. Full spectrum fluorescent light (just like natural sunlight) absorbs into the white paper with *no resulting glare* and allows the letters to stand out clearly. This factor results in higher grade point average (GPA) for students and easier reading for everyone.

Full Spectrum Lighting Requirements

Degree of Problem	Type of Full Spectrum Fluorescent Lights Required	Effective Distance from Lighting (Ft.)	Recommended Daily Exposure Duration (Hrs.)
Slight daily stress & irritation levels	Standard household lighting** (1100 LUX)	4-8	4-8
Moderate stress & irritation levels	Standard household lighting** plus Bright Light Box* (2500 LUX)	2-4	1/2 - 1
Reduced immune system	Bright Light Box* (2500 LUX)	2	1-2
Occasional depression	Bright Light Box* (2500 LUX)	2	2
Severe depression	Ultra-Bright Light Box (10,000 LUX)	2	2-4

* Or use new compact bright desk lamp (2700 LUX)

**Standard household lighting is obviously used during dark periods of the day.

Bright Light Therapy is better in the morning, but can also be done in the evening or even during the day.

Who's SAD and Why?

Although SAD occurs in both sexes, women in their 20s through their 40s are the group most vulnerable to SAD. There may also be a genetic-hormonal component in men and women that increases one's vulnerability to light deprivation, as SAD tends to run in families. It is unclear why women get SAD more often than men, but it is possible that it is related to the cyclical ebb and flow of the female sex hormones estrogen and progesterone. Once a woman goes through menopause, there is a major decrease of the secretion of the sex hormones, and then the incidence of SAD in post menopausal women is equal to that of men. Today it is unclear whether estrogen and progesterone replacement therapy has an effect on post-menopausal women's vulnerability to winter depression. Fifty percent of menstruating women with SAD also experience PMS symptoms. Other women who experience PMS all year round may notice increased symptoms or more acute symptoms in winter. The incidence of SAD among prepubertal boys and girls is similar until girls begin their menstrual cycles. It is possible that female sex hormones act on certain brain centers such that there is an increase in the incidence of SAD.

Light deprivation, whether it occurs in winter or any other time of year, precipitates SAD-like symptoms in people who have no previous history of winter depression. For example, it is common that an individual may experience adjustment difficulties related to light deprivation when they move from a sunnier location (such as Southern California) to a higher latitude and darker area (such as Seattle). Likewise, a change from a lighter to a darker residence or office location can precipitate symptoms of *light starvation.*

Ultimately illumination is the only thing that makes sense of life and for many there is an almost desperate need to obtain it. Illumination is associated with awakening and awakening may be described in terms of experience such as suddenly seeing things from a different perspective.

— *Pir Vilayat Inayat Khan*

DREAM

My body was made of crystal, so clear, so pure, so light. I was pregnant and lying on my back; my hands were clasped behind my head. I floated through the feeling of space. Within my pregnant belly was a prism. As I floated, light touched the prism/child within me and radiated throughout the Universe.

— *Bethany ArgIsle*

The Facts of Light:
Basic Light Concepts

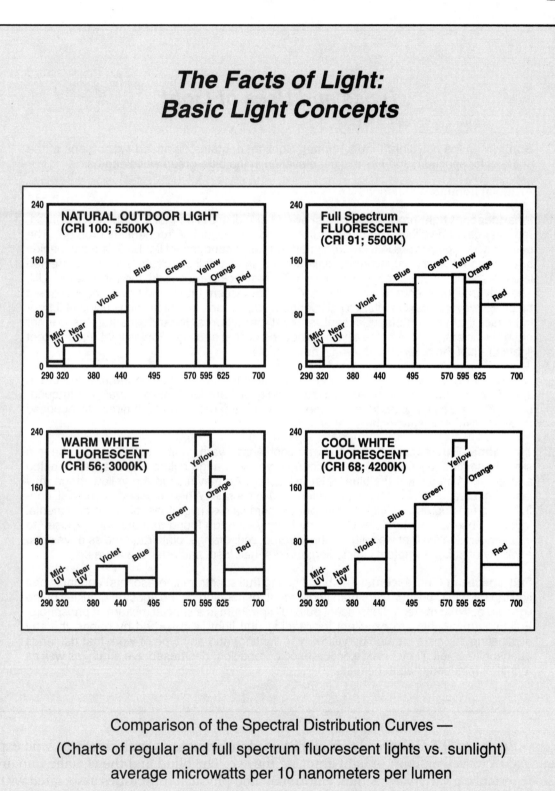

Comparison of the Spectral Distribution Curves —
(Charts of regular and full spectrum fluorescent lights vs. sunlight)
average microwatts per 10 nanometers per lumen

Types and Uses of Light

Sunlight is the only light that is normal. Sunlight contains balanced proportions of the entire color spectrum and has a slight elevation in the blue-green wavelengths.

Artificial lighting is abnormal.

Incandescent light produces a very skewed color distribution that is high in the infrared, red, orange, and yellow. The blues, purples and beneficial UV frequencies drop out. The blue end frequencies are least represented by most incandescent lights. Some companies advertising *full spectrum incandescents* are not, in fact, full spectrum but color corrected incandescents, such as the neodymium bulbs that lack certain reds, the far blue and UV. The only true full spectrum lights are made as fluorescent tubes and not as incandescent bulbs. However, John Ott offers a full spectrum fluorescent, complete with built-in electronic ballast that fits into incandescent (screw-type) fixtures. Incandescent lights are not energy efficient, as 80% of the energy produced is heat and only 20% is light. Fluorescent lights are just the reverse and remain much cooler.

Halogen lighting is unusually high in frequencies from the yellow to the red end of the spectrum. Its brightness can produce glare and even harmful levels of certain UV frequencies and should have glass in front of the exposed filament to be safe. Indirect, as opposed to direct, use of halogen light is better.

Traditional Fluorescent Bulbs such as cool white, warm white, soft pink, also have a skewed spectral distribution in which certain yellow-orange colors are over-represented and are missing a lot of the blue-violet frequency. An elevation in the yellow range may lead to hyperactivity of the nervous system and eye strain. When exposed to artificial, non-full spectrum fluorescent lights, some people complain of migraines, physical and mental fatigue. Observations by John Ott nearly thirty years ago found that animals exposed to imbalanced lighting that was high in the infrared, red, orange, pink frequencies developed a variety of stress symptoms, including: tumors, hair loss, and arterial plaques.

Full Spectrum Fluorescents: The best lighting (full spectrum fluorescents) and the worst lighting (non full spectrum) are both fluorescent, depending on the spectral qualities of the light used. What makes a fluorescent bulb full spectrum is a special mixture of phosphors. Full spectrum lights are excellent for reading (the light is absorbed by paper, thereby eliminating the glare created by yellow-type lighting) and any type of work that demands attention to detail. They provide accurate color rendition, decreased eye strain, as well as a host of mindbody health benefits.

Episodes of SAD have also been reported in individuals with cataracts who experience a decreased amount of light entering the eye. The blind and the visually impaired also experience a variety of mental, emotional, and physical difficulties associated with a decreased ability to take in and metabolize light. For example, visually impaired adolescents attain sexual maturity much earlier than their sighted counterparts.

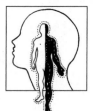

SAD Places

The Relationship Between SAD and Latitude

Estimated percentages of people who have seasonal affective disorder (SAD) and the milder "winter blues" at various latitudes in the United States, Mexico, and Canada:

SAD **10.2%**   WINTER BLUES **20.2%**

50°

45°

SAD **8%**   WINTER BLUES **17.1%**

40°

5.8%   **13.9%**

35°

3.6%   **10.6%**

30°

1.4%   **7.5%**

25°

A lack of light in winter causes decreased immune functioning and an increase in certain types of depressive illnesses, such as seasonal affective disorder (SAD) and the subclinical variety, winter blues. The farther north you go, the more common are both winter blues and SAD. The symptoms of SAD include depressed mood, difficulties in concentration, the need for increased amounts of sleep and the craving for carbohydrates. It is estimated by **Dr. Leora Rosen** that 6% of the United States population experiences SAD, while 14% experience winter blues.

SAD symptoms have their onset with the shortening of daylight in late fall and wane as the days grow longer in spring. In many areas of the United States there is a six hour difference in the amount of daily sunlight exposure from the shortest day of the year on December 22 until the longest day of the year on June 22. SAD symptoms tend to begin earlier and occur more frequently the farther north one lives.

Source: Dr. Norman E. Rosenthal, N.I.M.H.

Lifting the Winter Blues and Resetting The Brain's Clock with Light

Bright full spectrum fluorescent light is also effective with people suffering from the less severe form of winter depression, the *"winter blues,"* which affects twice as many individuals as SAD. Those people experiencing only mild winter symptoms may notice positive changes by merely increasing the amount of full spectrum environmental lighting in their home and office. People with both types of winter difficulties will benefit from increasing their amount of environmental lighting. Interestingly, those people who do not have SAD or winter blues may show no mood improvement from full spectrum bright light phototherapy (which uses 10,000 lux, more than 10-20 times the brightness of typical indoor lighting. For the sake of comparison, the midday summer sun obtains a brightness of nearly 100,000 lux). They may even experience some discomfort from the increased bright light exposure.

SAD Warning Signs Requiring Professional Consultation

Individuals should seek the advice of a mental health professional when they experience a significant impairment in their daily functioning, such as:

1. marked feelings of depression (prolonged sadness, pessimism, crying spells and a consistently negative outlook, including thoughts of suicide);

2. unusual difficulties with attention and concentration (i.e., difficulties completing previously manageable tasks);

3. difficulties awakening in the morning, and severe fatigue.

If light therapy is required, a competent professional (such as those listed in the *Resource List)* should be consulted.

The majority of research studies on the therapeutic effects of light with SAD have focused on full spectrum fluorescent lighting. There is less information on the effects of incandescent light. Although it is likely that incandescent light may have a therapeutic effect, its safety and effectiveness has not been thoroughly evaluated. **Unless one has access to a light meter, it is difficult to know how much light one is receiving from homemade phototherapy devices. The correct brightness is a crucial factor, as there is a therapeutic dose of light required to alleviate the symptoms of winter depression and SAD.** Individuals are better off with a professionally manufactured light box, such as the ***Sunray*™** by the ***Sunbox Company*** or the ***Ott Full Spectrum Light Boxes,*** and supplementing their living and working spaces with ample amounts of indirect light from full spectrum fluorescent light products (bulbs, tubes, and lamps), and finally, rounding out lighting requirements using halogen lamps or incandescent bulbs.

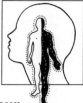

The best time for Bright Light Therapy is probably any time that you fit it in your schedule! Studies by **Drs. Lewy** and **Sack** have suggested that morning, as compared to evening, light was more effective in SAD patients, particularly those who have difficulty awakening in the morning. The lights could be attached to a timer at your bedside and controlled to come on before you wake. Some individuals may experience difficulty falling asleep if Bright Light Therapy is used late in the evening. Bright Light Phototherapy should be continued for at least several weeks of half-hour to four hours of exposure time, throughout the late fall and winter months.

Some individuals report experiencing an increase in mood and cognitive functioning after the very first treatment or within the first few days. There are no hard and fast rules for how long light therapy needs to be continued for the treatment of SAD. However, usually SAD symptoms return within one to two weeks after light exposure is stopped. If you are really depressed (and of course under the care of a therapist), you may need to be very disciplined about your use of the phototherapy equipment and your environmental light exposure. Most SAD patients are able to discontinue light exposure during the summer. More than three-quarters of individuals with SAD are helped by bright light exposure. They report experiencing an increase in energy, mood, and improved ability to concentrate and function as well as *joie de vivre,* as shown by an increased desire for sex, socializing and pleasurable activity.

Dr. Norman Rosenthal at the National Institute of Mental Health in Betheseda, Maryland, did the pioneering SAD research in the early 1980s. He and his colleagues contend that **winter depression is associated with disturbances in the hypothalamus, and particularly the role of the neurotransmitter *serotonin*.** The suprachiasmatic nuclei within the hypothalamus is the area associated with the body's *biological clock.* Nerve cells within this region contain high concentrations of serotonin. Interestingly, there's a seasonal variation in the amount of serotonin in this area of the brain, with the serotonin levels being at the lowest levels during the winter months. Patients with SAD have an abnormal response to a serotonin stimulating drug, and their levels of serotonin fall to abnormally low levels during the winter months. Their levels of serotonin normalize during the brighter and sunnier days of summer and after bright light phototherapy.

Full Spectrum Bright Light Boxes (10,000 lux) effectively alleviate the symptoms of SAD (within about four days) in approximately 80% of sufferers who expose themselves between a half hour and several hours a day to this light source. Bright Light Boxes alter our 24-hour internal rhythms, *circadian rhythms,* and may be useful in the treatment of a variety of other mood disorders both with and without antidepressant medication. For those SAD sufferers not fully helped by light therapy alone, anti depressants such as Prozac, Zoloft, and Paxil can raise the levels of serotonin and are effective both alone or when used synergistically with the lights.

Individuals who experience less severe forms of winter depression may not require a full spectrum light box but can benefit by supplementing their light exposure with full spectrum fluorescent tubes (which can be installed in standard fluorescent fixtures, mounted in and from the ceiling), full spectrum fluorescent screw-in bulbs which can be mounted in traditional incandescent light sockets, or special desk lamps using a compact fluorescent tube. **The Ott-Lite® Task Lamp** is a portable full spectrum desk lamp which provides an ideal light for reading. Full spectrum light boxes can be placed throughout the most frequently used home or office areas. Ideal locations for full spectrum light boxes include work-out areas, in front of a reading chair, or on a computer table.

An excellent method for maximum impact is to provide full spectrum lights in the bathroom; therefore, the body receives the same effect as natural sunlight in the morning. You wake-up quicker and with less morning shock. This is also the best period for altering your *biological clock*. (A row of 4-6 screw-in fluorescent bulbs mounted in a vanity fixture provides a dramatic yet calm environment, and you look "natural," as you do in sunlight.)

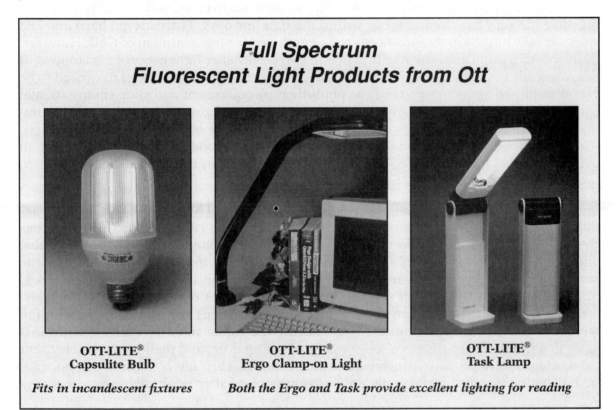

Full Spectrum Fluorescent Light Products from Ott

| OTT-LITE® Capsulite Bulb | OTT-LITE® Ergo Clamp-on Light | OTT-LITE® Task Lamp |

Fits in incandescent fixtures　　　*Both the Ergo and Task provide excellent lighting for reading*

Full Spectrum Bright Light is also prescribed for a variety of biological clock problems such as, the disturbed sleep of the elderly, jet lag, and the difficulties of night shift workers. More than a dozen space shuttle crews have utilized full spectrum bright fluorescent light to readjust their biological clocks to enable astronauts to effectively work the night shift (as well as adjust to seeing the sun rise and set sixteen times per day). **Dr. Charles Czeisler, head of the Laboratory for Circadian and Sleep Disorders Medicine at Harvard's Brigham and Women's Hospital,** has demonstrated since 1986, that light exposure can disrupt and reset the brain's biological clock. The doses of 10,000 lux full spectrum light can either advance or retard the biological clock depending on when it is delivered. At some times of the day bright light has little effect, while the biggest changes are evidenced when light is administered during the individual's habitual nighttime hours (as marked by minimum body temperatures). Light doses early in the night delay the clock to a later hour, while a dose late in the night advances it to an earlier

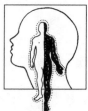

time. Research shows that circadian rhythms can shift about two hours per day with exposure from one to six hours of bright full spectrum light. Bright light used before the presumed minimum temperature was found to induce phase delays, while bright light administered after the presumed temperature minimum induced phase advances. Successful reprogramming of the biological clock, as measured by urine levels of melatonin, currently requires long hours of bright light exposure over a period of several days. Thus, this method of light exposure can not yet be effectively applied to travelers on long-distance airplane flights.

These phase-shifting procedures are now a permanent part of the space shuttle program, and the most recent models of the space shuttle include high intensity lighting in work areas, bathrooms, and exercise rooms. Astronauts also utilize dark color welder's goggles and black plastic over sleeping quarter windows to prevent inappropriate exposure to environmental sunlight during their "nighttime" hours. Near the end of the space shuttle mission, light exposure is gradually increased to shift astronauts' biological rhythms back to their normal daylight schedule.

A second theory and an effective treatment for SAD has been researched by **Dr. Alfred Lewy and his colleagues, Drs. Robert Sack and Clifford Singer, at the Oregon Health Science University in Portland.** They believe that there's a phase shift disturbance in the timing of the biological clock in people with SAD. Dr. Lewy's investigations have focused on the pineal hormone *melatonin* that seems to facilitate the synchronization of people's daily biological rhythms with the cycles of day and night. Pineal levels of melatonin are higher during the night and in winter months than during the day and summer months, as melatonin is only produced in the dark hours of nighttime. The precise role of melatonin in SAD is not yet understood; however, melatonin supplements (available without prescription in health food stores) are being investigated for their potential abilities to reset the biological clock in a variety of phase shift disorders, such as winter depression and jet lag. By timing the ingestion of melatonin, one may be able to set the body clock forwards or backwards. Other drugs which block the release of melatonin are being researched for their effect on SAD, including propanol and atenolol.

The biological clock may also be phase advanced or delayed by the timing of phototherapy. ***Dawn simulation* is another promising treatment for SAD. It utilizes Dr. Lewy's phase shift hypothesis by using very low levels of either incandescent or fluorescent lighting that is timed to come on one-and-a-half to two hours before daybreak.** At this time of morning the eyes and brain appear to be unusually sensitive to ambient lighting that enters through closed eyelids. **Dr. David Avery at Seattle's Harbor View Medical Center** has demonstrated that dawn simulation successfully reverses SAD symptoms and enables patients to awaken at their usual hours, even in the winter time.

Typically, with the decreasing daylight hours of late fall, these individuals sleep much later in the fall and winter — a sign that their internal rhythms are out of phase with society's early morning work schedules. Ironically, many cases of winter depression will lift if individuals are allowed to go to bed and awaken at a later time, in keeping with their internal body clock.

Dawn simulation reduces most SAD symptoms and is especially effective with individuals who have difficulty awakening during winter mornings. These low intensity (250 lux) bedside lights come on approximately two hours before dawn and, with the use of a dawn simulator computer chip, gradually increase in intensity to mimic the rising sun. As mentioned earlier, a relatively low brightness (30 lux to 6,000 lux) may also be effective in alleviating SAD symptoms, depending on how the light is used. For example, it may be that light of less intensity that is closer to the eye, as in a *Bio-Brite*™ *Visor* (see Resource List: Section Eight, page 374, Full Spectrum Light Products) or *Dawn Simulator,* which uses indirect light through closed eyelids, may be nearly as effective in alleviating SAD symptoms as the Bright Light Boxes (10,000 lux) placed several feet away.

Comparison of Different Sources of Light

Light Type	(Color) CRI	(Heat) Kelvin	Spectral Peak	Brightness Lux	Thousand (HR) Life	Price	U.V.
Sunlight	100	7500	Full Visible Range	93,000			Significant
Visible Spectrum Extra Bright Light Box	46	3700	Slight Yellow	10,000	10	$475	Slight
Full Spectrum Bright Light Box	92	5800	Near Sunlight	2500	30	$275	Moderate
Full Spectrum Tube (Fluorescent)	92	5800	Near Sunlight	1500	30	$20	Moderate
Full Spectrum Compact Desk Light	91	5000	Near Sunlight	2700	10	$90	Slight-Moderate
Cool White Tube (Fluorescent)	67	3700	Yellow-Orange	1500	5		Slight
100 Watt Bulb (Incandescent Bulb)			Yellow-Orange	1100	1		None
Ambient Indoors				400			
Dawn Simulator Unit with Standard Incandescent Lighting				100 - 250		$300	
Bio-Brite Visor® Krypton Incandescent				100-2500		$300	
Candle				125			

UV: Friend and Foe

Ultraviolet light has been used therapeutically in dermatology for nearly 100 years. In 1903, **Danish physician Dr. Neils Ryberg Finsen** received the Nobel prize for medicine and physiology for his discovery that UV light exposure could successfully treat a disfiguring form of tuberculosis of the skin. While some researchers claim certain frequencies of UV are beneficial or even necessary for physical and mental health, others maintain it is not. There is much research on UV that still needs to be done.

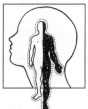

Today, the concern about ultraviolet light has reached almost phobic proportions. We commonly associate the word ultraviolet with skin cancers, wrinkles, and cataracts. **Dr. Jacob Liberman** in his book *Light: Medicine of the Future,* devotes an entire chapter entitled *"UV or not UV?"* about the therapeutic effects of ultraviolet light on the brain and nervous system. Liberman takes issue with the misconception of UV being a type of *death ray,* and presents a wealth of historic and current evidence of the *health promoting benefits* of ultraviolet light, such as: decreasing blood pressure, increasing cardiac output, increasing cardiac circulation, reducing cholesterol, improving metabolic efficiency via stimulation of thyroid, increasing the level of male and female sex hormones, as well as a skin hormone called solitrol, which plays a role in mood and immune system functioning and normalizes blood sugar levels.

Similarly, **Dr. Zane Kime** states that **ultraviolet is essential for optimal health and is the most "biologically active component of sunlight."** Ultraviolet increases the body's resistance to a wide range of infectious agents, increases the oxygen carrying capacity of the blood, and improves stress tolerance by increasing adrenaline. Laboratory experiments demonstrate that exposure to both sunlight and UV, at levels beneath those that cause burning and reddening of the skin, promotes an increase in lymphocytes and neutrophils.[2] Several studies from around the world show that as little as ten minutes of UV light exposure three times a week can reduce the frequency of winter colds and respiratory infections. Ultraviolet light has been used as an effective intervention in the treatment of a variety of diseases, such as: colitis, asthma, eczema, acne, herpes, gout, rheumatoid arthritis, anemia, and psoriasis.

John Ott, while warning that UV in overdose amounts can cause harm, has contended for years that we require minimal, though regular amounts of the entire spectrum of sunlight, which includes a natural proportion of UV exposure, both through our eyes and on our unprotected skin. The lack of ultraviolet during the winter months is suspected as a prime factor contributing to the SAD condition. Nonetheless, UV toxicity is a problem, as can be seen in the frightening geometric increases in skin cancer, in which decreasing levels of environmental ozone have been implicated. Individuals living or visiting in locations where there are documented holes in the ozone layer, such as in Antarctica, New Zealand, and the tip of South America, do need to exercise extreme caution and be prudent about UV protection. These areas have alarmingly high levels of vision impairment, and some people in these areas must wear special UV-shielding glasses to protect their eyesight. However, what constitutes appropriate caution may be less clear for individuals living in higher latitude cities such as Seattle, where ozone holes are not as direct an issue.

Joan Smith-Sonneborn at the University of Wyoming calls ultraviolet, "The Lady of Justice," because it both harms and repairs harm. Based on her laboratory results showing DNA damage during sunlight exposure and enzyme repair during the darkness period, she concludes that there is an optimum level of UV required for the human body — "the key word is balance."

---

2. Zane Kime, M.D., suggests that sunburning and skin cancer formation may be inhibited by supplementing the diet with beta carotene and an assortment of antioxidant vitamins (A, E, C,) and minerals such as selenium. Also a diet high in fats (both saturated and unsaturated) may increase the incidence of skin cancer.

Today, the majority of Americans use sunglasses or prescription lenses that block out much or all of the ultraviolet spectrum. **Undoubtedly, ultraviolet in large quantities is harmful. However, in smaller amounts it is beneficial to a variety of life functions, and we even have a minimum daily requirement for these wavelengths of light,** as UV light through the eyes stimulates the immune system. If lack of ultraviolet is a concern, then lenses which conduct a portion of the ultraviolet spectrum can be obtained.

Ultraviolet is not within the visible spectrum and is comprised of many different wavelengths. **Near ultraviolet (or shortwave ultraviolet) light,** called **UV-A** (320-380 nm), is the closest to the violet range of the visible spectrum and is responsible for tanning and sunburning. Generally, the longer UV wavelengths penetrate into the deeper skin layers and may be responsible for the systemic effects of UV. **Midrange-ultraviolet light, UV-B** (290-320 nm), catalyzes the production of vitamin D and the absorption of vital minerals such as calcium. **Far ultraviolet (or longwave ultraviolet) light, UV-C** (100-290 nm), is by far the most toxic and detrimental. It kills bacteria and viruses, though it only penetrates superficial skin layers and is filtered by the earth's ozone layer. In addition, the eye provides its own protection; the cornea filters UV-C, while the lens filters UV-B and the retina filters UV-A.

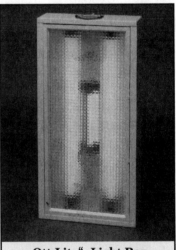

It is erroneously assumed that exposure to all wavelengths of ultraviolet are harmful. To light researchers such as Dr. Wurtman and John Ott, saying that *all* ultraviolet light is harmful makes as much sense as saying that all vitamin A is toxic. While too little of some ultraviolet wavelengths or too much of other ultraviolet exposure can produce problems, the correct amount of ultraviolet can have beneficial effects. For example, UV-A may be important for treating depression and UV-C kills airborne microbes in the environment and on the skin.[3,4]

The phosphors that produce these ultraviolet frequencies deteriorate more quickly than the other phosphors in fluorescent lights. Therefore, separate UV tubes that can be replaced more often are desirable in light boxes. The only full spectrum light boxes that contain separate ultraviolet tubes are manufactured by Ott-Lite® (*see Resource List*).

Ott-Lite" Light Box
With both full spectrum and UV tubes enclosed

---

3. The use of ultraviolet light in medicine has a long, rich, and successful history. Nonetheless, the improper use of sunlamps with UV-A can cause burns and damage chromosomes. Precautions must be taken regarding exposure duration, frequency, the possible need for protective goggles and distance from light source. Don't buy sunlamps that produce UV rays with frequencies less than 290 nm (UV-C).

4. UV-A phototherapy combines the use of psoralen medications in the treatment of various skin diseases such as: psoriasis, vitiligo (loss of pigment due to a decrease in number of melanin producing cells known as melanocytes) and mycosis fungoids (a type of blood cancer). Tanning and sunlamps produce UV-A and slight amounts of UV-B.

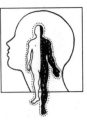

Harmful Radiation Effects from Fluorescent Lights

For nearly two decades, **John Ott** stated that the distorted spectrum of standard fluorescent lights was not the only factor that was detrimental to health. **Standard fluorescent tubes emit three types of harmful radiation: x-ray, radio frequency waves, and extreme low frequency (ELF).** These types of radiation can completely shut off the activity of the immune system. ELF is a form of magnetic radiation that is also emitted from power lines, electric motors, computer monitors, televisions, and a variety of household appliances. Research studies have implicated ELF readings above 2.0 milligaus with a variety of diseases such as leukemia and other malignancies. ELF dissipates quickly as one moves away from the source, and readings below 1.0 milligaus are recommended. If you are working under fluorescent lights for long periods of time, light sources need to be moved at least a foot away (and preferably 3 to 4 feet away) from the body. The Environmental Protection Agency (EPA) has categorized ELF fields as "B" carcinogens, which are in the same class as dioxin, formaldehyde, and PCBs. A 10-watt fluorescent lamp produces a magnetic field that is more than twenty times greater than a 60-watt incandescent bulb. Ceiling fluorescent fixtures with several 20-watt tubes can produce a field of greater than 1.0 milligaus near the heads of office workers below.

ELF is emitted in toxic proportions in older fluorescent boxes which utilize *electric* ballast (power transformer) as opposed to newer *electronic* ballast[5] (which are available in the latest light boxes by both Ott and Sunbox, plus the new Ott Capsulite screw-in bulb. *See Resource List).* Sinusoidal Electronic Dimming Ballasts increase the frequency of the spark in fluorescent lamps from 60 cycles per second to 20,000 cycles per second. This makes the frequency of the spark faster than the human eye can see, which eliminates the annoying flickering and hum of old type electric ballasts. These newer ballasts also significantly reduce ELF, while producing brighter light with less energy. This leads to longer bulb life as well as substantial energy and financial savings. The old electric ballast in standard fluorescent fixtures may be replaced with the new electronic ballast, which can be acquired from your local construction or electrical supply dealer.

John Ott, in his later studies, states that x-ray radiation from cathode-ray devices such as fluorescent tubes, television sets, and computer terminals causes blood cells to *clump* in persons exposed over a period of time, thereby contributing to tiredness, fatigue, and reduced alertness. Exposure to sunlight or full spectrum lighting resulted in *unclumping* of the blood cells. So if you are part of the rapidly growing number of computer users, get more sunlight periodically during the day or have full spectrum lights in your vicinity.

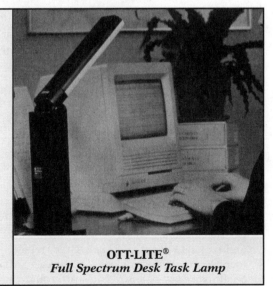

OTT-LITE®
Full Spectrum Desk Task Lamp

---

5. Ballast is a form of resistance used to stabilize the current in the circuitry of fluorescent lamps.

X-rays can be effectively stopped by lead tape shielding around the cathode portion of fluorescent tubes to decrease these potentially harmful emissions. Ott first observed that when geraniums were placed near the ends of fluorescent tubes adjacent to the cathode portion, they often withered and died. All full spectrum fluorescent products from Ott-Lite® are shielded.

All fluorescent tubes contain small amounts of mercury and should be disposed of properly. Call your local County Hazardous Waste Collection Program or recycling center.

Compact fluorescents can save you money on your electric bill and reduce energy consumption by 75%. Magnetic ballast fluorescents achieve the highest energy efficiency and weigh about 50% less than magnetic ballasts.

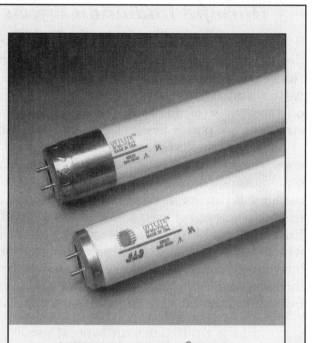

SHIELDED OTT-LITE® TUBES
The only Anti-Radiation Light

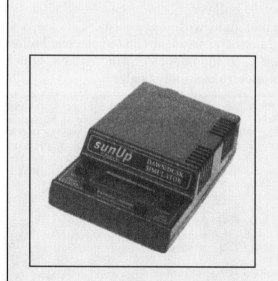

SUN-UP DAWN SIMULATOR™
Bedside incandescent lights plug into this unit and replicate dawn and dusk. Great replacement for radio/alarm clocks, and treats SAD. *See Resource List, page 376.* Available through the Sunbox Co.

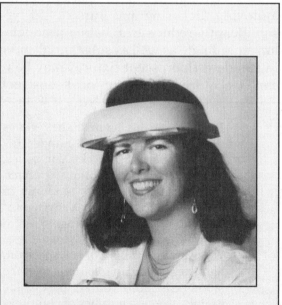

BIO-BRITE LIGHT VISOR™
Enables user to conveniently receive the benefits of SAD Phototherapy without having to sit in front of light box. *See Resource List, page 374.* Available through Bio-Brite and Tools for Exploration.

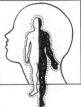

The Use of Lasers and Light Emitting Diodes in Acupuncture, Pain Management, and Tissue Regeneration

Our discussion of phototherapy now takes a quantum leap downward from the use of over 700 frequencies in full spectrum sunlight, to total mindbody health to utilizing only 1 frequency (monochromatic) for activating specific cell functions in damaged cell tissue and accelerating the body's normal healing process.

For the last 30 years, scientists in the United States, Eastern Europe, and Asia have researched the clinical uses of lasers. **Laser** is an acronym that stands for light amplification by stimulated emission of radiation. Better known are the surgical applications of so- called *hot lasers* to cut, cauterize, and destroy tissues. More recently, *cold lasers* or *soft lasers* (lower power) in a process called *laser photobiostimulation* have been researched for their ability to stimulate a variety of cellular functions in a nonthermal and nondestructive manner. Cold lasers are available in many clinics, research facilities, hospitals, and doctor's offices around the world. Researchers have used cold lasers to isolate the most potent individual frequencies or *monochromatic light* in their explorations of the effects of different wavelengths on human tissue samples. There are only two available methods for producing monochromatic single wavelength light beams. The first is with a laser. The second is with a **light-emitting diode, or LED.** Lasers produce *coherent light,* whereas light-emitting diodes emit *noncoherent light.* Human cell tissue has been observed to respond more powerfully to a single wavelength than when exposed to more than one wavelength at a time.

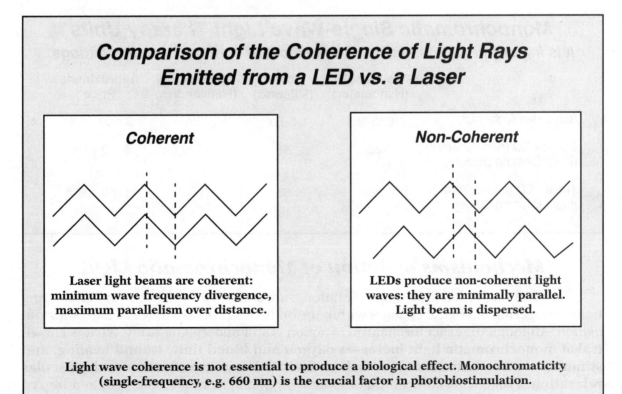

Comparison of the Coherence of Light Rays Emitted from a LED vs. a Laser

Coherent

Laser light beams are coherent: minimum wave frequency divergence, maximum parallelism over distance.

Non-Coherent

LEDs produce non-coherent light waves: they are minimally parallel. Light beam is dispersed.

Light wave coherence is not essential to produce a biological effect. Monochromaticity (single-frequency, e.g. 660 nm) is the crucial factor in photobiostimulation.

277

Much of the monochromatic light research has focused on isolating the most potent frequencies for the relief of acute or chronic pain and wound healing. Research demonstrates that **cell tissue responds best to certain frequencies which appear to be within the red and infrared spectrum,** such as 630 nanometers (nm), 660 nm, 880 nm, 940 nm, and 950 nm. The water and hemoglobin within the body's tissue restrict the full absorption of light frequencies outside the range of 600 to 980 nanometers. From the preliminary research it appears that one frequency of light may be a primary resonant frequency for the body, while the others may be harmonics. It has been demonstrated that **a single wavelength within the middle of the red spectrum (e.g. 660 nm) is the most resonant frequency to human tissue because it stimulates the production of cell tissue and rapidly promotes the regeneration of skin and blood tissue in the areas exposed to it.** For example, on a half dollar size wound the application of a 660 nm LED or cold laser for several minutes every two hours can, within one to two days, stimulate the generation of new skin without scabbing or the formation of scar tissue.

The recent phenomenon of red and infrared lasers and LEDs is just a rediscovery of the effect of red light on the body. Healing with red light was used in many ancient civilizations. In the 1890s, the pioneering **Dr. Neils Finsen** was curing smallpox lesions and variola using red and infrared rays. In the excitement of laser discovery and its concept of coherent light, we have overlooked this past knowledge. As we will soon come to understand, the coherency of light is not a necessary requirement for the healing process — *but being monochromatic is!*

Monochromatic Single-Wave Light Therapy Units
It is important all units have both pulsed and continuous wave settings!

	Wavelength (Nanometer)	Power (Milliwatt)	Illumination (Millicandles)	Approximate Price
Soft Laser (coherent)	630-950	5-50	N/A	$300 - 7500
Single-LED (non-coherent) (Light Emitting Diode)	660	55	7000	$140 - 170
Triple-LED (non-coherent) (Light Emitting Diode)	660	55	7000	$250 - 300

Mechanisms of Action of Monochromatic Light

It is thought that light quanta (photons) are absorbed by the skin and underlying tissue, triggering biological changes within the body in a process known as *photobiostimulation*. Although the exact mechanism of action is still undergoing study, what is known is that **monochromatic light increases oxygen and blood flow, wound healing, and stimulates nerve functioning, as well as facilitating pain reduction and muscular relaxation.** Proponents contend that monochromatic light in the blue, red, and far red regions enhance and speed up certain cellular metabolic processes, such as increasing the

278

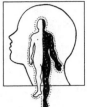

activity of the mitochondria (cellular organelles outside the nucleus that convert stored chemical energy into a more usable form), changing the electrophysiological properties of the cell membrane and activating enzymes which in turn activate key chemical reactions.

Tiina Karu, Ph.D., of the Laser Technology Center in Russia, and affiliated with the University of California at Berkeley, has extensively researched this process since the early 1980s. She believes that light is a trigger for the rearrangement of cellular metabolism. There are photo acceptors at the molecular-cellular level which, when triggered, cause a series of biological actions (e.g. increases in DNA-RNA synthesis, cAMP levels, protein and collagen synthesis and cell proliferation), resulting in the rapid regeneration, normalization, and healing of damaged cell tissue.

The exact photobiological effects of stimulation depend on the wavelengths, dose, and intensity of the light. **Although light penetration may be superficial, deeper physiological processes may be stimulated by the light. The stimulating effect of Laser Therapy has been observed to decrease healing time of wounds, ulcers, decrease edema, and facilitate the remineralization of bone tissue.**

Applications of Low Power Laser Therapy

The effectiveness and the method of application of Laser Therapy have been compared to ultrasound. In countries outside the United States, it has become an accepted extension to physiotherapy techniques which use other parts of the electromagnetic spectrum such as microwaves, shortwaves, infrared, and ultraviolet. Increasing clinical and laboratory data from around the world attest to the effectiveness of Laser Therapy. Although additional research is required concerning the success rates for treating particular conditions and the therapeutic protocols used (length of exposure time, frequency of treatments), low power lasers are winning acceptance for use in a number of bone, nerve, and soft tissue conditions.

Problem areas can be reached by applying the light beam directly to the skin where it penetrates as much as one inch into the soft tissue. If more extensive or deeper application into the body is required, the light can be applied to the acupuncture points. Using a combination of both direct application and acupuncture point techniques, most problems can be reached and treated by the light. Since 660 nm red light lasers penetrate only 8-30mm (this is deep enough to affect muscular tissue), it is most useful for superficial conditions such as scars, wounds, ulcers, and a variety of skin conditions (acne, psoriasis, eczema, tinea, nervous rashes). Local treatment with *infrared lasers* in the 830 nm and 950 nm range penetrate somewhat deeper, 30-40mm, and are used to treat conditions of the joints, tendons, muscles, and fascia, such as osteo and rheumatoid arthritis. They may be effective with conditions involving pain (both acute and chronic), swelling, and stiffness. Most effective results occur with tissues that have ample blood supply, such as muscles and soft tissue. Tissues with less blood supply, such as ligaments and tendons, respond more slowly to light treatment.

The application of lasers often seems contradictory, because it can: promote rapid skin regeneration *or* decrease scar tissue; reduce pain *or* promote increased sensitivity in damaged nerve tissue (numbness); reduce swelling and irritation *or* improve blood cells and the immune system.

There are several theories concerning pain reduction. One is that the light reduces the excitability of nerve tissue by interruption of the pain signal being transmitted by way of nerve fibers. Another is when there is pain, the tissue is in a state of tension. As the light is applied, the tissue relaxes, followed by muscular relaxation and a reduction in pain. Even traumatic and sports injuries, such as old fracture sites, tendonitis, torn ligaments, capsules, and chronic back pain have responded to laser treatment.

Circulatory conditions such as Reynaud's syndrome, respond well to local application of monochromatic red or infrared light over the vessels of the hands and feet. Light radiation causes enhanced capillary flow, as evidenced by increased temperature in the extremities. This increase in blood circulation to the damaged area promotes cellular detoxification.

The laser acupuncture publications are growing rapidly with more seminars, introductory classes, research papers, and textbooks. The FDA has increased its regulations governing the use of low-energy lasers and is issuing consent forms for acupuncturist research and practice. Laser acupuncture treatment protocols vary, because it is based upon the power of the laser (5-50 milliwatts) and the time applied. No units above 50 milliwatts should be used, and instant pain results when the power reaches 200-300 watts. There has also been considerable discussion concerning the use of *continuous* light beams for acupoint sedation and *pulsed* (intermittent on-off) beams for stimulation (tonification) of acupuncture points. This same concept applies to direct application of light to tissue where continuous beams are used for pain relief and pulsed light to cause rapid regeneration of cells. Several studies seem to correlate the use of pulse rates between 200-300 pulses per second with a 50%-on,-50%-off cycle. Pulse rates from as low as 1 per second, up to 20,000 per second, have been employed.

In summary, there are a staggering number of research and clinical studies concerning the uses of low-power lasers on health problems, using both direct application to damaged tissue and indirect application through acupuncture points.

The Use of LED Biostimulation: The Benefits of Monochromatic Light Without the Drawbacks of Lasers

The whole field of soft lasers in medicine and physiotherapy is new. There is a good deal that is not yet known, but preliminary indications are that they are effective, relatively safe, and a useful therapeutic tool. But the use of light emitting diodes (LED) as an even safer, longer lasting and less expensive alternative to low power lasers is growing. The majority of soft laser research is directly applicable to the use of the LED. It is the monochromatic single wavelength that is more crucial to evoking a cellular response than whether the light is coherent (laser) or non-coherent (LED).

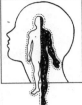

As mentioned earlier, **Dr. Tiina Karu** states in her studies that although laser biostimulation is a photobiological phenomenon, *coherent light is not needed!* Both coherent and non-coherent red light were clinically found to be effective in the treatment of peptic ulcers.

LEDs are increasingly replacing cold lasers, as they demonstrate comparable effectiveness without the laser's side effects. There is concern with the use of even soft lasers in terms of the potential for harm and negative side effects. They can be harmful if overused or if they come into contact with the eyes. The FDA classifies low power lasers as Class III, nonsignificant risk medical devices for investigational purposes only. Acupuncture seminars held at the University of Washington, cautioned that cold lasers can detrimentally affect or damage a particular acupoint if used for a prolonged period and can lead to reduced effectiveness. Overuse of soft lasers can occur. Laser treatment is calculated based upon the power of the laser and the duration of time that it is applied. Either one of these components can be overdone. Since photostimulation has a triggering effect, non-coherent light allows the photoacceptor mechanism and the cellular functions to be in greater control than with the more powerful coherent laser. With lasers you need to know the exact location of the acupoint. **LEDs give a larger light dispersion beam and allow a greater margin of error in locating and activating the acupuncture point — a great advantage for the average person using acupuncture at home!** Soft lasers are not readily available for home use, as they are more expensive with shorter life spans (4 years) and are approved for use only by licensed physicians, health professionals, and clinical technicians.

LEDs have been researched and used by thousands of practitioners internationally. In the United States, the use of low power lasers are considered acceptable practice in states that sanction physiotherapy with light, heat, water, sound, and electricity. In Israel, monochromatic red light LEDs are commonly used by medical doctors in a variety of specializations. **LED biostimulation has been applied in the fields of dermatology, neurology, physiotherapy, dentistry, as well as cosmetic applications.** Recent technological advancements in LEDs make monochromatic photostimulation more readily available to professionals and lay people. The LEDs used in phototherapy are primarily manufactured in Southeast Asia and are similar to the indicator lights frequently seen in electronic equipment, such as the ones on your stereo or smoke detector, although the therapeutic LED is 200 times brighter (8,000 millicandles). In sum, the advantages of using LEDs include the lower cost, longer life (50 years at 2000 hours per year), increased safety and ease of professional and home use. Because LEDs are diffused light, they can be used anywhere on the body without side effects, such as damage to the eye. Finally, the LED phototherapy units can be used on a much wider range of problems than the soft laser.

Application of Lasers and LEDs in Tissue Regeneration

Monochromatic lights have been used to promote tissue regeneration with such physical problems as wounds, burns, cirrhosis, rashes, tendonitis, herpes, torn ligaments, arthritis, circulatory conditions, organ and tissue degeneration, and sinus problems. Radiation of local areas can have systemic effects. A recent study reported in the January

1992 edition of *The Journal of the American Geriatric Society,* by Israeli medical researchers at the **Schmuel Harofe Geriatric Medical Center in Ber Yaakof,** found that pulsed monochromatic red light helped relieve pain and disability from knee osteoarthritis, suggesting that it can be a useful addition to medication. **The monochromatic light was applied on both sides of one knee for 15 minutes, twice a day. After ten days, the group getting red light scored 50% lower on pain tests and 40% lower on tests demonstrating a reduction in disability than a group that used a placebo light treatment.**

Preliminary Research and Clinical Trials with Monochromatic Light

The following uses represent those problem areas where a significant number of proven results have been recorded, as measured by clinical results, research techniques, and reported testimonies.

Pain Relief	Accelerated Wound Healing
Ulcers	Relaxation of Muscle Tension
Reduced Swelling	Acupuncture Point Stimulation
Food Allergies	Reflexology Point Stimulation
Sinus Relief	Emotion and Stress Release
Headaches	Facial Toning (wrinkle reduction)
Arthritis	Strengthening the Blood
Meridian Balancing	Improved Circulation
Skin Conditions	Addictive Habit Reduction:
Teeth and Gums	(Tobacco, Food, Drugs, and Alcohol)
Eyes & Ears	Insect Stings and Bites
Asthma	Whiplash and Low Back Pain
Burns	Sprains and Pulled Muscles
Herpes	Energy Balancing and Stimulation

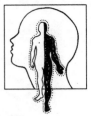

The Use of Lasers and LEDs in Acupuncture

The acupuncture system contains twelve meridians on each side of the body and two master meridians along the center line. Each meridian contains from twenty-five to one-hundred fifty acupuncture points (acupoints) and terminates at the end of a finger or toe. The meridians are named for the specific vital organs they traverse (e.g. lung, heart, stomach). Energy (or chi) flows through the meridians in a predictable manner. Health problems in the body are reflected as abnormal conditions in the meridians. Acupuncture treatment is directed towards restoring the energy flow and balance, thereby improving the health problem.

Acupuncture points can be photoactivated. In acupuncture, lasers and LEDs are being used instead of needles to stimulate the flow of life energy in the meridian system. **The benefits of light being used in place of needles is that the laser and LED is non-invasive, painless, achieves quick results, and is safe from transmitting infection (HIV, Hepatitis) to either the patient or the acupuncturist.** LEDs and soft lasers can achieve the same results as acupuncture needles, sound, low voltage electricity, or other acupuncture modalities. Since the LED has a wide dispersion, there is a larger margin of error for hitting the acupoint than with a soft laser or needles, (anywhere within a range of three quarters of an inch can be effective because of scatter of the beam). There is much more comfort when the LED is used to treat sensitive acupuncture points around the face, such as sinus and ear points.

Use the light that is within you to regain your natural clearness of sight . . . Seeing into darkness is clarity. Knowing how to yield is strength. Use your own light and return to the source of light. This is called practicing eternity.

— Lao-tzu

Acupuncture Points and the Meridians

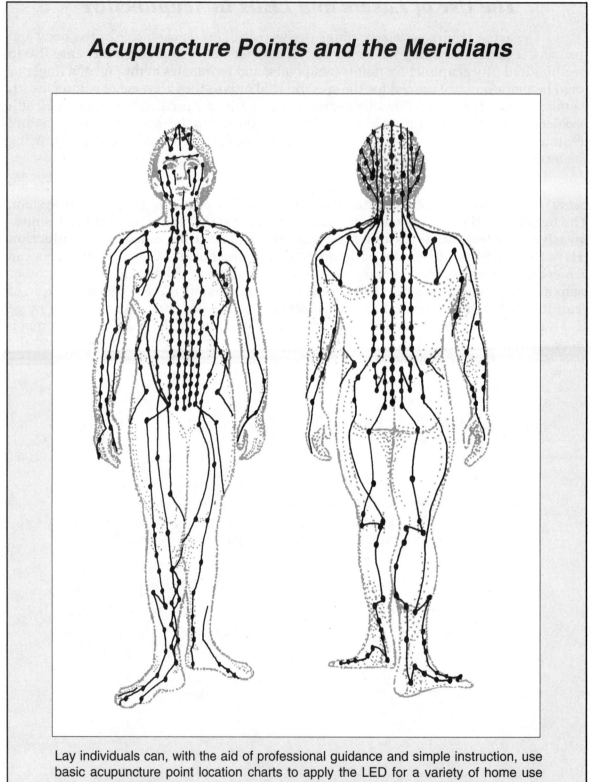

Lay individuals can, with the aid of professional guidance and simple instruction, use basic acupuncture point location charts to apply the LED for a variety of home use self-care applications.

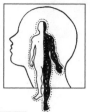

World Health Organization: Diseases that Lend Themselves to Acupuncture Treatment

In 1979, in an international seminar on acupuncture, acupuncture anaesthesia, and moxibustion held in Bejing, China, the World Health Organization enumerated a provisional list of diseases that respond favorably to acupuncture treatment. The list is based on clinical experience. The use of light in acupuncture has many potential applications. It is effective in those conditions treated by needles and shows similar benefits, requires less skill, and shows fewer side effects.

Upper Respiratory Tract
Acute Sinusitis
Acute Rhinitis
Common Cold
Acute Tonsillitis

Respiratory System
Acute Bronchitis
Bronchial Asthma

Gastro-Intestinal Disorders
Acute Bacillary Dysentery
Diarrhea
Hiccough
Gastric Hyperacidity
Chronic Duodenal Ulcer (pain relief)
Acute Duodenal Ulcer
    (without complications)

Neurological and Musculo-skeletal System
Nocturnal Enuresis
Intercostal Neuralgia
Cervicobrachial Syndrome
"Frozen Shoulder"
"Tennis Elbow"
Sciatica/Low Back Pain
Osteoarthritis
Sequelae of Poliomyelitis (early stage)

Disorders of the Mouth
Toothache
Post Extraction Pain
Gingivitis
Acute and Chronic Pharyngitis

Disorders of the Eye
Acute Conjunctivitis
Central Retinitis
Myopia (in children)
Cataract (without complications)
Constipation
Paralytic Ileus
Acute and Chronic Gastritis
Spasms of Oesophagus and Cardia

Migraine/Headache
Trigeminal Neuralgia
Facial Palsy (early stage)
Pareses following a stroke
Peripheral Neuropathies
Meniere's Disease
Neurogenic Bladder Dysfunction

The soft laser is usually held close to the skin and applied for a determined period of time to produce the desired energy treatment for a specific condition. Treatments generally range from 1 to 12 joules of energy. (A joule is a unit of energy equal to 1 watt for 1 second.) If you know the energy output of a soft laser in milliwatts, and you know the energy required for the treatment, you can calculate the number of seconds of treatment time.

The LED is applied with gentle pressure on the acupoint for approximately 30 to 90 seconds. The gentle pressure also provides a rough diagnostic technique, since the degree of acupoint sensitivity gives a relative evaluation of the status of the health problem. As the condition improves the acupoint sensitivity reduces. **Whereas lasers can only stimulate an acupoint or meridian, the LED device can either sedate with the use of continuous light or stimulate (tonify) with the use of pulsed light.**

Additional Uses of Light in Acupuncture

Research led by **Russian Olympic Team psychologist Dr. Gregory Raiport at the National Research Institute of Physical Culture in Moscow,** describes the use of laser acupuncture to treat organic problems, as well as depression, anxiety, and addictions. The cosmetic industry has used both low powered lasers and LEDs on acupuncture points on the face to help give a "facelift," as point stimulation helps tone slack muscles, ease lines, and improve blemishes. This method of light stimulation encourages the production of collagen and elastin and gives the skin tissue greater elasticity and a healthier and younger appearance. Today, there are many acupuncturists in America using light in addition to needles.

Dr. Pankratov of the Institute for Clinical and Experimental Medicine in Moscow, has verified that the **acupuncture-meridian system conducts light, particularly in the white and the red spectral range, when the light source is held against or within 1-2 millimeters of the acupoint.** This means that the body's meridian system acts as a biological fiber optics system for the distribution of light. By using the meridian ending points, an avenue exists for applying light deeper into the body than the normal red and infrared penetration depth of 4-80 millimeters, literally providing a conduit into specific organs and tissues.

With the light conductive properties of the acupuncture system now being studied more fully, it appears that the increased effectiveness of acupuncture treatments, using monochromatic light may be due to the effect of two modalities at work simultaneously: (1) the stimulation of energy (chi), and (2) the "triggering" effect of light on the photo acceptors in the problem area, resulting in accelerated tissue regeneration from the molecular level.

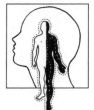

Meridian Points on the Hands and Feet Can Be Easily Treated with LED Phototherapy

Each of the twelve meridian systems is associated with a specific organ and can be easily reached by LED application to points on both sides of the fingers and toes at the base of the nails.

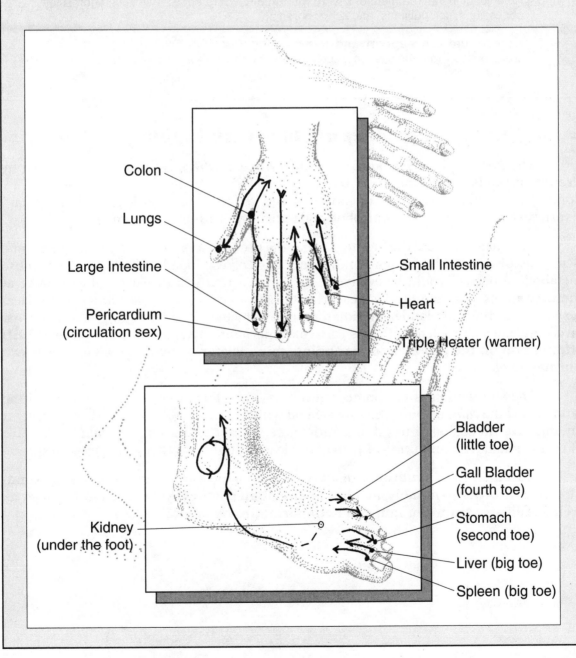

More Recent Applications of Acupuncture

1. **Environmental illness** such as poisoning from pesticides, air and water pollutants, and radiation sickness.

2. **Substance** (alcohol and chemical dependencies) **and process addictions** (relating to gambling, sex, work, and eating disorders).

3. An adjunct in the treatment of severe **mental disorders** such as anxiety, depression, obsessions, compulsions, and schizophrenia.

4. Acupuncture can **support and improve immune functioning** in patients with compromised immune systems, such as those with CFIDS, HIV, and AIDS.

Ear Acupuncture with Light

The system of ear acupuncture, called *Auriculotherapy,* was first developed by **French physician Paul Nogier, M.D.,** in the early 1950s. Auriculotherapy is traditionally done with acupuncture needles and is used in the treatment of chronic pain, dyslexia, and a variety of addictions such as alcohol, cigarettes, and withdrawal from opiates.

The Russians were the first to pioneer the use of lasers on ear acupuncture points. Scientists discovered that points on the earlobes corresponded to bodily organs whose metabolic processes could be evaluated by the measurement of electrical resistance at these earpoints. For example, by measuring the galvanic skin response (GSR) or electrical resistance at the gall bladder meridian point on the ear, a GSR reading below normal levels indicates a problem with this particular meridian. **After several minutes of LED stimulation on the gall bladder ear point, skin resistance readings change to more normal levels.**

The stimulation of ear points affects the body. For example, in pain control the point called the *valium point* when stimulated with a monochromatic red light LED, gives an objective effect similar to valium. Patients report noticing a sense of calming, a wave of relaxation and a diminution of pain and release of tightness in areas of muscle spasm.

Adrenal stress syndrome displays some of the same symptoms as seasonal affective disorder — namely, an altered circadian rhythm cycle. Auriculotherapy as well as full spectrum sunlight can help normalize this condition.

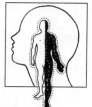
Ear Acupuncture (Auriculotherapy) Points for Treating the Adrenals

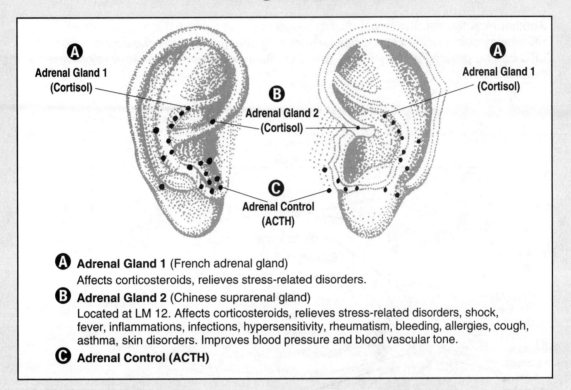

Ⓐ Adrenal Gland 1 (French adrenal gland)
Affects corticosteroids, relieves stress-related disorders.

Ⓑ Adrenal Gland 2 (Chinese suprarenal gland)
Located at LM 12. Affects corticosteroids, relieves stress-related disorders, shock, fever, inflammations, infections, hypersensitivity, rheumatism, bleeding, allergies, cough, asthma, skin disorders. Improves blood pressure and blood vascular tone.

Ⓒ Adrenal Control (ACTH)

Procedure to treat the Adrenals and Glands with LED Light

- The Adrenals (and other glands) will also benefit from the Full Spectrum Bright Light treatments by simply providing more full spectrum light through the eye.

- The Monochromatic Single-Wave Light Therapy units can provide a trigger to the acupuncture point which directly affect the adrenals. They can be applied as follows:

Method:	Minimum Application:	Notes:
1. Direct penetration through the skin in the area of the kidneys	5-7 minutes, daily	
2. To the auriculotherapy (ear) acupuncture points shown here	30-60 seconds per point with slight pressure, daily	Method 2 and 3 also can be accomplished by applying standard acupuncture or acupressure treatment techniques, as well as using the light stimulation process.
3. To the kidney meridian either at the base of the foot (K1) or on the collar bone before head of clavicle (K27)	3 minutes, twice a day	

- Progress can be monitored with the GSR, the Adrenal Stress Index Test or other circadian measurement methods.

Reflexology of the Hands

Another reported effective application of monochromatic light LED is the stimulation of the reflexology points located on the palmar surface (bottom) of the feet and on the hands. The LED can be pressed directly on the reflex points and tightly rotated slowly clockwise for several minutes.

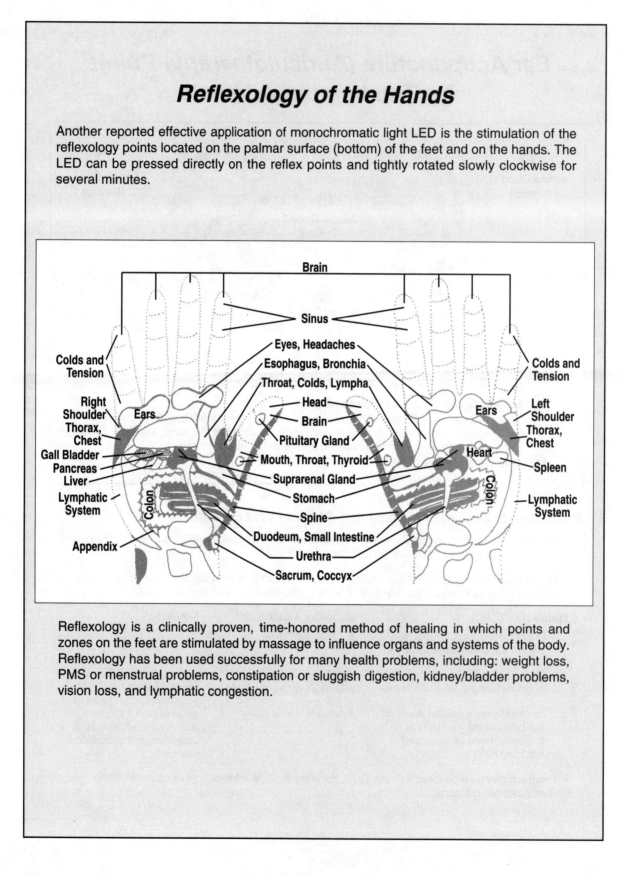

Reflexology is a clinically proven, time-honored method of healing in which points and zones on the feet are stimulated by massage to influence organs and systems of the body. Reflexology has been used successfully for many health problems, including: weight loss, PMS or menstrual problems, constipation or sluggish digestion, kidney/bladder problems, vision loss, and lymphatic congestion.

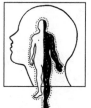

Reflexology of the Feet

Research is now being attempted to determine if monochromatic light conducts through the reflex system in the same manner as it does in the acupuncture-meridian system. If so, then light and pressure provide two modalities for results instead of just the one using energy flow.

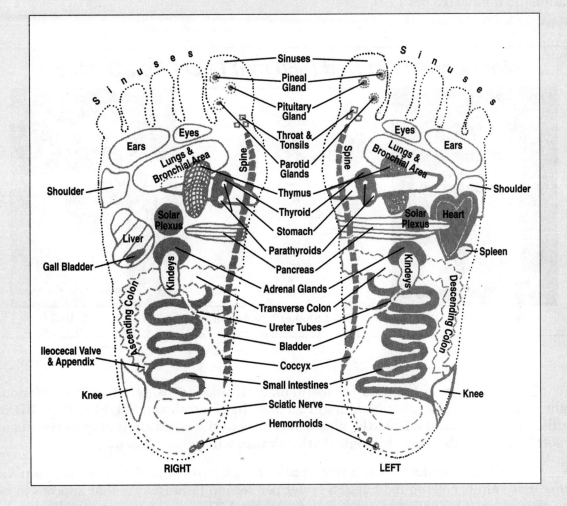

The Reflexology Zones are located on the bottom of the feet. The chart is read as if the feet are facing you.

Light Emitting Diode(LED) Phototherapy Units

LED Phototherapy devices such as the *Light Shaker*™ and *Tri-Light*™ are small, portable, battery operated units which can fit into a pocket, briefcase, or purse. **These portable units have been successfully used by acupuncturists, chiropractors, physiotherapists, massage therapists, naturopaths, and other health professionals.** LED devices are primarily designed for meridian acupuncture point applications and for surface area coverage. Both the Tri-Light™ and Light Shaker™ produce the same single monochromatic frequency (660nm) as expensive helium-neon soft laser technology. They use safe, non-coherent, light-emitting diodes that emit 6,000 to 8,000 millicandle illumination (55 milliwatts) per LED.

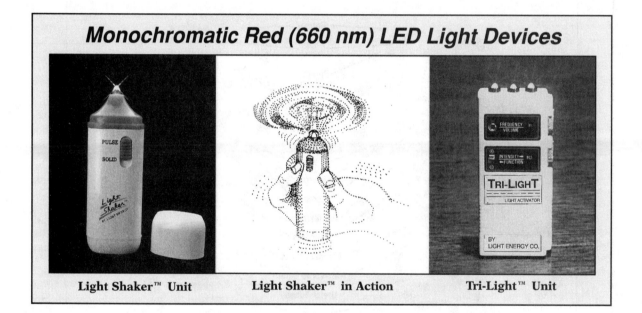

Monochromatic Red (660 nm) LED Light Devices

| Light Shaker™ Unit | Light Shaker™ in Action | Tri-Light™ Unit |

Their operation includes photostimulation function using either a continuous light (sedating) or pulsed (stimulating) function. **In general, the brighter the LED in millicandles of illumination, the closer it comes to the equivalent energy results of a soft laser, and the more biological stimulation will be produced.**

The **Light Shaker**™ has a three-position slide switch. In the upper position the *pulse mode* emits 660 nm light at 266 cycles per second (a pulse rate that appears to be the most compatible with the body's nervous system). The *continuous or solid light* is the down position, while off is in the center position.

The **Tri-Light Model II**™ was designed for faster coverage of large surface area applications on the skin, and can still be used for meridian acupuncture point applications. It is a larger version of the Light Shaker. This unit can also be used in a pulsed or continuous light mode. The **Tri-Light**™ is identical to the Tri-Light Model II™, except that this model contains five pulse rates that can alter the pulse frequency from a low of

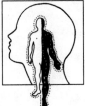

2.5 cycles per second to a high of 17,024 cycles per second. Both models can be operated with batteries or with an adaptor to use standard house electricity.

The present trend is to develop larger models with more LEDs to facilitate light application over larger areas of the body more quickly.

David and Pamela Olszewski are the owners of Light Energy Company in Seattle, Washington, which carries the products in this chapter. See *Resource List: Section One, page 342, Light Years Ahead Authors* for their address and phone numbers.

Shadow and sun — so too our lives are made — here learn how great the sun, how small the shade!

— Richard Le Gallienne

And life is colour and warmth and light and a striving evermore for these . . .

— Julian Grenfell

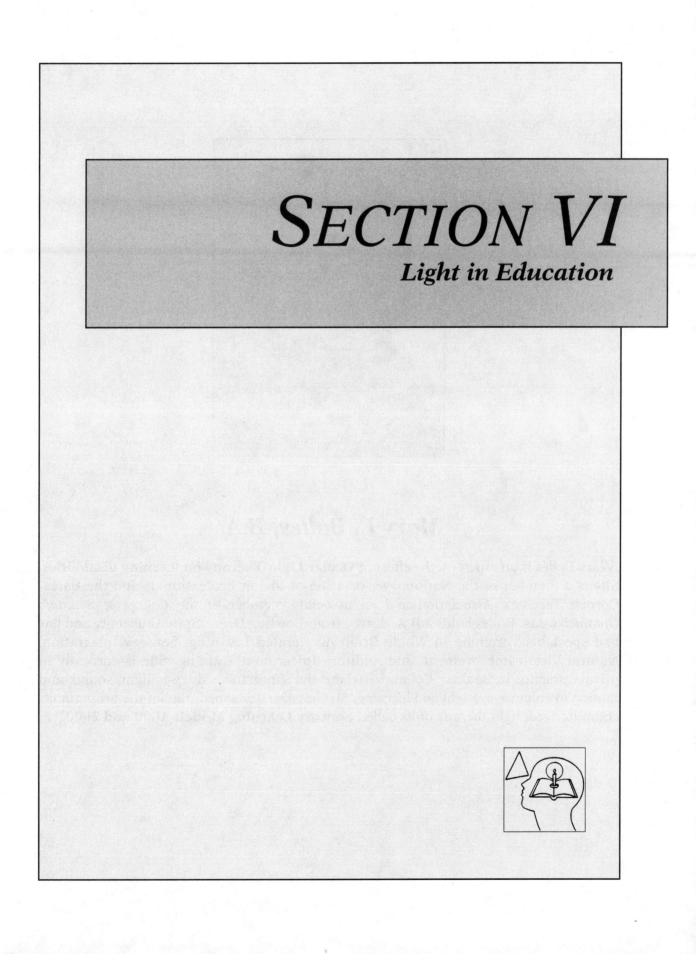

SECTION VI
Light in Education

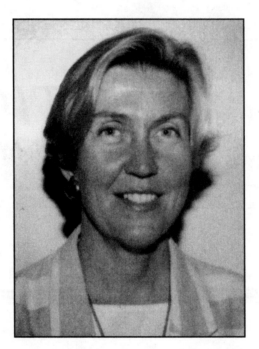

Mary L. Bolles, B.A.

Mary Bolles is an expert on the effect of **Ocular Light Therapy on learning disabilities.** She is a member of the National Association of Vision Professionals and the Bates-Corbett Teachers' Association and an associate member of the *College of Syntonic Optometry.* Ms. Bolles holds a B.A. degree from Bowling Green State University and has had specialized training in Whole Brain Accelerated Learning, Sensory Integration, Natural Vision Improvement, and Auditory Integration Training. She is currently in private practice in Boulder, Colorado, where she simultaneously uses light, sound, and motion to enhance eyesight and learning. She has also developed state-of-the-art portable, computerized, light therapy units called **Sensory Learning Models 1000 and 2000**™.

CHAPTER THIRTEEN

Learning Abilities' Dramatic Response to Light, Sound, and Motion

Mary L. Bolles, B.A.

The journey into light and color is really to "know thyself," and the end of this quote, actually, is "to be divine." An emotional tone scale that I discovered in my training is that the emotion of the pineal gland is enthusiasm. Enthusiasm means literally, "the act of bringing God within."

I'd like to relate this idea now to the area of learning disabilities, starting with *dyslexia*. I passed out these **Heart-Shaped Eye Charts** to give us a little background, to give us a feel for the dyslexic person. I'd like you to pick up the eye chart and hold it about seven inches away and choose one of the middle hearts. If you can share, sit really close together and look at the same eye chart. What you'll be doing is looking at the eye chart while I talk, and then, when I give you the signal, look up at the plain white screen or look over at the plain wall, whichever is easier for you. Remember to keep looking at the very same place.

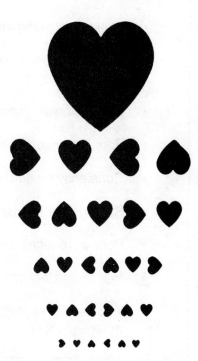

Symptoms of Dyslexia

Dyslexia involves every part of a person's existence and may include the following problems:

- Difficulty with reading, writing, and mathematics

- Difficulty with understanding words in normal conversation

- Difficulty with relating to people in groups or in understanding their conversation

- Getting lost easily (a poor or nonexistent sense of direction)

- Little or no concept of time

- Difficulty with following sequential instructions or events

- Difficulty with following motion or moving objects, such as balls, people, or traffic

- Host of different phobias, including those which are height-and motion-related, such as escalators, elevators, or bridges

- Difficulty with making decisions

- Feelings of being inferior, stupid, or clumsy

- Inability to concentrate, even when involved in an enjoyable activity such as a game

- Disequilibrium or balance dysfunction

- Poor motor coordination

- Constantly bumping into things or dropping things

- Stuttering or hesitant speech

- Poor word recall, such as the inability to remember names

- Inappropriately intense emotions or mood swings

- The need to repeatedly reread the same word or phrase to get any meaning out of it.

I can think of specific positive responses to ***phototherapy*** involving each of these facets of learning in dyslexia. Yet, **what I see most consistently in clients of all ages is that after the light, sound, and motion treatments they have less fear**. **Fear may actually be *the* learning problem. Fear actually causes a breakdown in the connections between the various brain centers. Thus, the major change I've witnessed in most people after light therapy is a lessening of fear and an accompanying increase of peace within that person.**

So, now look up at the wall or the screen. The hearts may be coming up as white now and the background as black. You may even see some color. The color you see indicates the nerve plexi from which you're operating. If you see yellow, you're operating from your solar plexus. Maybe you saw blue, pink, or green around the edges. Then that is the color which would most help your memory. Use that color of paper or index card to write things down that you want to remember, and use that color of highlight pen.

Each level of sensitivity in the body is correlated to a part of ***The Seven-Tiered Brain,* a concept which was conceived by Bruce Lipton, Ph.D., at Stanford University, and Christopher Hills has also written about it. The physical areas of the Seven-Tiered Brain all have their own learning mode.** On the chart on the following page we see the different plexi and the seven parts of the brain. This model is how we conceptualize the seven brain centers and their different functions. They start at the lower brain stem and come up to the cortex at the top of the brain. Each of these areas has its own learning mode.

I shall remold my consciousness. In this new year I am a new person. And I shall change my consciousness again and again until I have driven away all the darkness of ignorance and manifested the shining Light of Spirit in whose image I am made.

— *Paramahansa Yogananda*
AFFIRMATIONS FOR REMOVING BAD HABITS

The Seven-Tiered Brain

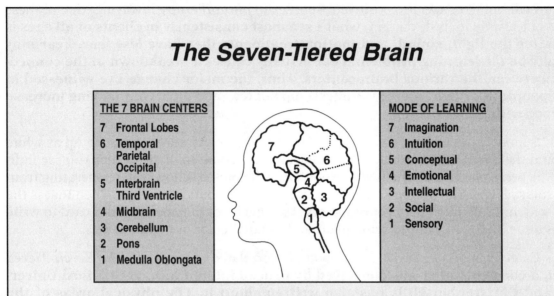

THE 7 BRAIN CENTERS	MODE OF LEARNING
7 Frontal Lobes	7 Imagination
6 Temporal Parietal Occipital	6 Intuition
5 Interbrain Third Ventricle	5 Conceptual
4 Midbrain	4 Emotional
3 Cerebellum	3 Intellectual
2 Pons	2 Social
1 Medulla Oblongata	1 Sensory

1. **The Medulla Oblongata** is concerned with the **senses** and expresses itself physically in activities such as walking and dancing.

2. **The Pons** is the area involved with **social instincts** and use of social skills.

3. **The Cerebellum** is the part of the brain that makes someone an **intellectual**, operating like a computer, scanning, categorizing and selecting, as it is cross-referenced and coded with all the signals entering into the first two brain parts; this third brain area dissects things piece by piece.

4. **The Midbrain** is the fourth part of the brain, and this is where the *hypothalamus, pineal,* and *pituitary* are located. This part of the brain **correlates with the heart** in the body; the midbrain integrates the lower functions which gives one the **emotional sense** of being secure within their environment. This **feeling** sense is important, because when we think of ourselves, what we're really doing is thinking of how we feel. The midbrain also relates the past to the future. **The midbrain's function is to connect the three lower levels with the three higher levels of the brain.** Looking at these seven centers in relation to the whole body, the heart would be in the midbrain center, because no matter what part of the brain we're talking about, it's all going to loop back to our heart center, which includes our feelings and our sense of security.

5. **The Interbrain** (in the third ventricle) is the fifth part of the brain. It operates opposite to the third brain, the cerebellum; its function is **conceptual** — it puts things all together in a meaningful way. This area forms a concept, then looks at the environment to see if the whole is present.

6. **The Temporal, Parietal and the Occipital Lobe.** These three lobes control our sixth level of experience of **knowing**; using this part of the brain, we listen to the voice of our own **intuition**.

7. **The Frontal Lobe** is concerned with the most complex abilities of the mind: **imagination, creativity, and creating through foresight** (making positive images about our future).

Next, we come to the problem of *learning disabilities* in children. We all know that the parents of the learning disabled child get behind their bedroom door every night and say to each other, "What are we going to do about him/her?" One of them may say, "Well, I don't know. This problem didn't come from my side of the family!" When there is a learning problem in a family, it's often a tense situation. **Dyslexia is a broad term that includes a number of disorders affecting people's ability to read. It is believed to affect 4 to 5% of the population, or some 12 million Americans.** The majority of investigators have determined that this complex disability is a bewildering combination of processes leading to a disorganization of responses within the central nervous system.

Parents usually do not realize that their child's learning and behavioral problems are often the result of mental processing problems which the child can't control. Many times the child seems completely normal except for difficulties with school work, so no one suspects that the child is experiencing inefficient and irregular sensory processing.

The learning disabled child's major problem area is perception. Perception is the major key to reading. *Visual Perception* has nothing to do with visual acuity.

Five Areas of Visual Perception

1. Perception of position in space

2. Perception of spatial relationships and sequences

3. Perception of constancies such as size, brightness, and color

4. Visual-motor coordination

5. Perception of figure/ground relationships

Likewise, **Auditory Perception** is a problem, for dyslexics cannot break down words to their basic sounds, and they have lasting problems with the sound system of language, even if their reading problems improve over time.

Joseph Chilton Pearce, author of *The Magical Child* and *The Crack in the Cosmic Egg*, says:

> *Right before birth there is a major housecleaning that has to take place in the neurons of the brain. Certain functional neuronal structures that are appropriate only for uterine experience have to be deconstructed or they would be excess baggage.[1]*

---

1. Many dyslexic, school-age children still show evidence of infant level reflexes such as *tonic neck reflex* and *tonic labyrinthine reflex*, which normally children outgrow in their development.

In *The New York Times* (Sunday, September 15, 1991), there was an article in which the lead sentence read, "A new finding about dyslexia suggests that the disorder may not be a malfunction in the way people understand language, but rather a brain abnormality that involves the sense of vision, and perhaps also hearing and touch."

It has recently been thought that ***the visual system*** is composed of two major pathways:

1. **The magno-cellular system,** which evolved in animals to help them see predators move in the dark. It is composed of *large cells that carry out faster visual processes.* For example, if these cells were runners, they would be the sprinters, those with the fast-twitch muscle fibers.

2. **The parvo-cellular system** probably evolved to help primates see brightly colored fruit while swinging through the trees in broad daylight, it is composed of *smaller cells that carry out slower visual processes.*

For a person to be able to read, the information from the magno-cellular system must precede the information from the slower, parvo-cellular system in exactly the right time sequence. **Dr. Mary Williams of the University of New Orleans,** has found that when children read through blue plastic gel filters, the timing of the cells between the magno system and the slower parvo system becomes more finely synchronized. When enough of the red is removed from what the dyslexic sees, these cells are allowed to work normally.

Dr. Albert Galaburda, Director of the Dyslexia Neuroanatomical Laboratory at Beth Israel Hospital in Boston, says, "Scientists have found that animals can form antibodies that destroy a protein found only in a magno-cellular system." This suggests that dyslexia could even be an autoimmune condition or a predisposition acquired before, or soon after, birth. Abnormally processed sights and sounds might begin to shape the infant's brain and cause it to be wired differently from the start.

Joseph Chilton Pearce speaks of various conditions in modern life which can seriously impede the development of a child's intelligence. When there's a separation of the mother and the infant immediately after birth, a psychic shock is produced. A connection or link is made between the two hearts while the child is in utero that must be re-established after birth. Immediately after birth each heart sends a signal to the brain, and the brain shifts its functioning accordingly. This bond is then carried over to the new environment, giving a foundation of unity within the new diversity between the mother and the child. If that connection doesn't happen immediately after birth, there can be a buildup of adrenal steroids which, after about 45 minutes, causes the infant to lose consciousness from the overload and go into shock. It then takes an average of three months for nature to compensate for this damage. In our modern-day-hospital-birth-culture we see it as "natural" that there are few signs of consciousness in the child until somewhere around the tenth to twelfth week after birth.

When **Paul McClean** was **Director of the National Institute of Mental Health's Department of Brain Evolution and Behavior**, his theory of *The Triune Brain* described the functions of our three separate brains. He looked at our three-part brain as evolutionary. It's as though we see the world through three different evolutionary perspectives, three quite different mentalities, two of which communicate not with words, but with motions or emotions.

The Triune Brain

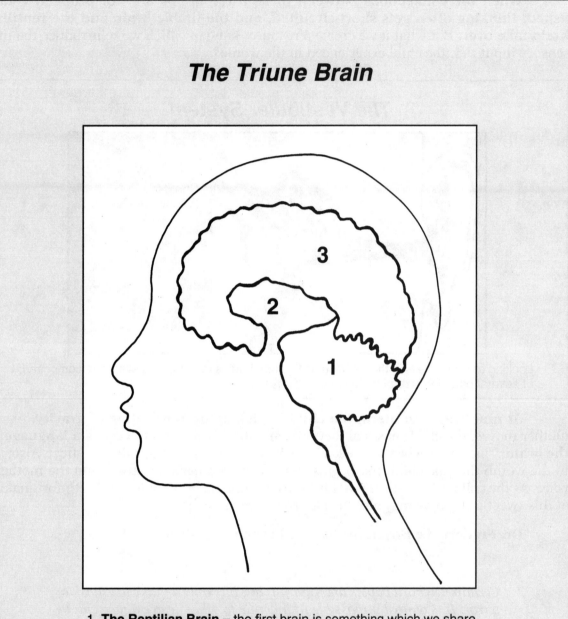

1. **The Reptilian Brain** – the first brain is something which we share with all animals, reptiles, and amphibians. Among other things, it incorporates **bodily movement, motor skills, and sensory impressions.** In a fully functioning human there is a perfect integration and balance between the three brain systems. The reptilian brain involves itself only with **physical activity.**

2. **The Limbic System** – the second brain, is concerned only with **feelings and emotions.**

3. **The Neocortex** – the third brain, relates to what we call **thinking.**

When the connections between these three brains are not properly established, thinking often gets short-circuited, and the limbic brain and the reptilian brain take over. But what if we create a resource state in which we reintroduce the first sensory input that the child experienced in the womb?

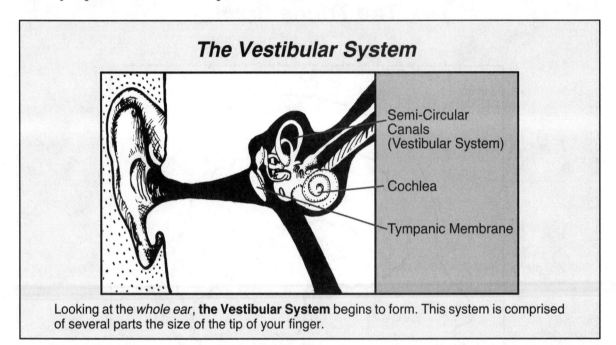

The Vestibular System

Semi-Circular Canals (Vestibular System)

Cochlea

Tympanic Membrane

Looking at the *whole ear*, **the Vestibular System** begins to form. This system is comprised of several parts the size of the tip of your finger.

At nine weeks in utero, the child is picking up the feeling of gravity. As the mother moves, the child senses all her movement. This **motion becomes a language of the brain**. That's why when we rock a baby it has a very quieting, calming effect. Also, it's in the womb that the child first begins to hear the mother's heartbeat and the mother's voice. As the child is born there is a third sensory input, a bright white light. Unfortunately, at this sweet time there may also be a lot of trauma and fear.

Dr. Frederic Le Boyer, the famous **French pediatrician,** says:

> *Certain newborn babies are frightful, but it is only a mask the mask of terror. It is almost impossible to imagine to what degree a face can be deformed, disfigured by this terror. Once fear is exorcised, the mask falls away and the most repellant child changes; unrecognizably.*

When I first see children, I look right at their faces and into their eyes and at the way they hold their facial muscles. You can see how their brains are working and how their hearts are feeling. The one thing I really watch is their facial changes, it's the way I can tell what's going on.[2]

---

2. The carriage of the face and body posturing change dramatically after Ms. Bolles' therapy, indicating a deeper state of nervous system relaxation.

Case A – Head Injury, Learning Disabled Child

The first case, ***Case A,*** is that of a kindergarten child with a *head injury,* who had taken a dive into the corner of a sharp piece of furniture and opened up the top of his forehead. Amazingly, nothing changed in either the behavior or the *learning ability* of the child until about a year-and-a-half later, when everything precipitously changed. This is when I did a ***visual field test*** on him. He was in the middle of the first grade by then and he couldn't learn the spelling words; they'd be there one minute, and then some cloud would pass over his mind and that spelling word would disappear. So, he was put in a learning disability class, and the teachers were afraid he would not be able to pass the proficiency test to go into second grade.

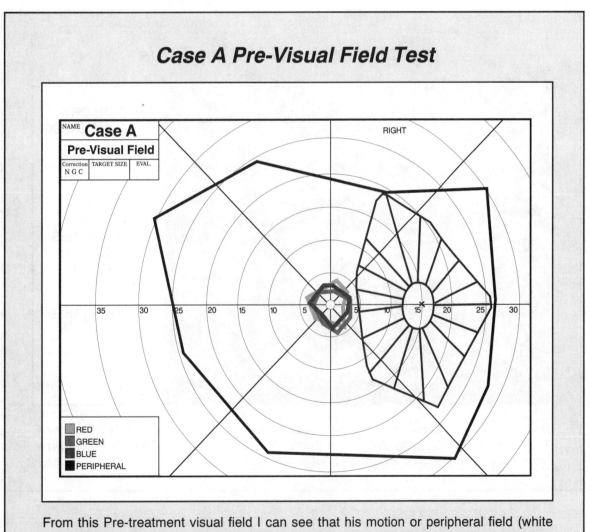

Case A Pre-Visual Field Test

From this Pre-treatment visual field I can see that his motion or peripheral field (white markers) had collapsed somewhat. The blind spot (the oval that begins at approximately 15 degrees) is constricted around the edge of the optic nerve, and these color fields (red, blue, and green markers) are constricted as well.

Therapeutically, **I work with simultaneous motion and light stimulation,** and until recently, that was all I worked with.[3] So, at the time of this case I had the child lie on a *Motion Table* (called a *Graham Potentializer*) in a darkened room. If there was a dinner plate on his feet, he would be moving in a seven inch circle on the Motion Table, and sometimes it would go counterclockwise, and then sometimes the circle would go from his head to his feet. In my office the light stimulator hangs above the table. This is a light instrument I've manufactured called the *Sensory Learning 2000*™, which will soon be for sale (see *Resource List*). One knob changes the colors automatically so that you can go through six colors, with the ability to project either constant or oscillating (flashing) color. Colors include: magenta, ruby, red, yellow, green, blue-green, and purple. The child continues to look at the light while on the Motion Table.

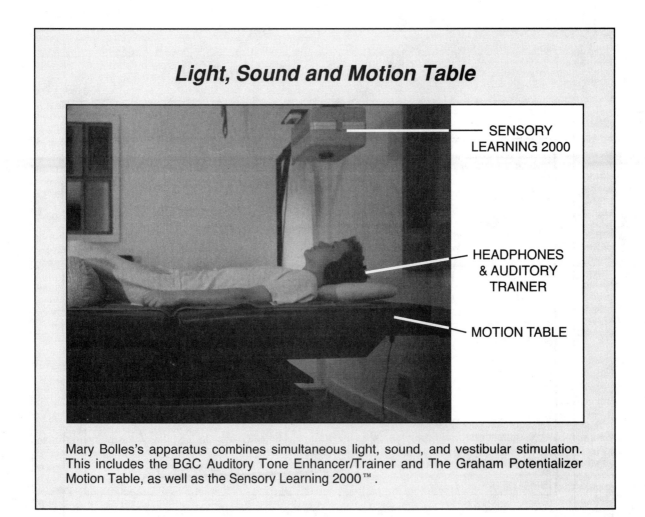

Light, Sound and Motion Table

SENSORY LEARNING 2000

HEADPHONES & AUDITORY TRAINER

MOTION TABLE

Mary Bolles's apparatus combines simultaneous light, sound, and vestibular stimulation. This includes the BGC Auditory Tone Enhancer/Trainer and The Graham Potentializer Motion Table, as well as the Sensory Learning 2000™.

---

3. Mary Bolles has recently added *sound* to her repertoire via the BGC Auditory Tone Enhancer. She simultaneously stimulates the client's visual, vestibular, and auditory systems.

Case A Post-Visual Field Test

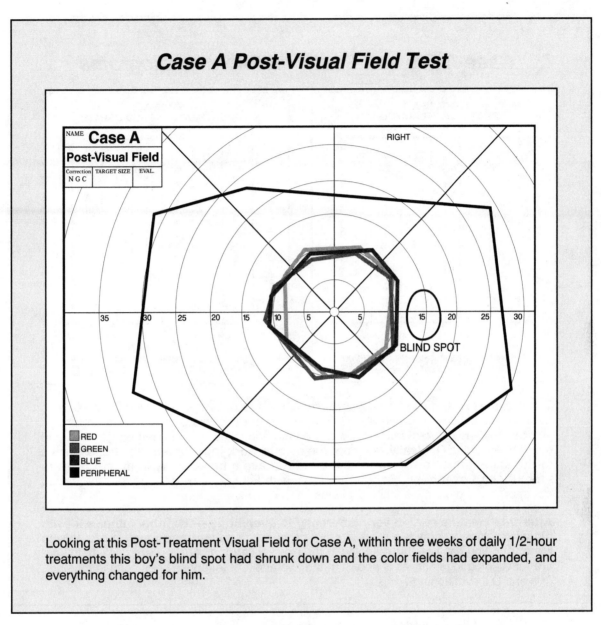

Looking at this Post-Treatment Visual Field for Case A, within three weeks of daily 1/2-hour treatments this boy's blind spot had shrunk down and the color fields had expanded, and everything changed for him.

You can't behave differently until the eyes perceive things differently.

— *Suzan Dallé*

"... the fire of the eye causes a gentle light to issue from it. The interior light coalesces with the daylight, like to like, forming thereby a single homogeneous body of light. That body, a marriage of inner light and outer, forges a link between the objects of the world and the soul. It becomes the bridge along which the subtle motions of an exterior object may pass, causing the sensation of sight."

— *Plato*

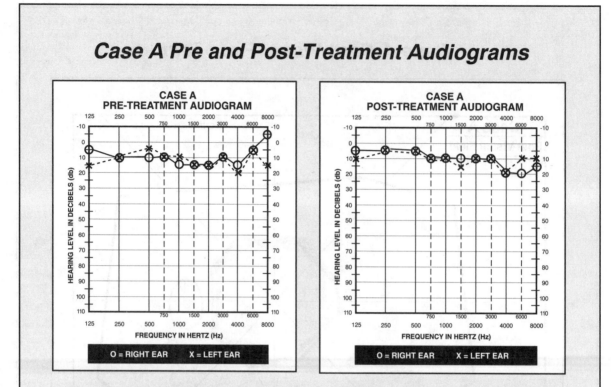

Case A Pre and Post-Treatment Audiograms

This was the ***Pre and Post-Test Audiogram for Case A.*** We were looking for the sounds to which the child is sensitive. As you can see from the audiogram, *decibels* are on the vertical axis, the different *frequencies* are on the horizontal axis, the left ear is the X and the right ear is the O. **Ideally, we want the ears to work together so the sounds arrive at the same time, and we want the child to have a nervous system that reflects stability and evenness**. So, I treated him with light, sound, and motion; the sound treatment filtered out the sensitive sounds for that child.

After treatment he related very differently to everybody — with his father and with his whole family. Now his mother says he is much calmer and much more able to cope. And you can see this reflected in the ***Post-Treatment Audiogram.*** Now both ears are functioning together, as is shown in the two auditory response lines coming together, (X's and O's overlapping).

    The children who have learning problems are actually *overly* sensitive to certain sounds. Autistic children can actually hear snow hitting the ground; to them it's as loud as breaking glass!

    You may have seen **Dr. Guy Berard's** work. **He's a French doctor who specializes in auditory therapies** and he appeared on the television program "20/20" this past summer. I combine his sound work with the light and the motion. Sound work is very hard for children to do. *The sound therapy component* consists of musical selections — some with words, some without, played on a CD through headphones. Then it is put through another piece of equipment the **BGC Auditory Tone Enhancer/Trainer,** *(see photo page 318)* which filters out the frequencies to which the client is most sensitive. After treatment I do another audiogram and watch the sensitivities flatten out.

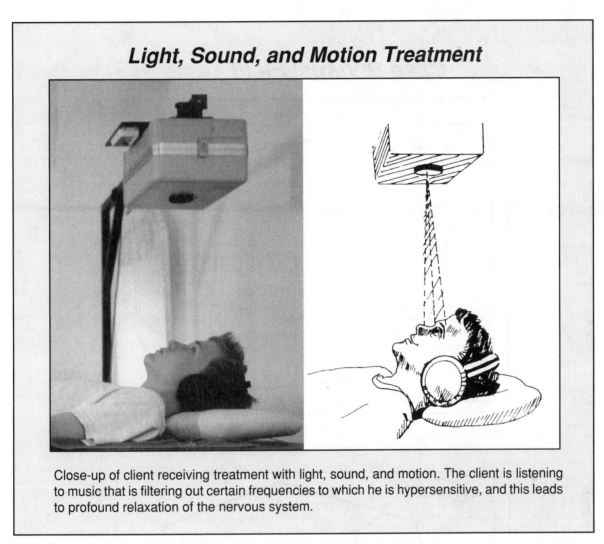

Light, Sound, and Motion Treatment

Close-up of client receiving treatment with light, sound, and motion. The client is listening to music that is filtering out certain frequencies to which he is hypersensitive, and this leads to profound relaxation of the nervous system.

Dr. Albert Tomatis, a French doctor who has also worked with sound, believes that the ear is one of the first organs that forms in the fetus. The nervous system takes its cue as to how it forms and functions from the ear. The tiny hair cells of the inner ear are all frequency-specific, as are the nerve cells. Yet, the ear is considered to be a rather primitive part of the brain because it and the way we hear hasn't changed much during thousands of years of evolution.

Case B – Dyslexic Adult

Next, we have the case of a thirty-five year-old dyslexic male, Case B, who is a chiropractic student. He had some extremely difficult times. He was a Cesarean birth. His mother, a woman with a genius IQ, is in Mensa, and his brother is a medical student. There were never any hereditary signs of a learning disability in this family. Added to this pressure, he'd always had a difficult time with his relationship with his father.

Case B Visual Field Tests

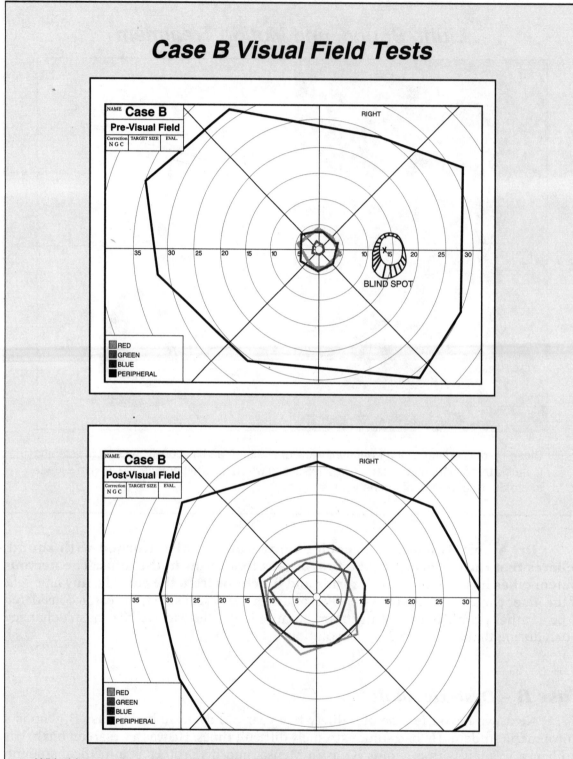

With this case there is a definite improvement between his Pre and Post-Visual Field tests, as can be seen in the expansion in client's Post-Treatment Visual Field.

Case B Pre and Post-Treatment Audiograms

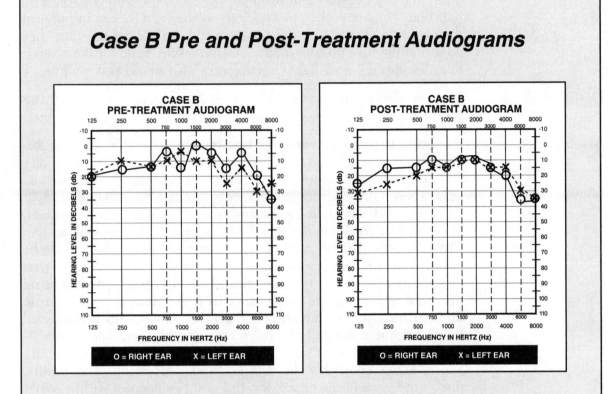

Notice that on this ***Pre-Treatment Audiogram*** sensitivity is in the high end. Also, he is very sensitive in the middle frequencies. Not coincidentally, the mid-range frequencies are those by which we hear language. So, he had to tape all of his lectures. He absolutely could not learn things verbally or auditorily. On the ***Post-Treatment Audiogram*** for Case B, look at the nice improvement in auditory perception that he attained. **Afterwards, this man had a very different sense about himself. He's excited about life and learning. He feels more confident and is passing all of his tests now. He is better organized; he prioritizes his work better; he feels better about himself; and he doesn't get so angry any more.**

QUESTION: Would a perfect score on the audiogram be marks all along the zero line?

Ms. BOLLES: We're looking mostly at the configuration here. It should be more flat than up and down, and the ears should work together.

QUESTION: Do you work this way with the adults also?

Ms. BOLLES: Yes. With children I do a half-hour in the morning and a half-hour in the afternoon. Remember, that the way that I work is incorporating all three of these modalities together. I do light, sound, and motion daily for two weeks. They go on the Motion Table for a half

311

hour, and the Ocular Light Stimulation and the sound goes on for a half-hour concurrently. The children do the light for ten minutes at the beginning of that session; then in the middle ten minutes they do something like puzzles on the Motion Table. Then for the last ten minutes they do more light concurrently with sound and motion.

QUESTION: Do you also notice sensitivity to motion sickness in learning disabled people?

Ms. BOLLES: It's all tied in with the visual and vestibular systems. The table movement is very slow; it's eleven revolutions a minute, which is very calming, and the sessions themselves do not create any motion sickness. There's one characteristic I see no matter how well they cover it up, and that is in their hearts they have a low self-image. If you go to the **Orton Dyslexic Society** and you hear these people come in and talk, one of them may be a very famous judge, but inside he doesn't have that image of himself. Instead, he has an image that he's always having to be bolstered. **Actually, with the learning disabled, self-image is often more of a problem than academic difficulties.** As an educational therapist, I work in a darkened room, helping these children to go through their fear and their self-doubt. With feelings it's always the same. First, it's the denial and anger, and second, it's the sadness and depression. And finally, there's the joy and the peace of mind that lies deepest within. What we're working toward is that master gland, the *pineal*. There are billions of us; each of us has a different type of intellect. The brain is diversity. We are impelled outward by our curious intellect. Yet our brains are diverse — despite our differences, we are all alike.

Beyond our identities and desires, there's a common core of self, and it is in that place which **T.S. Elliot** calls *the still point* that resides the intelligence of the heart. There is always that thread back to the unified state of things where we feel safe and non-threatened. **Light really does seem to open us up to love and to feelings of security that may have been obscured by trauma in the womb or birth or by recent or past emotional or physical trauma. When this is replaced by a feeling of security, you cannot stop a child from learning!**

QUESTION: Is the point of filtering out the sensitive areas of sound simply to make that treatment acceptable or comfortable for the patient or the client at that particular time, or does it make some sort of permanent change in their hearing patterns?

Ms. BOLLES: The sound affects them on every level, just like light. It's a powerful sensory input, and they're dealing with the way they receive sound all the time, twenty-four hours a day. They're actually hearing something too well, and this is how they're hearing it differently after treatment. **When we make a particular sound one hair frequency**

less sensitive, there's a long-term change, a relaxation that happens in the whole system; it's permanent. It's a little hair that is just very, very sensitive; and when that relaxes, everything changes for those children. Typically, as they go through the sessions, they get more and more tense because they're hearing all this sound, but they're not getting that sharp pain. Then, gradually, **fear and tension just drain out of the body and they relate in a wholly different way.**

QUESTION: Mary, do most children have some kind of problem that would benefit by going through this?

Ms. BOLLES: For learning enhancement? Yes. Yet I always like to do all the testing so that I know exactly where I'm starting and continue with both auditory and visual monitoring. And yes, the treatments are enhancing. One person just asked, "Is this good for *any* child?" There's a sensitive period in every child's development, so when there's any hesitation there, it seems most natural to me to intervene and to make this developmental period really easy and fun. **Learning really occurs in the unconscious mind.** Learning goes on all the time; it isn't something we have to put effort into. It should just be that socially and emotionally everything's fine with the child so they will automatically learn all the time.

I work with a lot of children who come to me because visual problems are their primary difficulty. And I work with a lot of children with *wandering eyes*. **We have such good response with the *Motion Table* and with light; it's working all those extrinsic eye muscles.** I also have had lots of children who have been in glasses for five years or more, and they have been able to walk away from them and maintain their functioning very, very well. This treatment really goes a long way. I work with families and children in a basic way. I also have the children's progress monitored by an optometrist.

QUESTION: What kinds of different motion exercises do you use?

Ms. BOLLES: The Motion Table that I have is called a *Graham Potentializer*™. It was designed by **David Graham,** although it's not being made by him now. It is a table that moves in a seven-inch circle, eleven revolutions a minute. He didn't design it for this work really. I use this table, because I'm working from **Gene Ayer's** theories. He was an occupational therapist who had the child roll over and over like a log on the floor.

The man in this chart is moving around in circles, and what this *vestibular movement* is doing is making the fluid in the *inner ear canals* move. The movement of that fluid excites the brain at the levels of the pons, and that makes all the messages, including the visual messages, get around the body more easily.

QUESTION: What is benefitted?

Ms. BOLLES: Everything changes for these children. You can't even see that it's the same child. Everything gets better for these children. The parents come to me just looking for a little bit of improvement, and they are so amazed that they go out telling everyone about it. They almost oversell it. There's really no limit to the changes that can happen. As I described the list of dyslexic symptoms *(see chart page 298),* I read all those different things that dyslexic people feel when they are stressed. We all pick up some of these same symptoms from time to time. Yet, all of those symptoms can just float away with the use of light, sound, and motion.

QUESTION: In **Joseph Chilton Pearce's** latest book, *Evolution's End,* he includes the idea that cranial sacral manipulation, including the temporal mandibular joint (TMJ), affects the inner ear canal and helps place the eyes in the proper position.

Ms. BOLLES: Yes, and going through the birth canal is also molding this area. It's very important.

QUESTION: Okay, does body position on the Motion Table make a difference? Do you use a flashing light sometimes, rather than a solid light? And do you ever change the sequence? And what is the sequence?

Ms. BOLLES: **The light source on the light, sound, and motion table has an oscillation to it.** The light is always on in the center of the Motion Table; first it comes on bright and then fades. If this were sound, it would be getting louder and softer. I find this works better than the flashing light; it seems more alive, more natural, and more in tune with breathing and in resonance to the color. As for position on the table, these kids often require tactile stimulation, and a lot of times, they're around three-and-a-half years-old. When they look at the color, I may hold their hands or I may put my hand on their body or the child may hold onto my earlobe. You can just feel that the child becomes one with the light. If they become really scared, they just pinch my earlobe really tight. Then often the child asks, "Could I have a hug?" So, you do whatever you can to stay with them, to help them to go through their experience of the light. Some of these kids just can't get a whole sentence together or can't remember the names of their playmates. However, when they're under the light, and they're moving, they say everything perfectly. Then things really begin to work better, and they begin to develop more evenly.

I start the session with *magenta,* and I may have to start with it in small increments of time, like five minutes, and build up from there. **I always try to start treatment on the *red end of the spectrum*. That color represents the lower brain stem area, and it also is going to stimulate activity in the lower part of the chakra system. The brain stem area is where the thoughts and traumas are that they've held onto the longest.** They will need to stay with that color, even though another color might be easier; but I still go for the red. **Red is opening**, and the **magenta is more balancing**. Magenta is a perfect blend of the violet and the red. So, red is where we start, and then we just look for a change in the child. I look for a calming and then move on to the next colors another day. Usually, every session will begin with *red* or *ruby*. **What I'm trying to put into this child is an organization of their perceptions and an ability for them to have flexibility within their system. Gradually, they will be able to comfortably move from one color to the next all the way through the spectrum**.

Some adults are really sensitive, but still I want to try to begin with light from the red end. If I'm working with a child in the morning, it probably would be *red.* If we had used red in the morning and we were going to use *blue-green* in the afternoon, we would begin the second session with a little *red,* then a little *yellow-green*, and then we'd use *blue-green.* **I always start with the base color and go in.**

Dr. Levinson learned a lot from his dyslexic patients. He uses a drug that has worked with vestibular problems and motion sickness. It also helps children with learning problems. This drug also works on the pons, that lower part of the brain stem. I haven't personally had experience with it, but I've studied his work. I believe that by stimulating the vestibular system, drugs might be unnecessary. The system of light, sound, and motion treatment may titrate out what's being masked with drugs.

QUESTION: On a practical level, have you had any trouble, since you don't come from a medical background, with authorities in any way? Using this as an educator, have you had difficulties about that?

Ms. BOLLES: No, I have really gotten respect and cooperation from a lot of medical people, and, of course, I wish more educators were ready for it. But we're really moving. It's coming.

QUESTION: Have you noticed a significant increase between using light alone versus light, sound, and motion together? Is there synergy?

Ms. BOLLES: Yes, I started out using sound and motion. We would hold a child in our arms. We had a small round platform that moved around slowly like they use at Sea World for the seals. We would hold this child in a darkened room where we had thirty-two speakers positioned all around the room, and we overwhelmed them with all kinds of sounds. Great things happened for these children! Then we'd take a flashlight and we'd shine it in their eyes; their eyes would start to track. They would just make all kinds of wonderful progress.

Next, I moved on to working with light, sound, and motion. Now that I have found where I can go with the audiograms, I know exactly how to filter out the specific frequency of sound that's exactly right for each child. **After ten days of using light, sound, and motion, we follow up with two more weeks of just light; that's the protocol.** Now I'm working with really difficult children, and I know that this synergy is a lot easier on the children than working with one modality alone. I also now know that **had I used sound earlier with some of the children, rather than only light, I would have been able to have a greater impact on them**. In our daily life we've got light, sound, and motion going on all the time, and to separate it out makes it more difficult to use as an enhancement tool. It makes sense that we should keep it all together, and it really works like a resource state from which that child may draw.

QUESTION: How do you test the visual field?

Ms. BOLLES: The *visual field testing device,* also called a *Campimeter*™ *(see page 31),* is a well-lighted, slanted apparatus that the child sits about a foot away from. How do we check for the visual field? We move in from the corners a half-degree-sized round target in the different colors, the same colors as the cones, the eyes' color receptors. For example, first I'd move in a red target, a pointer with a tiny red tip; then I'd move in a green target; and then I'd move in a blue target. *The blue color cone* is thought to correlate with the physical part of the person, the **lower reptilian brain,** or the part involved with movement and motion. *The red color cone* is thought to correlate to the **limbic system's activity**. So, this gives an idea of how much light is coming in and touching these parts of the brain. *The green* *color cone* correlates to the **neocortex,** the thinking part of the brain, which is the last part to develop in the child. **We normally expect the blue field to be the largest, the red field to be next, and the green to be the smallest.** After treatment we always see such a lovely expansion, so you know more light is touching the green, the cortex; the red, the limbic system; and the blue, the reptilian brain. Both objectively and subjectively, you see wonderful things going on.

QUESTION: What is the device you use to filter out those sounds?

Ms. BOLLES: The instrument[4] I'm using is made in San Diego, and it's the only one made in this country. It's called an ***Audio Tone Enhancer/ Trainer,*** made by ***BGC Enterprises*** *(see photo on following page),* and it supports **Dr. Guy Berard's** work and **Dr. Tomatis'** work. Dr. Tomatis has French-made sound filtering equipment. Dr. Berard also has sound filtering equipment that's made in France, called the ***Kinitron.*** There are about three different filtering devices that I know of, and I'm using the BGC.

QUESTION: How could we all learn to do what you're doing?

Ms. BOLLES: I'm willing to share however I can. Doing a traveling show with the Graham Potentializer, the Motion Table, would be very difficult. It's a $13,000 piece of equipment that's very large and very heavy. You have to break it all apart, but I've broken it all apart and taken it in a van to chiropractic offices. I mean I have done whatever it takes, and I am willing to do it all, if there's an interest to learn about it.

QUESTION: Would you show us your light instrument?

Ms. BOLLES: The instrument comes on and changes colors. The instrument is portable and computerized. It holds 999 programs and is able to make whatever changes you'd like in light exposure time, flicker rate, and light intensity. I wanted to make something portable that the family could take into the closet or bathroom or laundry room, or wherever they could make it dark in their home. When families do the light work together, there often is a real bonding. This is a great opportunity for parents to learn how to really help their children!

---

4. For information on Mary Bolles' phototherapy instrument and sound filtering devices, See *Resource List: page 373, Colored Light Therapy Instruments, and Section Ten, page 378, Other Instruments Mentioned in this Book.*

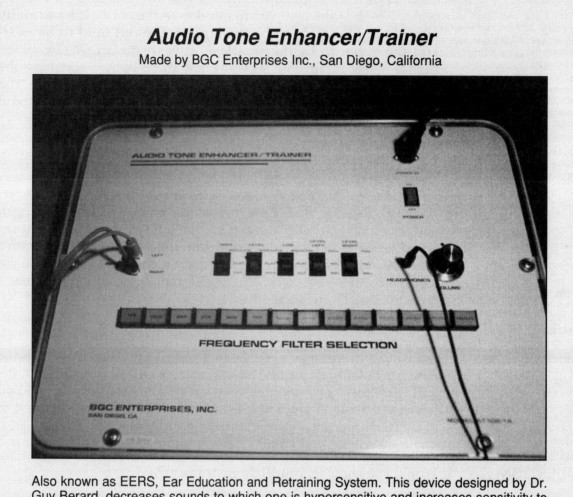

Audio Tone Enhancer/Trainer

Made by BGC Enterprises Inc., San Diego, California

Also known as EERS, Ear Education and Retraining System. This device designed by Dr. Guy Berard, decreases sounds to which one is hypersensitive and increases sensitivity to those frequencies to which one is hyposensitive.

You are light in the Lord; walk as children of light.

— Ephesians 5:8

Be joyful, for joy lets in light.

— Motto from Human Service Alliance, Winston-Salem, N.C.

SECTION VII
Light in Spiritual Awakening

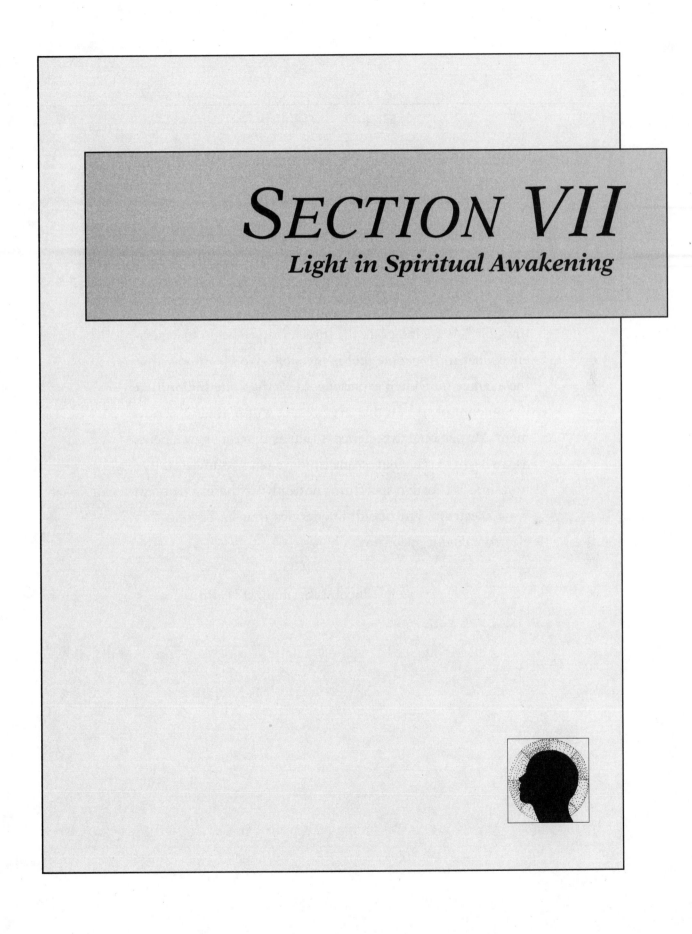

Jonathan Swift said, "Real vision is the ability to see the invisible." As we integrate the three eyes, we begin to experience what most people feel is invisible. We now know that the average individual experiences less than one-billionth of the amount of stimuli that are present within their environment. My personal experience is that as that *inner eye* opens, as we begin to see what at one time we felt was invisible, we tune into a broader spectrum, not only of the electromagnetic spectrum, but of subtle energies that lie beyond this electromagnetic spectrum.

Jacob Liberman, O.D., Ph.D.

CHAPTER FOURTEEN

From Light to Enlightenment

Jacob Liberman, O.D., Ph.D.

Norm Shealy **said that the only negative emotion is fear.** I just want to share with you that, **from my experience, there are no negative emotions; there are only unexpressed emotions**. A few moments ago something came to mind about negative responses. I've never experienced any negative responses. The only thing that I have experienced is when an individual I'm working with has something surface and I have that same thing within myself. Then I act as a "tuning fork" in relation to their "tuning fork," it resonates in that same place within myself. If I am not in touch with that, to the point that I cannot be with it and allow that to be a learning experience for me, then I become uneasy, and I might say, "The patient went off the deep end." What I'm really saying is: I have found no negative responses.

First, I don't believe God makes any mistakes; and secondly, **I find that negative responses tend to occur mostly within the person acting as the *guide*, not within the individual in the role of the *client*.** And that only occurs when the guide has not yet done their own healing to the level that either they've cleared that piece of themselves or they can just be present with it and allow whatever there is to just be. I've also heard at this conference things like, "Well, I'm not a therapist, and I can't do this, and I can't do that."

When an individual is re-experiencing something that was painful for them in the past, in most cases, unless I am asked, or unless I have an incredible insight, there is nothing for me to do. All I have to do is just be present with them. When we were children and we had painful events that surfaced, our parents, to protect themselves, did one of several things, but it all resulted in the same thing — our expression was cut off. Either they became caretakers and sort of embraced us with our mouth against their chests so we couldn't say anything; or they babied us; or they did something that cut off our expression. Because our expression was resonating with their own unexpressed, painful, and unresolved feelings, they became uncomfortable, so they did something to cut it off within us. If our parents could have only been present with what we needed when we asked for it, most people would get well all by themselves.

If you look at **the nature of diseases, about 92% of them are chronic, which means that they are related to lifestyle** — how one is living one's life. There are about 8% of diseases that are acute. So, the ones that are chronic have to do with people's life-style and are healed by changing their lifestyle, while the 8% that are acute are self-limiting. If you did nothing at all, they would heal. So the point is, we have this idea that we have to do something most of the time. I find I have to do nothing unless I am asked or I have some deep desire to share something. If I am just present for what's happening within me, as this is occurring within them, then we come into communion, and they feel supported.

One of the problems that I see in the typical relationship between doctor and patient is that a *hierarchy* exists. One is the doctor; the other is the patient. This same thing we experienced in our families of origin. We had our parents; then we had the kids; we had the teachers; we had the students; we had the employers; we had the employees; and, until recently, we had men and women. Where did that hierarchy come from? What I find is that when I play doctor and they play patient, they think they have something wrong, and then they have the illusion that I can fix it. And if I'm not careful, I get sucked into the same illusion — they've got something wrong that I can fix.

What I notice is as long as *I* played doctor and *they* played patient, *we* never got fully well. There was always this difference. They were always below; I was always above. The truth is, we are all suffering from an array of "nonexistent incurable disorders." And as we come into communion and we all come out of the closet, if you will, and share what is really going on, we find out that we all have the same stuff going on. Well, if we all have the same stuff going on, then we all go, "Oh, thank God, I'm not the only one." And then what happens is, rather than feeling like we've jumped off a cliff into a big abyss in the middle of the night, we feel like we are in a partnering situation where your best buddy comes up, takes a hold of your hand and says, "You know, this is really scary; let's jump together." What a difference! **So I try to use every situation as an opportunity for my own healing.**

Now, one of the other things that has come up at this conference today is *my technique* versus *your technique* versus *their technique.* So, what I thought I would talk about this afternoon is what I perceive as *nature's technique.* The body has it's own wisdom, and it is a microcosm of a larger macrocosm called nature and the universe. If we could understand something about the way nature does its little healing trick, the way nature works — the larger picture, if you will — then we have a much greater understanding of how we work within ourselves and in relation to others.

This phenomenon came to me many years ago, and the way it appeared was this. You see, *the old materialistic paradigm* **had the idea that the body was a piece of equipment with replaceable parts,** and we had this solid thing that we called a body, and then we had this little tiny thing that we called the mind. And since there wasn't that much we knew about it, we didn't mess with the mind very much. When things happened within an individual that we felt had something to do with their mind, we called it a *mental disorder.* They'd just lost their mind; they went insane; and we would take them away in white jackets. You remember the old paradigm? **The old paradigm was built on the illusion of hierarchy.** This illusion, I believe, was built into the body because we

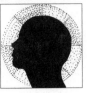

dealt with the world as if we were separate from everything within it. So, there were always the doctors, the patients, the teachers, the students, and so on. There was always this hierarchy. So, based on that I believe that we developed a superstition about how the body worked and how healing worked.

What we believed about the way the body worked was that we had these senses, and the senses picked up whatever was out there and fed that information into the brain. The brain mixed that information with old information, and then it told another part of the brain what to do. And that other part of the brain told the nervous system and the endocrine system what to do, and those systems passed it down to the muscles and the nerves, and so on and so forth. Wasn't that the view that we were all told about, that that's the way the body worked? So, we had an idea that the body worked as a hierarchy. We had an idea that primarily we had a body and then we had this thing called the mind which we didn't understand.

If you look at all the original approaches to light and color, whether it was the ancient rishis in India or the seers of Egypt, they understood something more about nature. But in modern times, within the last couple hundred years, it's clear we've forgotten about this connection with nature, so we've developed this separateness, and out of that came a hierarchy. So, if you look at some of the modern approaches to utilizing light and color, they use light on the body to treat conditions. The body had conditions; you alleviated conditions. That was *the old hierarchical paradigm,* **and our family structures and everything were built like that.** Thus, our view of reality followed that same idea.

Today we have started seeing shifts happening. Remember, if you looked at old movies, you never really saw people having emotional expressions of a deep nature. It just wasn't part of what was going on then. As my parents said, "It just wasn't in vogue." You didn't hug in public. I really never understood how my sister and I were born. I never heard my parents making love. When did it happen? See, It wasn't "in vogue." I can remember. When I said to my mother — my mother is seventy-nine and my dad's almost eighty-two — when I was going through a lot of my own healing, I said to my mom, "Why was it that I never remember dad hugging?" And she pulled me into the room and she said, "How do you think I felt? He's never hugged me." They were married fifty years at that time! **So this is part of** *the old paradigm:* **expressionlessness.** Boy, that's hard work!

We've recently seen changes. It used to be when we got to the point that people allowed themselves to express feelings openly, we'd say they were "losing it." When they lost it in the movies, the next scene was that they were usually taken away to a mental hospital. They were medicated; they were given shots; and they were taken away in the white coats. That was our old view. The mind was a dangerous thing. The paradigm has been shifting.

Next you had a *paradigm* **called** *psychosomatic.* That was sort of an interesting way of saying the person was crazy. You know, what it actually means is merely that the psyche affects the soma, the body. But the way we used it was, "They're really crazy; it's all in their imagination." That was a big word, the imagination. **Then we went into the**

area of *mindbody integration*, and then people like **Norman Cousins**[1] expressed his own experience of . . . well, supposedly he was going to die of a certain illness, and then he watched funny movies and laughed himself into health. See, it's hard to die while you're laughing. So, what's happened is the old paradigm has gradually transformed into a new paradigm.

Now, a lot of the ***new paradigm*** is based on work that probably began a long time ago; but in terms of current scientific work to validate this, you'd have to go back to 1977. At that time, some very, very important discoveries were made by a friend of mine, **Dr. Candace Pert**, who at the time was working at the **National Institute of Mental Health**. Candace Pert is someone whom I feel may, in the next two or three years, win the Nobel prize. She also has a book coming out next year called *Molecules of Emotions*. There is a good possibility she may have discovered a cure for AIDS as well. Candace Pert and her colleagues at N.I.M.H. **discovered a group of *informational substances* called *neuropeptides*.**

Now, in the body we have many informational substances. Some of them are called *neurotransmitters*; some of them are called *hormones*; some of them are called *neuropeptides*. Anyone who really understands endocrinology will tell you there's no difference. We used to think they were different. Now, those who really know will tell you they're all in the class of informational substances, they take information into or transport it around the body.

The old thought was that when something happened in the body, a reaction occurred in the mind. That's why they called them neuropeptides, "neuro" meaning "within the mind." And then the mind would create these chemicals. The chemicals would be secreted in a hierarchy throughout the body, and that's the way the body knew what it needed to do. **What Pert discovered as she was looking at the immune system was that when these neurochemicals, these informational substances — neuropeptides — were secreted in the brain, they were simultaneously secreted by the immune cells**. Then what she found was that the secretion of these informational substances — or, let me change that, **the materialization of these informational substances came about in response to a feeling or thought or an intention or an emotion or a belief.**

Thus, when you felt something or had a thought, an appropriate chemical messenger would come from invisibility into materialization and would express throughout the body what that feeling was. We used to think it happened as a hierarchy. What she discovered was that the way this occurs, **the way informational substances are felt throughout the body, is as a network, not as a hierarchy, as a field within a holographic field.** So what was discovered was whenever you have a feeling, emotion, intention, whatever it is, simultaneously you have the materialization of these chemicals throughout the body. It started out as something we discovered about the immune system. We now know there are about sixty different neuropeptides, each associated with different states of mind and emotions. What has now been discovered is that these are manufactured by every single cell in the body at the same instant of time as you have a feeling.

---

1. Since Dr. Liberman delivered this talk, Norman Cousins passed away. His interest in the powers of the human spirit in mindbody healing inspired many individuals during his lifetime. His journey into wellness using laughter therapy is chronicled in the book *Anatomy of An Illness, As Perceived by the Patient* (New York, NY: Bantam, 1991).

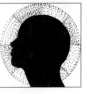

So, what I'm saying is **the mind has essentially escaped the brain**. The mind is no longer in the head, as we thought. We used to say, "up here," being in your head, but it's not in your head. **What we now know is that the mind exists throughout the body, and the way that the body works is directly related to your state of consciousness**, what's going on through that inner chatter. **John Bradshaw**[2] says that there are approximately twenty-five thousand hours of "tapes" in your mind, your mental chatter. We know that each person experiences about sixty thousand thoughts per day. Unfortunately 95% of the thoughts you're having today are the same ones you had yesterday and the same ones you'll have tomorrow. Now that was a very profound discovery in the area of mindbody medicine.

Then another discovery came about in the early 1980s, and a new set of *informational substances* was discovered. The reason we hadn't thought about it before or hadn't seen it before was that it seemed to be predominantly researched within the insect and plant kingdoms. These informational substances were known as *pheromones*. Now, pheromones are informational essences, energetic essences that are secreted by the body. They are also in response to your state of mind, your state of being; and these are secreted into the environment.

When your mind is going through whatever it goes through every microsecond, the body responds by creating the appropriate chemical informational substances. **The entire body knows and feels simultaneously, as a field, what's occurring; and concurrent with that the same energy is being transmitted out into the atmosphere as a field of information.**

So, where's the mind? Not in the head. Not in the body. So, where's the body? The body is inside the mind. It's not the body that creates the mind, as we used to think. It's a *mind field* of energy, a nonlocalized area of intelligence, that creates what appears as a physical entity. This was a big shift in paradigms! Now, that's really the basis for a lot of what we now call *bodymind,* one unit. It doesn't work anymore to separate mind and body. They are both the same thing. Quite honestly, **there's no treatment that just treats the mind, and no treatment that just looks at the body.** We've been talking about all these different modalities. They all affect everything at the same time. There's no way to separate them.

The real question is, "At what level do you enter?" We all enter at the most appropriate level for who we are and what we want to do. Someone may wish to treat it at this level, because that is what's comfortable and appropriate for them; and someone else may want to treat it at another level. Just like **Mary Bolles**[3] utilizes a table that moves as she's simultaneously giving the light, sound, and motion treatments, this is her particular approach. It isn't right or wrong. The bodymind is being affected. It's just a different way.

2. Internationally acclaimed author and television personality, John Bradshaw, is a pioneering light within the 12-Step Recovery Movement. In his television series, books, and tapes, he demystifies and clarifies key concepts of academic psychology and psychotherapy to make it accessible to lay people for their own healing. His books and tapes are not to be missed! Look for these titles: *The Family* (Deerfield Beach, FL: Health Communications, 1988); *Healing the Shame That Binds You* (Deerfield Beach, FL: Health Communications, 1988); *Homecoming: How to Champion and Heal Your Inner Child* (Deerfield Beach, FL: Health Communications, 1988); and *Creating Love: The Next Great Stage of Growth* (New York, NY: Bantam-Doubleday, 1992).

We are all different, we all bring in a different gift. All of these approaches affect everything, but the reason I wanted to contrast the old paradigm against the new paradigm is to give us an understanding of what I'm going to share with you.

The way that it came into my awareness that nature does the healing was not through reading a newspaper or reading some scientific literature, but through my own experience. I'll share the experience with you, because I think that most of you have had similar experiences. When I was a youngster, I used to have a lot of daily interactions with my father. We used to bang heads. I didn't think that those things that happened to me as a child would in any way affect me as I became older, that is, until I was about twenty-five and I ended up marrying my father dressed as a woman. I guess I'm the only one in this room who has had that experience! Then after six or seven years of being married, I went through a very, very difficult separation and divorce.

There is nothing that anyone has spoken about here — whether it is major *anxiety attacks*, deep *depression* or wanting to commit *suicide* — that I haven't experienced. I used to have thirty or forty major anxiety attacks every day. I had them for about six and a half years — 911 was my favorite number! I can laugh about it now. I was frightened to death continually. My body would shake and I couldn't catch my breath; my color would be gone. In fact, that's why I do what I do now, that was my schooling. If you haven't had that experience, it's scary! This is an area that I know "by heart" out of my own experience. As John Downing said about me, "I'm not a psychologist. I probably could be, but I don't care to be."

Within a couple of years of my divorce, I once again got into a relationship with my father, this time dressed as a different woman. I thought this was interesting. However, this time it didn't take seven years; this was a three-and-a-half year relationship. I was beginning to get smarter. So, at some point I started looking at that phenomenon, and I said, "My goodness, it's so interesting that I keep attracting into my life women that are energetically like my father," until I realized that all my close male friends were just like my father, too. Then I looked at all of my close friends, male and female, since I was a little kid. Sixth grade was the first time I fell in love with the first girl; and every single one of them, without exception, was just like the parent — my dad in this case — that I had unresolved issues with. Even my teachers, with the exception of Mrs. Williams in the fifth grade, were just like my dad. I mean, I looked at this really carefully. Now this may sound odd, but **look at your own life and see if nature does not, in fact, feed you anything in your life that's unresolved.** Now when I first heard that, people said, "Well, that's karma." You know, "What goes around, comes around."

At that time I identified myself as a scientist, and I needed to have a greater objective understanding. I wondered if this was just something that was in my imagination, or did this have any validity at all? Because if there was something to this, **if in fact we are each other's "homeopathic remedies" running around being attracted to each other for very specific reasons, then everything we need for healing is within our relationship dynamics. The problem is we are all in relationships, but we don't know how to relate!**

---

3. Mary Bolles uses Phototherapy as part of a comprehensive treatment program working with children and adults with learning disabilities. For Ms. Bolles' presentation entitled "Learning Abilities Dramatic Response to Light, Sound and Motion," see *Chapter Thirteen, page 297.*

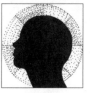

So, I look at the human relationship phenomenon as a series of "tuning forks." You know how a tuning fork works. You hit this one here; the one over there will buzz. What do you think happens when we get together? We resonate with the part of each other that's like the part of ourselves. So, how does that actually work? Or is that just an illusion, something I'm just passing on to you? If we go back to the Periodic Table of Elements — because everything comes down to those elements — and you take any element in the periodic table — let's say you're dealing with iron. The way that the chemist determines the difference between one element and the other is just the same way that the police department knows Bob Dubin from me — fingerprints. This is my signature; he has his own. Well, if you look at an element, every element has a fingerprint. Because if you take two rocks out of the ground, they only look like two rocks. How do you know which is the iron and which is the mercury if they don't look different? Well, the way they do it in science is to take this element and heat it up; then they put it inside an instrument called a ***Spectroscope,*** and that element will give off an energetic essence. It will give off light. You remember **Bob Dubin** said this morning, **"Whenever there is change within a system, the electron jumps states; it jumps to a different orbital ring." And when it does, photons are given off; light is given off. The photons are the informational substances. So, when you look deeply into the body, the way that the body communicates within itself is that every time there's a change in state, each cell gives off light. Light is the way the cells communicate. These are informational photons**. When you take an element, you heat it up — which means you are activating it — it starts giving off its fingerprint, its vibrational, *electromagnetic signature.*

If you look through the spectroscope, you can see that each element is giving off light in different portions of the visible light spectrum. If you take an element, let's say you have a rock here — it's being heated up — you look through the spectroscope and you see here's violet, the violet end of the spectrum. Here's the red end of the spectrum, right? And you notice that the element all of a sudden has a peak here. It's giving off something in the blue or indigo range, and then it's flat, and then there's another peak over here in yellow. That's the energetic signature of the element when it is in a state of excitement, which is what happens when something gets heated; it gives off energy, let's say in the blue violet and yellow portion of the spectrum. In science we call those *Fraunhoffer emission lines*, but in real terminology it's just the energetic signature of the element. What I'm saying is, **every element has a signature, an energetic signature, which is within the visible light spectrum**.

Now that in itself is important, but let's get to the real guts. You take this element; you heat it up; you're looking at its signature; and now you do something — you shine white light into the space, into the environment that this element is excited and where it is giving off energy. Then what you notice is that the element will attract to itself from the white light an exact mirror image of what energy it is giving off. Let me repeat that, because **this is really crucial to the understanding of how nature works. You take any element; you excite it by heating it; it'll give off an energetic signature. You put it into an environment of white light, and it will attract to itself an exact mirror image of what it is giving off.**

What is this body? On one level the body is made up of all of these elements, everything. You take this body and, except when we're sleeping — and we're still excited then — but when we're awakened, we're also excited; and **when we're excited we, too,**

are giving off an energetic vibrational signature. You can call it an aura. You're walking around with this aura in an environment of light. So what do you do? You attract from the "quantum soup" of life experience "out there" an exact mirror image of where you are at, at any particular instance of time. How can there be a negative effect?

The doctor and patient are being attracted for a reason. The therapy you're giving is absolutely appropriate. The experience is appropriate. Now we could go back to the initial paradigm that there is right and wrong. But there is no right and wrong in the world; that's just what our mind has done. There just "is." If you look at it carefully, you will notice what your piece is in the interaction. So the experience nowadays is: There are no accidents. Things don't "just happen." The world has as much knowing as our mind does.

The importance of this surfaced for me when **I started noticing that I was attracting into my life things that were unresolved,** and I wanted to know how that related to this energetic essence. **My sense is that we are biological or physiological prisms**. You know what happens when you take a glass prism? It's very pure, and you take invisible energy called light and you shine it in through one end, and then out the other end comes all these colors. But have any of you seen auras? Have you ever seen anybody walking around that looked like a rainbow? No.

What makes us different than the prisms? **The only thing that makes us different from the glass prisms is that the prism doesn't have a mind.** What comes in just flows through. But we do something with our minds, and when we do it, it's as if you had a hose and water was running through it. Now, if you didn't touch the hose, the full flow of energy would come through. But if you took your hand and you gripped that sucker, the more you squeezed, the less water would come out. This is the mind; **that's one of the things that the mind does; it strangles the flow of energy as it comes in.** Because we want to be in control, so we control it. We put a wrench in the works, unfortunately. When we do that, the light that's emitted is not the rainbow. It's something less than that. What was being emitted from me were the weak links in my chain, the sensitive spots. Why?

Our mind knows what it *wants*, but it doesn't have any idea what it needs. The **body knows just what it *needs*.** So there is the mind saying, "Give me what I want." And there's the body saying, "Well, for the species to evolve, we're going to need to do it differently." That's called evolution of the species. **We attract just what we need in order to continually expand.** If we didn't, we'd probably self-destruct. And some people have the idea that we're going to keep doing that. People throughout history have always thought the world was coming to an end — but it hasn't. It just keeps going. And it keeps getting just what it needs for the evolutionary process to keep shifting. So, what I noticed was that we attract just what we need. I also noticed what happened with the clients that came into my office. Always they had a gift for me. They thought I had a gift for them. They didn't realize they also had a gift for me.

The reason I'm sharing this is that I want to take us into *the newer paradigm,* but I needed to lay a little bit of a foundation about the old paradigm for the new paradigm to create the newer paradigm. This is going to be the subject of my next book. What we know is that **the body is encapsulated by a field, a non-localized field of intelligence**. Remember when Norm Shealy showed us the book entitled *The Visionary Art of Alex*

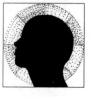

Grey? If you would have looked at all of his paintings, they all had something in common. In several of his paintings the body was radiating energy, and if you looked at the body and the field, there were little things throughout the field — what were they? Eyes. Remember yesterday when I told you about my experience in the early 1970s, that I felt like I was seeing from everywhere at the same time, that we don't see from our eyes? I've had that book for years, but I never looked at it . . . until about two weeks ago. I opened it up; I was unpacking some boxes and I opened it up; and I said, "My God!" Now, one of Alex's pictures, the one that Norm Shealy said he loved the most, was of an individual sitting in a lotus position, and he was situated within an energetic net, and the netting went out everywhere. That's the way that I view how we're all connected. **When we are not in our mind, our** *local mind*, **when we are in** *non-local mind, Universal Mind*, **we are without thought, if you will; we are infinitely connected to everything. Everything!** So I make that statement, and you say, "How do you know that?" Well, I'll tell you how I know it. I've been having parapsychological experiences, metaphysical experiences, for years.

There was a man in the field of optometry who was a very dear friend of mine, named Dr. Elliot Forest. We were very connected, and one day I was in the shower, and all of a sudden — I don't know what happened — I started sobbing. I just started sobbing. I mean it was like one of those real deep sobs when you knew you couldn't quite catch your breath. All of a sudden I had this feeling that Elliot had died. I stepped out of the shower — I was soaking wet — and I picked up the phone and called New York. I said, "Libby, when did it happen?" And she said, "How did you know? He just died." So, how did I know? What was I picking up? I felt it. Was I picking up something in the radio wave frequencies? Was I picking up something in the waves that create television?

What happens when the phone rings, and you know who it is? What are you picking up? Are you picking up the same fiberoptics that U.S. Sprint uses? What happens when a healer lays their hands above your body and you feel this intense heat? What's coming out? Is it infrared? I mean what is going on here? What are we picking up and how are we picking it up? Does the body have a field that's like a radar screen? You know what a radar screen is? It's a device that the armed forces or the airports use to pick up things, planes, let's say, before your physical senses can pick them up. **Well, we know that the physical senses are very poor devices for evaluating reality. After all, we pick up less than one-billionth of the information that is available. Yet we think that what we are seeing through that little peephole into life is what really exists.** We pick up less than one-billionth of the stimuli of what's actually going on out there — one-billionth of all that's potentially available to us. And you know what we're picking up? **We're only picking up the stuff that fits our picture of what reality is.**

When I was in optometry school, people would say **"Seeing is believing."** But it's not true. **If you don't believe it, you won't even see it!** When I was in optometry school between 1969 and 1973, some interesting experimental research was being done at **Harvard Medical School** by two neurobiologists, **Dr. David Huble** and **Dr. Torsten Wiesel, who eventually received the Nobel Prize in physiology for their research in the process of visual information.** They reared kittens under two separate conditions. In one condition the kittens were reared in rooms of horizontal, alternating black and white stripes; and the other kittens were reared in rooms that had alternating vertical black and white stripes. When these cats had grown old and finally died of natural causes, their brains were examined. It was found that the actual connections between the neurons, the stuff that was sending the information, was such that the cats reared in the horizontally striped rooms could only see a horizontal world; they could only see the horizontal aspect of things. Conversely, the cats reared in a room with vertically oriented stripes could only see a vertical world; they couldn't see anything horizontal.

There is also **Rupert Sheldrakes' theory of *Morphic Resonance*, or *Morphogenetic Fields*. Along with the information received genetically, there is information within the field of the individual that has to do not only with the physical structure of the body, but also with the belief systems of our predecessors.** So, we don't come into this world as blank slates. Look at babies; they're all different. When my two kids were born, my daughter came out just breathing like a lark, and she still is. My son came out holding his breath to the point that I thought he would die, and I think to this day he's still holding his breath. What I'm saying is that morphogenetically we bring in certain beliefs along with our genetics. Combined with the initial experiences we energetically attract, these experiences sculpt our neurology in such a way that all our subsequent experiences are automatically, unconsciously edited out of our consciousness unless they conform to the same beliefs that were created from our first experiences. You get what I'm saying? When we say you create your own reality, what are we really talking about? You are only seeing it your way.

Each of you is an artist, and there is a blank canvas here within a frame. As you are observing me you are each individually creating me on your slate. Each of you thinks it's me, but it's not. Each of you sees me in a different way. Some of you came up to me today and shared some really wonderful things. I'm sure there are some of you who think I'm a pain in the ass. Well, I'm neither a pain in the ass nor am I wonderful. I just am. You make me what I am to you based on your experiences. You hear what you hear, but not what I'm saying. You are creating this experience.

How is it that we see what's going on? When I went to school, we had the idea that the way that vision worked was that information entered the eye, went back into the computer, and the computer inverted the picture. Professors made the eye sound as though it were something like a camera and then, through some magic, we saw. We all understood the neurology, physiology, and so on, but we were never told how it is we see. What I discovered quite a few years ago is something about how it is that we see. The eyes are always making these micromovements. The eyes are situated right at the helm of this system. **The eyes are not a separate entity from the brain — they are the brain. The brain has two frontal extensions called eyes. When light strikes the eye, it simultaneously strikes the brain. The eyes and the brain are the same.**

So, the eyes are at the helm of this system. They're the navigational system. How do they work? Well, when I went to school, I was led to believe that when I looked at what we call experience, there were some things more important than others. Isn't that what you were taught? It was something called *"the figure."* The figure was the main thing. Then the other things that were less important were called *"the ground."* In education they call it *figure/ground relationships.* I was led to believe that this actually existed in the world, that there was something that was important and the rest of it less important. I didn't realize that this was the way our minds worked; it had nothing to do with reality.

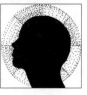

What I discovered that really improved my vision was that this quantum soup of energy doesn't in reality have a figure and a ground. It's a constantly changing figureless ground.

If I could view reality, if I could look at this experience here and see everything equally, then there's no difference between anything out there and me. I become part of the experience, not an observer of the experience. If you allow your eyes to see that way, you notice a few interesting things. The first thing is that in order to do that you have to give up your point of view. You have to see with fresh eyes. You have to see from nowhere. And if you do that, you'll get into **spontaneous remission** with your vision, and probably every other part of your body at the same time. Now, I know that sounds a little weird.

Those of you who wear glasses, take off your glasses sometime, because you can't really see with your glasses on, and I'll explain that a little later. Take off your glasses, close your eyes, and get yourself relaxed. Then open your eyes, and you'll notice a very interesting phenomenon. As soon as you open your eyes, just for a quick second everything is very clear. How many of you who wear glasses have ever had that experience? When you had your eyes closed, regardless of your prescription, you opened your eyes, and everything was crystal clear — and then it got fuzzy. What do you think was going on between the point of crystal clarity and the point of bluriness? As soon as you opened up you saw from no point of view. Within microseconds every filter stepped back into place, and then you were viewing this quantum soup through all of these filters. **You don't really see what's truly going on; you just make of it some distorted thing based on your own experience.**

What I noticed is that if I could see from nowhere, or if I could see from everywhere at the same time, then my vision became clear. I still have a significant prescription. For those of you who are optometrists here, one diopter-and-a-half *myopic*; and I have two-and-a-half to two-and-three-quarters diopters of *astigmatism*, which means — for those of you who are not optometrists — my vision should be, at best, maybe 20/50 and, at worst, maybe 20/300, or worse. But it's nowhere near that. I saw everything that was projected on the overhead screen here today. So, where am I seeing from? Perhaps **Alex Grey** was right on the money; the eyes are within the field. These in my cranium are only the *windows of the soul*. The eyes are out here all over the place.

As I started to understand something about how this phenomenon of field occurs, I began to realize that our field can be endless, infinite, which means that our intention touches everything. And you say, "How's that possible?" Well, I was always led to believe that the way our vision worked was that light entered the eye; we've all agreed upon that the last two days, right? Light enters the eye, and then all this stuff happens. But something else is going on. You see, **light affects the body, but consciousness determines how we take light in and what portion we take in**.

Forget about what's out there. If all we needed to do was get *full spectrum light*, then every farmer in the country who's using pesticides and killing you at the same time should be very conscious, because they're getting the full spectrum of everything. **But it isn't about just getting full spectrum *light*. It's about having a full spectrum *life*. It's being able to receive what is present.**

Dr. Bob Dubin can do all the chiropractic adjustment he wants; it won't do anything unless you're open to Bob. Unless your receptivity opens up, your treatment is nothing. **We are the major pharmacopoeia. We are the major healing energies**. We have an infinite field of intelligence. I used to think that the way we saw was by light through the eyes, but have you ever been in a bus or somewhere out in the public in a group of people and all of a sudden you "got the feeling" somebody was staring at you? And you turned around and, by God, they were looking at you. What were you feeling? Were they sending beams of light out of their eyes? Is that possible? They looked at you with their eyes, with their intention, and zap. Something goes out of their eyes. And that's the way I think intention works. It goes out holographically in every direction and dimension simultaneously. **We have this field of energy we live in, and the field is a big radar screen that picks up information before our senses pick it up.**

We call that *precognitive experience*, or *psychic experience*. We know children have that, right? That is until they grow up, or what I call the process of "adulteration." We adulterate them; and their field collapses. But what causes the field to collapse? Because the field can stay expanded, or the field can stay collapsed, which means you have a dynamically shifting radar screen. Now, you know, if the radar screen is infinite, then you can pick up everything that's going on, can't you? **In reality we know everything that's going on. But for some reason we seem to block out a lot of it. Why? The field collapses**. The radar screen gets small; and when it goes to its extreme, **if you evaluate the visual field, which is the physical manifestation of this larger field, it will shrink. When consciousness opens up, the visual field expands. And it can happen in a microsecond, because this field is not a static thing; it's a constantly breathing kind of phenomenon in every direction there is; and it changes with states of mind, your breathing and so on. What causes the field to collapse?**

In 1974, when I first was able to see *auras*, I noticed something interesting. You can really see the aura brightly until people start thinking. **The moment they think, the field collapses.** We were led to believe that thinking was necessary for learning, weren't we? Thinking supposedly made us higher than the other members of the animal kingdom. That's what allowed us to use animals for cruel experiments if we wished to, or eat them or whatever we wanted to do. Isn't that so? We could think; they couldn't. Yet, we are the only animals on the planet that have a concept for being "unemployed" or needing to "exercise," as I mentioned in my earlier presentation *(Chapter One, Light: Medicine of the Future)*. What we call thinking is just a fancy word for something I call worrying. **Most of our thinking is really worrying** — but it's not really even worrying; it's the most sophisticated cheating ever created. I used to think that cheating was the thing you did when you looked over someone's shoulder to see what was happening on their test because you didn't study. That's obvious cheating, like obvious addiction, drinking, or drugging. But the real addiction, **the biggest addiction in this country is thinking. It's what we all do to avoid whatever we're feeling — we go into our minds**. What I've noticed is that what we call thinking is really just a process of rehearsing continually. It's what we do to try to guarantee that things come out our way. And we do that because we've never developed an authentic security about our own functioning. So, we do this cheating as a way of trying to appear in the world the way we think we're supposed to. **The moment we think, we can't learn. The moment that we start thinking, we stop breathing.**

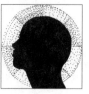

It was **Freud** who said, "When a parent yells, the baby holds its breath." When we get scared, we hold our breath. Why do we think? Because we're scared. We're afraid to be spontaneous. We're afraid that we won't be accepted; we won't be loved. They'll say we made a mistake; we'll be embarrassed . . . whatever the hell happened to us as children. **I find that fear and thinking, for the most part, are identical.** Now, your minds won't like that, but that's been my direct experience. The moment you start thinking it's impossible to learn. Whatever you want won't come until you stop thinking. While you're thinking it gets to the tip of your tongue. That's it. Then it stops, and it won't pop out until you stop thinking. So, the idea of thinking, trying harder, totally screws you up. That's what meditation is about: get out of your head; get out of your thought processes; and then magic happens!

So the real question is, how do you take the magic into the world? How do you keep the field expanded? When I started working with light, I noticed that if I put colors into the system, I could intuitively feel what was going on, and the person could also subjectively tell me what was going on. I could even monitor the physiology to determine what was going on. **There were several different ways that I would know energetically what portion of the *life's experience* — which is the same as the *light experience* — the person was not receiving.**

Some people said we were making comparisons between *allopathic* and *homeopathic* uses of light. **John Downing** used the word *antagonistic*, referring to a method of light treatments. We're not antagonizing anything; the system has what it has. You feed the light in, and through either one of the ways I just mentioned the body tells you, "Gee, this doesn't feel comfortable." Why? Because **the light is an energy "tuning fork," and it's awakening a "tuning fork" just like it that's lodged in your body. This uncomfortable feeling represents the part of the light that never exited your prism. This is the part of your life's experience that you couldn't digest when you ingested it, so you held onto it. You couldn't express it. It was too scary to say how you felt, so you held onto it**.

Well, you know, **Bob Dubin** said that everything is light. **All matter is frozen light. You take in energy; you slow it down; it becomes solid. You take the energy of emotionality and you slow it down by not expressing it, and it becomes a biological resistor; it crystallizes in the body and becomes a lump, if you will.** And then what happens is — well, you know how they crack kidney stones now? They use wave sound to shatter them. This is the same phenomenon. You have this crystalline energy, this stagnant energy that's been held onto emotionally because it wasn't safe to express it or to release it; **then you put light into the system, and it "homeopathically" awakens it.** The person starts feeling. When Margaret, in Steve Vazquez's demonstration, was exposed to the light, he asked her, "What do you feel?" She said, "I feel some energy moving." Margaret said, "My heart is pumping a little fast." The soma (the body) was where she first felt the energetic buzzing. If you sit with it for awhile, just sit with it, something surfaces, and you get an insight or an intuitive flash.

I'll give you an example of a flash. I woke up this morning and did some yoga. In the process of doing some yoga, I hurt my back. And then I did what I typically do; I needed to fix it because it was too uncomfortable to sit with it. So, I went to Dr. Lamb here and said, "Ward, could you do a little magic?" So, Ward did a little magic; he tried to fix it; but I still had it. It wasn't to the same degree, but it was beautiful because it was just there as a reminder, right? Then I sat down, and I started writing. I wrote in my journal, "I notice that I get frightened when physical things like traumas, even minor ones, have decked my body, for example, this lower back stuff. It seems to resonate with a prior feeling of helplessness."

At that moment I knew I had some things coming up, so I walked out of the room — some of you may have noticed — and I went over to a spot in the lobby where the phones are and sat down. The next thing that came was a feeling of helplessness, a feeling of loss of control, a feeling of being all alone . . . and then the next things that came out were: "I don't want to be left alone; it's lonely. It's scary; it makes me cry; my body shakes; my shoulder is shivering." I actually felt something. I visualized something happening in the past that made my shoulder shiver — a cramp in the upper right shoulder close to my neck. Where's my mother? I hurt my head; I cracked it on the right side. Where is she? Am I going to die? What's going on? Where is my dad? Where is my sister Eva? Now, when I was a young boy, I cracked my head open twice. I had a lot of physical stuff. I cut my face open, my chin three times, my head twice, and so on. Then a little later I wrote on the bottom of the page — and, by the way, right after that some tears started surfacing — "I hurt myself a lot as a child. I wanted their love. Where were they?" Homeopathy, *human homeopathy*. Something happened; it resonated an old event. I could go for the immediate fix, the "bandaid on the melanoma," or I could sit with it; and then I start to reel.

This is the same way the light therapy works. You energetically simulate something that the person is unreceptive to. Initially they're unreceptive to it because it's unfinished business. They keep attracting "this irritant" into their life. But it's not an irritant, it's a *gift*. So we put light into their mindbody system, into the area where they are least (or most) responsive. You just do that from your intuition, as well as from their feedback. I don't have any method. My method is I just trust myself. That's what I'm doing right now in front of you, just trusting myself. What a wonderful opportunity. I have all of you here to love me. At the same moment it's a little scary, but let's go for it. I do the best I can to just go for it.

Well, that's the way I am with people. I trust this piece of technology, the Lumatron™. What presents symptomatically I just use. The session may start at violet or it may start at red; I don't know how it's going to start . . . or even if it's going to start. I just do whatever comes up. That's just the way that I happen to work. It doesn't mean that anyone else has to do it this way. It's just the way I need to do it; it's my particular medicine that I need to help me evolve. Any way you use this technology will be appropriate for what you need, and that's what needs to be trusted.

I'm starting a new book called *Take Off Your Glasses and See*. As I approached the end of my first book, *Light: Medicine of the Future*, I became aware that the process of writing the book had transformed my awareness. I realized that the last section about the healing power of relationship was the essence of what I really wanted to communicate. As the book was almost finished, I didn't rewrite the previous chapters, but I could see that another book would be necessary to do justice to this topic.

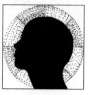

As I went into the world to promote the book, these ideas became even clearer. The first book was largely a product of my mind; it had been written by thinking, planning, and organizing words on paper. I realized that the next book would have to come from a more organic level of knowing. I wanted it to be a creation of the spontaneous wisdom that arises in each moment. I wanted it to share what I know by heart. **The real message is not in the material; it's in ourselves. We ourselves are the only healing remedy. Through the transformation of the self this remedy becomes more and more potent.**

My goal is to be a living example of this process. When I share or present my work, I don't prepare it in the usual way. I don't do an outline of what to do first, second, and third. I allow myself to follow and trust the intuitive impulses that arise out of the spaces between my thoughts, because the information that comes out of that gap has its own innate organization and perfection. To capture that intuitive flow, I decided to base this book on transcriptions of an intensive workshop that I gave in the fall of 1992. We called this workshop "An Experiment in the Workings of Our Mind," meaning, we allowed it to evolve spontaneously without a superimposed structure. I'm hoping that as you read this book you will feel as if we're having a heart-to-heart conversation that reaches deep inside you and stimulates your own fundamental knowing.

That knowing arises out of the magical gap between our thoughts, which **Dr. Deepak Chopra**[4] calls *"the pregnant emptiness."* We think of it as nothing until we experience it, and then we realize its incredible fullness. It contains both nothingness and allthingness, together. My friend Truth says that it is like the Zen concept of *"no mind"*— that place of emptiness where the mind is not constructing things, where all things originate and exist. It is true creativity. In this book I would like you to be able to feel the essence of that magic and discover your own creativity. **We have all learned to suppress our feelings, which suppresses the essence of our humanity, our creative power. When we ask for emotional support, most people don't understand that we are not asking for their advice; we are just seeking a safe place to express who we truly are.** How often do you really hear, "I'm so glad that you're sharing your feelings with me?"

Like most people, I grew up thinking that I was imperfect, that it was not okay to trust my intuitions and express my emotions. Our parents learned from their parents that love means telling someone what they're doing wrong. We got the message that we were inadequate and unlovable and others expected us to be perfect. So, we tried to look perfect to satisfy their expectations. In the process we totally skipped over being ourselves. Then we'd go from one emotional extreme to the other, feeling inadequate and trying to appear perfect. When I began writing my first book, I wanted it to be perfect, to convince the reader of my expertise. It's easy to trace how my perspective was transformed.

---

4. Deepak Chopra, M.D. is the bestselling author of numerous books exploring the leading edge of the new paradigm of mindbody medicine. As a practicing endocrinologist, Dr. Chopra integrates allopathic and classical Indian medicine called "Ayurveda." His books include *Quantum Healing: Exploring the Frontiers of MindBody Medicine* (Bantam, 1990); *Ageless Body, Timeless Mind* (Crown Publishing, 1993); *Perfect Health: The Complete MindBody Guide* (Crown Publishing, 1991); *Return of the Rishi: A Doctor's Search for the Ultimate Healer* (Harmony, 1991); *Creating Health: How to Wake Up the Body's Intelligence* (Harmony, 1991); *Unconditional Life: Mastering the Forces that Shape Personal Reality* (Bantam, 1992).

The book moves from objectively reporting other people's work to an intuitive flow describing my own experience.

Since then I've continued the process of learning to follow my inner promptings. That's why I'm basing this book on my spontaneous self-expression. I don't want its contents to be more important than its message. I don't want it to be an escape from life, which is the reason that many people read books. I want it to resonate with my life force, speaking a language that your life force will also recognize. Reading only confirms what you already know, and I want this book to touch the part of you that already knows everything. **For so long we've been told to ignore our gut feelings unless their validity could be proven in a laboratory with a double-blind study. Now we're beginning to realize that these feelings may be as, or even more, accurate than the chatter in our minds.** As Chopra says, "The only difference between a gut cell and a brain cell is that the gut cell has not yet evolved to the level of self-doubt."

There was a time when humans were completely attuned to their inner selves and were able to read the language of nature as a reflection of their own inner harmony. They could sense what was happening within another person and what remedy to use for every disease. You can still see this today in so-called "primitive cultures." In our modern world we have forgotten that natural ability. Instead, we dismiss it as "witchcraft" or the "imagination." But now science itself is proving that this "imagination" may be the organizing principle of our body and that this "witchcraft" may be our most potent healing remedy. We are fundamentally connected to everything in the universe, just as the ancient people knew.

In our lifetime we are seeing the convergence of three healing paradigms, three different ways of understanding reality. To discover and transform ourselves, we will move through all three perspectives. **The *first paradigm* is the world view that we learn in childhood.** It structured our formative experiences, the past causes of our current patterns. In medicine it was based on the scientific principle of ***Cartesian dualism*. We split the mind and the body apart.** The body was a machine which could only be understood and treated mechanically. All of the mind and the emotions which could not be explained in mechanical terms were dismissed as not real, as imaginary. **This separated the individual from their only true source of healing, the gut knowing of the belly brain.** These healing powers were then projected outside the self, turning the medical doctor into the "medical deity."

The *second paradigm* is the place of expanding awareness and integration. Working from this perspective, we have created a new view of reality that connects ancient wisdom with scientific discoveries and reintegrates our fractured selves. **It recognizes that our mind and body are one and that consciousness on all levels consists of wholes within wholes. *Mindbody medicine* strives to reawaken our connection with the healer within.** In the process we are demystifying the "medical deity" and turning the doctor/patient relationship into a partnership.

In the *third paradigm* we try to apply these insights to our daily lives. Can we achieve and maintain ***bodymind integration,*** not just during meditation or in therapy, but throughout the day? Can we maintain full self-awareness during our daily activities

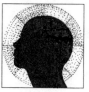

and interactions? Can we become aware of how we magnetically attract certain life experiences? Can we consciously expand our opportunities for growth and self-awareness? We can do all these things, but not by learning a perfect technique or by having a great personality. We do it by becoming so aware and so directed that our full awareness flows spontaneously like magic. This is both very easy and almost impossible. Life is a process of becoming aware, a constant practice.

Today we're at the threshold of a *new healing paradigm*, but the new medicine turns out to be the same as the oldest medicine, *The Healer Within*. Nature's innate intelligence knows exactly how to heal ourselves and others. We are the most potent remedy in the world, a healing pharmacopeia that energetically attracts the transformative experiences we require next, and life's little irritations are often precisely the medicine that we most need to assimilate. Not so long ago scientists would have laughed at these ideas, but now our beliefs are changing.

Deepak Chopra, Larry Dossey,[5] and **Bernie Siegel,**[6] all three of them medical doctors by training, are **well-known pioneers in the movement to integrate scientific research with the insights of mindbody medicine and quantum physics.** They show us scientific studies that validate our intuitive knowings. Awareness is not limited to the mind, and healing is not limited to the body. Let's really look at the healing effect of the placebo. For years we thought that medications created healing. First paradigm doctors had considered the placebo to be literally "nothing," so its effect was invisible to them. Now we are wondering if the most powerful medications may in fact be the placebos, the "nothings." It is only a matter of time before even skeptical scientists confirm that **we are the most powerful medicine in the world.**

What will the FDA do then? How will it regulate us when we become the doctors, the healers? — when we talk to each other and healing occurs, when we touch each other and healing occurs. Everywhere I travel I see that this is already happening, but don't take my word for it, create your own healing shifts.

My new book is designed to help you create those shifts in consciousness to provide you with information, techniques, and technology. It will guide you in retraining your vision, enhancing your color receptivity, releasing blocked emotional traumas, and healing your relationships. It will show you exercises that help you get out of your own way and learn without effort. These are all valuable techniques, but I've learned that the exercise and the technology play only a minor role in the healing process.

---

5. Larry Dossey, M.D. retired from a practice of internal medicine in Dallas, Texas and is actively engaged in clinical research. He has written several books including: *Recovering the Soul: The Meaning in Medicine* (Bantam, 1989); *Healing Words: The Power of Prayer and The Practice of Medicine* (San Francisco: Harper, 1984); *Space, Time and Medicine* (Shambala Publications, 1982); and *Beyond Illness: Discovering the Experience of Health* (New York, NY: Random House, 1985).

6. Bernie Siegel, M.D. is a retired general and pediatric surgeon who is now actively involved in humanizing medical care and medical education. He and his wife Bobbie and their family travel internationally to speak and run workshops sharing his techniques and experiences. Bernie's acclaimed book titles include: *How to Live Between Office Visits: A Guide to Love and Health* (Harper Collins, 1993); *Peace, Love and Healing: BodyMind Communication and the Path to Self-Healing* (Harper Collins, 1990); *Love, Medicine and Miracles: Lessons Learned About Self-Healing from a Surgeon's Experience with Exceptional Patients* (Harper Collins, 1990).

When I was an optometrist, I had many tools and techniques, so when I sold my practice in 1986, I felt naked. I had lost all those little gadgets. Eventually I realized that I could still do everything I had done before, only now I was using my head, my hands, and my heart. Since then I've been cultivating my own instrument, the healer within. **As we expand our awareness, we need fewer and fewer external techniques and technologies. True healing can only be triggered by the core energy that flows between the guide and the seeker. Our only real training is self-transformation; that's how we become vehicles for guiding others.**

Someone recently asked me, "So you use light; that's your main technology, right?" And I responded, **"You only need to use the light until you see the light." Tools, techniques, and mental constructs are just ways to return our consciousness to the lost parts of ourselves**. Once this awareness is integrated, the whole world becomes our tool for healing. As we move from "light to enlightenment," every light experience becomes an opportunity to further expand our self-awareness, to realize more fully who we really are.

The eye through which I see God is the same eye through which God sees me; my eye and God's eye are one eye, one seeing, one knowing, one love.

— Meister Eckhart

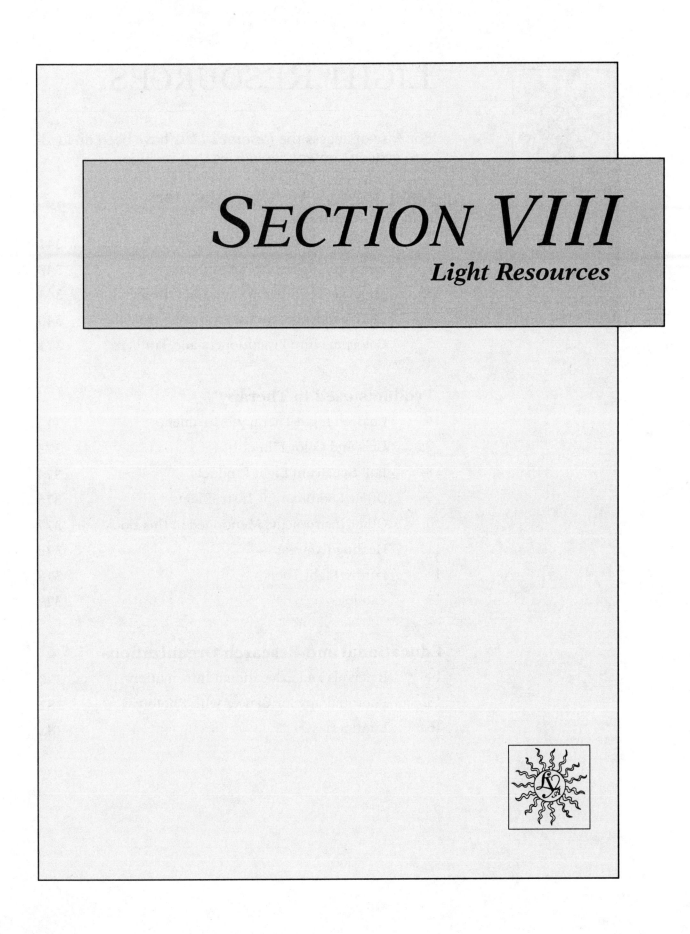

SECTION VIII
Light Resources

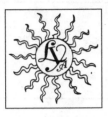

LIGHT RESOURCES

For ease of access the *Resource Lists* have been divided into sixteen content categories that include:

Light Therapy Authors, Educators, and Practitioners

Products used in Therapy

Educational and Research Organizations

LIGHT THERAPY AUTHORS, EDUCATORS, AND PRACTITIONERS

1. LIGHT YEARS AHEAD AUTHORS

Mary L. Bolles, B.A.
Sensory Learning
1705-14th Street, Suite 344
Boulder, CO 80302
(303) 530-4911
Specializes in light, sound, and vestibular stimulation to potentiate increased *learning abilities*. Developer of light, sound, and motion instrumentation, portable computerized light therapy instruments appropriate for home or office use.

Brian J. Breiling, Psy.D., M.F.C.C.
Light Years Ahead Productions
21 Main Street
P.O. Box 174
Tiburon, CA 94920
(415) 435-1578
FAX: (415) 435-3195
E-Mail: bbreiling@aol.com
Light-Assisted Psychotherapy Conference and Training Seminars, publisher and co-editor of the book *Light Years Ahead.*

Gabriel Cousens, M.D.
Tree of Life Rejuvenation Center
P.O. Box 1080
Patagonia, AZ 85624
(520) 394-2060
FAX: (520) 394-2099
Gabriel Cousens, M.D., director, holistic physician, family therapist, and author of *Spiritual Nutrition and the Rainbow Diet; Sevenfold Peace* and *Conscious Eating*. He is co-director with his wife, Nora, of Tree of Life Rejuvenation Center in Patagonia, Arizona, a spa, healing center, and wellness lifestyle community.

For appointments in Arizona and Petaluma, California, call:
(520) 394-2520

Manohar Croke, B.A.
Colorpuncture & Kirlian Photography
1705 14th Street, #198
Boulder, CO 80302
(303) 443-1666
Certified colorpuncture practitioner and trainer specializing in use of colorpuncture and other energetic subtle vibration therapies.

Akhila Dass, O.M.D., L.Ac.
Licensed Acupuncturist
P.O. Box 3013
San Anselmo, CA 94979
(415) 461-6641
Teaches and practices acupuncture and colorpuncture internationally. For sessions, equipment, information and training. Distributor of Esogetic oils and sound tapes based on the teachings of Peter Mandel, M.D.

John Downing, O.D.
1055 West College Drive, #107
Santa Rosa, CA 95401
(707) 525-4747
Optometrist, inventor of the Lumatron Ocular Light Stimulator' . Founder of The Downing Technique of Ocular Light Therapy' , worldwide teacher.

Robert Dubin, D.C.
802 Bonita Way
Petaluma, CA 95952
(707) 763-0947
Chiropractor. Integrates The Downing Technique of Ocular Light Stimulation' with both chiropractic and *cranial sacral therapy*. Specializing in treatment of *trauma*. Radio show host.

Jerry A. Green, J.D.
Medical Descionmaking Institute
20 Sunnyside Avenue, Suite A-200
Mill Valley, CA 94941
(415) 383-6437
Professional consultations, seminar trainings and the independent study-consulting program Medicine and Holistic Practice.

Light Years Ahead Authors—Continued

Elson M. Haas, M.D.
Preventive Medical Center of Marin
25 Mitchell Boulevard
San Rafael, CA 94903
(415) 472-2343
FAX: (415) 472-7636
An innovative practitioner in the fields of nutritional and preventive medicine, who specializes in *integrated medicine*. He is the best-selling author of *Staying Healthy with the Seasons* and *Staying Healthy with Nutrition*, and *A Diet for the Seasons*.

Lee Hartley, Ed.D., M.F.C.C.
Light Years Ahead Productions
21 Main Street
P.O. Box 174
Tiburon, CA 94920
(415) 435-1578
FAX: (415) 435-3195
Conference Director for **Light Years Ahead** 1992. Director of Educational Services for Light Year's Ahead Productions and consultant for the treatment of *depression, seasonal affective disorder, and PMS*.

Ward Lamb, D.C.
14817 Alderwood Way
P.O. Box 2129
Nevada City, CA 95959
(916) 478-0448
Chiropractor. Specializing in Chromotherapy, the integration of simultaneous light treatment through the eyes and on the body to correct *neuromuscular and subtle energy imbalances*.

Jacob Liberman, O.D., Ph.D.
Universal Light Technologies, Ltd.
P.O. Box 520
Carbondale, CO 81623
(303) 927-0100
FAX: (303) 927-0101
1-800-81-LIGHT
Optometrist, inventor, and author of *Light: Medicine of the Future; Take Off Your Glasses and See*. Director of Universal Light Technologies specializing in *natural eyesight improvement*, light, and color therapy and the psychospiritual basis of personal transformation. Audio and videotapes of Dr. Liberman's seminars are available.

David Olszewski, E.E., I.E.
Light Energy Company
1056 NE 179th Place
Seattle, WA 98177
1-800-LIGHT-CO
1-800-544-4826
Electrical and industrial engineer, lecturer and consultant on the effects of artificial light and radiation and light therapy applications. Mr. Olszewski is president of Light Energy Company, which carries the majority of the light therapy products mentioned in this book.

Samuel Pesner, O.D.
133 Second Street
Los Altos, CA 94022
(415) 948-3700
Optometrist. Editor of *The Journal of Optometric Phototherapy*. His special interests include: the history of light therapy and the use of light in the treatment of *developmental, visual, and learning problems*.

Norman Shealy, M.D., Ph.D
Route 1, Box 216
Fair Grove, MO 65648
(417) 865-5940

The Shealy Institute
1328 East Evergreen
Springfield, MO 65803
(417) 467-3102
1-800-692-0536
Offering on-site intensive programs, evaluations, and treatment of *depression, chronic pain, psychosomatic disorders*. Research on the neurochemical/neurohormonal effects of light therapy. Bestselling author of nine books, including: *90 Days to Self-Health* and *The Creation of Health* with Caroline Myss, *Third Party Rape*, and hundreds of professional articles.

Steven Vazquez, Ph.D
The Health Institute of North Texas
1225 Precinct Line Road
Hurst, TX 76053
(817) 589-9100
Medical psychotherapist specializing in Brief Strobic Phototherapy for the treatment of *life threatening illness and dissociative disorders*. Developer of Confluent Somatic Psychotherapy. Internationally acclaimed lecturer. A unique blend of psychotherapy and subtle energy healing.

2. LUMATRON™ MASTER PRACTITIONERS

John Downing, O.D., Ph.D.
1055 West College Drive, #107
Santa Rosa, CA 95401
(707) 526-1881
Founder of the Downing Technic® of Neurosensory Development. Creator of the Lumatron Ocular Light Stimulator™ has spent more than twenty years researching the optometric applications of strobic colored light.

Samuel Berne, O.D.
1405 Luisa Street, #7
Santa Fe, NM 87501
(505) 984-2030
Specializing in behavioral optometry and vision therapy and *psychoemotional aspects of vision improvement*. His private practice is in Santa Fe, New Mexico. He is a workshop facilitator and author of *Creating a Personal Vision: A Mindbody Guide to Better Eyesight*. Dr. Berne was trained at the Pennsylvania College of Optometry and is a Fellow in the College of Optometrists in Vision Development and a member of the College of Syntonic Optometry.

Brian Breiling, Psy.D., M.F.C.C.
21 Main Street
P.O. Box 174
Tiburon, CA 94920
(415) 435-1578
Light-assisted psychotherapy, conference training, seminars, and publications.

Suzan Dallé — Seeing The Light
7839 North Pershing
Stockton, CA 95207
(209) 954-7644
Ms. Dallé uses Lumatron™ light therapy to address *binocular vision dysfunction*, an important reason for the *lack of brain integration*. Monocular visual-perceptual techniques are used to promote bilateral fusion in clients seeking improved visual functioning, learning ability, and emotional well-being.

Robert Dubin, D.C.
802 Bonita Way
Petaluma, CA 94952
(707) 763-0947
Experimented with the Lumatron™ for *learning disabilities, PTSD*, and *SAD*.

Ellen Eatough
Light Impact
205 Camino Alto #155
Mill Valley CA 94941
(415) 388-6766
Colored light therapy techniques for adults and children, addresses *learning disabilities, hyperactivity, attention*, and *concentration problems, stress, migraines, head trauma, negative emotions*, and *underlying emotional issues relating to illness*. The Lumatron™ is used in this office and portable units are available for home use.

Norm Einhorn, O.D., M.B.A.
613 10th Avenue
Belmar, NJ 07719
(908) 681-2320
Experimental use of the Lumatron™ for vision training for *learning disabilities, improving athletic performance*, and *closed head trauma*.

Dominic Greko, Ph.D.
7808 North El Cajon Blvd.
Building #11
La Mesa, CA 91941
(619) 469-4444
Experimenting with the use of Lumatron™ for *learning disabilities*.

Deiter Klinghart, M.D., Ph.D.
1468 South St. Francis
Santa Fe, NM 87501
Experimental use of the Lumatron™ for pain control and psychosomatic illness.

Dan Lippman, Ph.D.
1807 South Washington, #106
Naperville, IL 60565
(708) 460-5877
Experimenting with the use of Lumatron™ for *post traumatic stress disorder* and *attention deficit hyperactivity disorder*.

Carol J. Rustigan, M.S.
668 4th Avenue
Sacramento, CA 95818
(916) 443-7673

Is a Lumatron™ practitioner who integrates music, tones and focusing techniques with colored light to enhance client's mind, body and spirit connections. Additionally, she offers left/right brain strategies for clients seeking enhancement of learning abilities.

Charles and Conseicåo Solis
450 Siskiyou Boulevard, Suite #4
Ashland, OR 97520
(503) 488-3700
FAX (503) 488-1906

Experimenting with the use of Lumatron™ for neurosensory development work with *developmentally delayed* and *educationally challenged children and adults.*

Steven Vazquez, Ph.D.
The Health Institute of North Texas
1225 Precinct Line Road
Hurst, TX 76053
(817) 589-9100

Founder of Brief Strobic Phototherapy. Experimental use of the Lumatron™ for *dissociative identity disorder, post traumatic stress disorder, attention deficit disorder,* and *chemical dependency.*

Mary Ellen Visconti, M.A.
85 East India Row, #19H
Boston, MA 02110
(617) 367-0101

Experimental use of Lumatron™ for maximizing performance, creativity, and intuition.

Nancy White, Ph.D
4600 Post Oak Place, #301
Houston, TX 77027
(713) 961-5243

Psychotherapist. Director of the Neurotherapy Center in Houston, Texas. Her work encompasses individual, group, and *marriage and family therapy,* where she has excellent success with the experimental use of light therapy with *affect disorders, alcohol/drug abuse, learning disabilities,* and *attention deficit hyperactivity disorder.* Dr. White has been a presenter at many conferences and symposia. She is a licensed marriage and family therapist, sex educator, an art therapist and a chemical dependency counselor. She is on the Board of Advisors of the Lumatron™ Corporation. She holds a Master's degree in Behavioral Science and a Doctorate from Union Institute in Clinical Psychology.

3. MEDICAL PHOTOTHERAPY AND LIGHT RESEARCH

U.S.A.

Dr. Daniel Kripke
Scripps Clinic
10666 N. Torrey Pines Road
La Jolla, CA 92037

Dr. Barbara Parry
UCSD Medical Center, T-004
225 Dickinson Street
San Diego, CA 92103
or Department of Psychiatry
P.O. Box 0804
La Jolla, CA 92093

Dr. Robert Skwerer
1650 S. Osprey Avenue
Sarasota, FL 34239

Dr. Charmane Eastman
Biological Rhythms
Research Laboratory
Rush-Presbyterian
St. Luke's Medical Center
1653 West Congress Parkway
Chicago, IL 60612

Dr. Henry Lahmeyer
Sleep and Seasonal Affective Disorders
Clinic
University of Illinois
912 S. Wood Street, M/C 913
Chicago, IL 60680

Medical Phototherapy and Light Research—Continued

Dr. Edward Goldenberg
Behavioral Medical Group
1401 Harrodsburg Road, #A-420
Lexington, KY 40504

Dr. Norman Rosenthal, Dr. Thomas Weir
National Institute of Mental Health,
Bldg. 10
9000 Rockville Pike
Bethesda, MD 20892

Dr. Gary Sachs
Wall 815
Clinical Psychopharmacology Unit
Massachusetts General Hospital
Boston, MA 02114

Dr. Noel Hermele
73 State Street
Springfield, MA 01103

Dr. Richard Depue
Department of Psychology
University of Minnesota
75 E. River Road
Minneapolis, MN 55455

Dr. Oliver Cameron
Department of Psychiatry
University of Michigan,
Riverview Building
900 Wall Street
Ann Arbor, MI 48109-0722

Dr. A. Pande
Department of Psychiatry
University of Michigan
Medical Centre
1500 E. Medical Centre Drive
Ann Arbor, MI 48109-0118

Dr. Robert McGrath
Department of Psychology
Fairleigh Dickinson University
Teaneck, NJ 07666

Dr. Richard Kavey
Department of Psychiatry
Crouse-Irving Memorial Hospital
725 Irving Avenue
Syracuse, NY 13210

Dr. Michael Terman
Columbia University
College of Physicians and Surgeons
722 West 168th Street
New York, NY 10032

Dr. Alfred Lewy
Department of Psychiatry
University of Oregon
Oregon Health Sciences
Portland, OR 97207

Dr. Mark Bauer
Department of Psychiatry
University of Pennsylvania
Philadelphia, PA 19104

Dr. Karl Doghramji
Sleep Disorder Centre
1015 Walnut Street, #316
Philadelphia, PA 19107

Dr. William Sonis
Philadelphia Child Guidance Clinic
2 Children's Center
34th Street and Civic Center Blvd.
Philadelphia, PA 19104

Dr. Michael Thase
Department of Psychiatry
University of Pittsburgh
School of Medicine
3811 O'Hara Street
Pittsburgh, PA 15213

Dr. Frederick Jacobsen
Transcultural Mental Health Institute
1301 20th Street N.W., #711
Washington, DC 20036

AUSTRALIA

Dr. Stuart Armstrong
Department of Psychology and
Brain Behaviour Research Institute
La Trobe University
Bundoora,
Victoria 3083

Dr. Philip Boyce
School of Psychiatry
Prince Henry Hospital
Little Bay
New South Wales 2013

Dr. Peter Marriott
140 Church Street
Richmond 3121

Dr. Iain McIntyre
Department of Psychiatry
University of Melbourne, Austin Hospital
Heidelberg,
Victoria 3084

AUSTRIA

Dr. Margot Dietzel
Department of Psychiatry
University of Vienna
Wahringer-Guntel 18-20
A-1090 Vienna

Dr. Christian Neudorfer
Department of Psychiatry
Innsbrucker Universitaets Klinik
BEDA-Webergasse 8
A-6020 Innsbruck

Dr. Josef Schwitzer
DeparTment of Psychiatry
Innsbrucker Universitaets Klinik
Anichstrasse 35
A-6020 Innsbruck

CANADA

Dr. Gail Eskes
Department of Psychology
Dalhousie University
Halifax, NS B3H 4J1

Dr. Raymond Lam
Department of Psychiatry
University Hospital, UBC Site
2255 Wesbrook Mall
Vancouver, BC V6T-2A1

Dr. Levitt
Affective Disorders Clinic
Mood Disorders Program
Clarke Institute of Psychiatry
250 College Street
Toronto, Ontario MST 1R8

Dr. C. Shapiro
Department of Psychiatry
Toronto Hospital
399 Bathurst Street
Toronto, Ontario
MST 258

Dr. V.P.V. Nair
Douglas Hospital Research Center
6875 Lasalle Blvd.
Verdun, Quebec H4H 1R3

ENGLAND

Dr. Chris Thompson
Department of Psychiatry
Royal South Hants Hospital
Grayham Road
Southampton SO9 4PE

Dr. Stuart Checkley
Institute of Psychiatry
London SES 8AF

Medical Phototherapy and Light Research—Continued

FRANCE

Dr. Jean Foret
Etude du Sommeil
CNR5 UNA 1159
Hopital de la Salpetriere
47 Boulevard de l'Hopital
F-75651 Paris Cedex 13

ICELAND

Dr. Andres Magnusson
Department of Psychiatry
National Hospital
101 Reykjavik

IRELAND

Dr. Philip Carney
University College Hospital
Department of Psychiatry
Galway

ITALY

Dr. Alfredo Costa
Neurological Institute C. Mondino
University of Pavia
Department of Neurology III
Via Palestro 3
Pavia 27100

Dr. Alessandro Meluzzi
1st Medicina Psicosomatica di Torino
Corso Dante 53
1-10126-Torino

JAPAN

Dr. Hishikawa
Department of Neuropsychiatry
Akita University School of Medicine
Hondo 1-1-1 Akita 010

Dr. Kiyoshisa Takahashi
Div. Mental Disorder Research
National Centre of Neurology
and Psychiatry
4-1-1 Ogawahigashi
Kodaira, Tokyo 187

THE NETHERLANDS

Dr. Anton Coenen
Department of Psychology
University of Nijmegen
P.O. Box 9104
6500 HE Nijmengen

Dr. C. Van Houwelengen
Psychiatric Clinic
University Hospital
P.O. Box 30 001
9700 RB Groningen

SWITZERLAND

Dr. Anna Wirz-Justice
University of Basel
Wilhelm Klein Shasse 27,
Psychiatrische Universitaetsklinik
CH-4025 Basel

WEST GERMANY

Dr. Henner Giedke
Psychiatrische Universitaets Klinik
Osianderstrasse 22
D-7400 Tubingen 1

Dr. Siegfried Kasper
Universitaets-Nervenklinik Psychiatrie
Sigmund Freud Str 25
D 5300 Bonn 1

Dr. Wilfred Kohler
Zentrum der Psychiatrie
Johann-Wolfgang-Goethe
Universitaet
D-6000 Frankfurt am Main 71

4. SCHOOL OF SYNTONIC OPTOMETRY MEMBERSHIP

U.S.A.

ARIZONA

Al Balthazor, O.D.
8003 E. Apache Trail
Mesa, AZ 85207
(602) 986 1601

Robert W. Brooks, O.D.
P.O. Box 10103
Prescott, AZ 86304
(602) 778-4402

Bruce D. Burns, O.D.
5806 West Camelback Road
Glendale, AZ 85301
(602) 937-1655

Pamela S. Golden
3366 E. Evans
Phoenix, AZ 85032
(602) 971-1207

Susan Gordon
1440 W University Drive
Tempe, AZ 85281-7219
(602) 921-9988

Billie M. Thompson, Ph.D.
2701 E. Camelback Road
Phoenix, AZ 85016
(602) 381-0086

ARKANSAS

John D. Miller, O.D.
P.O. Box 926
Jacksonville, AR 72076
(501) 666-2020

Lyman Squires, O.D.
P.O. Box 424
Berryville, AR 72616
(501) 423-2576

CALIFORNIA

Moses Albalas, O.D., Ph.D.
12732 W. Washington Boulevard #A
Los Angeles, CA 90066
(213) 306-3737

Beth Ballinger, O.D.
833 Dover Drive #9
Newport Beach, CA 92660
(714) 642-0292

Donald L. Barniske, O.D.
260 Main Street, #1071
Brawley, CA 92227
(619) 351-2020

Curtis Baxstrom, O.D.
3636 N. Blackstone
Fresno, CA 93726
(209) 226-8161

Laszlo Belenyessy, M.D.
12732 Washington Boulevard #D
Los Angeles, CA 90066
(213) 822-4614

Anna Bergstrom, D.C.
1222 Boulevard Way
Walnut Creek, CA 94595
(510) 944-9201

Elliott Brainard, O.D.
2562 State Street #E., Plaza Flores
Carlsbad, CA 92008
(619) 434-5025

Elliott Brubaker, O.D.
917 Eye Street
Los Banos, CA 93635

Syntonic Optometry Membership—Continued

Douglas L. Chase, O.D.
1342 E. Chapman Avenue
Fullerton, CA 92631
(714) 526-5338

Stephen Chase, O.D.
22850 Crenshaw #104
Torrance, CA 90505
(213) 539-1210

Dennis Chinn, O.D.
5074 N. Palm Avenue
Fresno, CA 93704-2201
(209) 224-8302

Steven Cohn, O.D.
833 Dover Drive, #9
Newport Beach, CA 92660
(714) 642-0292

Andrew Delany
73 Ross Avenue
San Anselmo, CA 94960
(415) 454-8415

Kenneth Ethiersea, O.D.
1150 A Coddingtown Center #223
Santa Rosa, CA 95401
(707) 573-1548

Joe Falzone, O.D.
8950 Villa La Jolla Drive, #1114
La Jolla, CA 92037
(619) 453-0442

Michael Farrar, O.D.
Box 818
Cottonwood, CA 96022

Dale A. Fast, O.D.
1111 Howe Avenue #235
Sacramento, CA 95825
(916) 688-2295

Melvin B. Fox, O.D.
35 Maria Drive, #860
Petaluma, CA 94954

Curtis M. Froid, O.D.
111 Dakota Avenue, #4
Santa Cruz, CA 95060
(408) 423-5844

Clifford A. Fukushima, O.D.
5501 Hillsdale Drive, #D
Visalia, CA 93291
(209) 625-5464

Mr. Nicholas Harmon
626 York Street, P.O. Box 7633
Vallejo, CA 94590

C. William Harpur, O.D.
1288 Camino Del Rio N.
San Diego, CA 92108
(619) 692-1781

Leslie Hassman, O.D.
5555 Reservoir Drive, #300
San Diego, CA 92120
(619) 286-3711

Rick Ideta, O.D.
4747 N. First Street, #133
Fresno, CA 93726
(209) 225-7908

Larry A. Jebrock, O.D.
1702 Novato Boulevard
Novato, CA 94947
(415) 897-9691

Keith Kajioka, O.D.
2505 Van Derk Circle
Modesto, CA 95356-0376

Stan Kaseno, O.D.
2020 N. Waterman Avenue, #C
San Bernardino, CA 92404
(714) 886-4945

Louis J. Katz, O.D.
4009 Governor Drive
San Diego, CA 92122-2591
(619) 453-0444

Syntonic Optometry Membership—Continued

Benjamin J. Kohn, O.D.
5051 Canyon Crest Drive #102
Riverside, CA 92507
(714) 686-3937

Peter J. Krupocki, O.D.
P.O. Box 38
Mountain View, CA 94042
(415) 967-2612

Jeff D. Lester, O.D.
135 Monte Vista Avenue
Watsonville, CA 95076
(408) 724-1164

College of Syntonic Optometry Library
c/o Betsy Hancock, O.D.
21 East Fifth Street
Bloomberg, PA 17815

Max Lund, O.D.
1424 Lloyd Place
Escondido, CA 92027

Jim Mayer, O.D.
1329 E. Thousand Oaks, #120
Thousand Oaks, CA 91362
(805) 495-3937

Steve McMurry, O.D.
1032 Hollywood Way
Burbank, CA 91505
(818) 845-3549

Cornelius Mietus, O.D.
1125 Coast Village Road
Montecito, CA 93108

Bradford Murray, O.D.
1556 Meridian Avenue
San Jose, CA 95125
(408) 445-2020

Wayne Nishio, O.D.
1735 Minnewawa Avenue #103
Clouis, CA 93612
(209) 299-3179

Carl Olson, O.D.
1685 Peony Lane
San Jose, CA 95124-6427
(206) 782-6071

Dennis L. Olson, O.D.
3315 Almaden Expressway, #31
San Jose, CA 95118
(408) 448-1444

Sheldon B. Pitluk, O.D.
11243-183rd Street
Cerritos, CA 90701
(213) 924-0950

Marianne D.L. Prak, M.D.
1815 Highland Place
Berkeley, CA 94709

Richard Rishko, O.D.
6319 De Soto Avenue, #410
Woodland Hills, CA 91367-2612
(818) 889-9177

Eldon Rosenow, O.D.
817 Coffee Road, Bldg. D
Modesto, CA 95355

Gary Scheffel, O.D.
3958 Cambridge Road
Cameron Park, CA 95682-8933

Marvin I. Schwartz, O.D., F.C.O.V.D.
3811 Florin Road, #9
Sacramento, CA 95823
(916) 421-3311

Robert L. Severtson, O.D.
121 S. Del Mar Avenue, #A
San Gabriel, CA 91776
(818) 287-0401

Lawrence G. Simons, O.D.
9701 W. Pico Boulevard, #215
Los Angeles, CA 90035
(213) 284-8033

Phillip B. Smith, O.D.
3636 4th Avenue, #200
San Diego, CA 92103
(619) 297-4331

Syntonic Optometry Membership—Continued

Dennis Spiro, O.D.
11311 La Mirada Boulevard
Whittier, CA 90604
(213) 946-3311

Gilbert Stocks, O.D.
321 W. Yosemite, #300
Madera, CA 93637
(209) 674-0039

Daniel R. Taketa, O.D.
611 E. Ocean Avenue
Lompoc, CA 93436
(805) 736-7010

Sintau Two
1514 South Chapel Avenue
Alhambra, CA 91801-5139

Daniel Ulseth, O.D.
200 Vera Avenue
Ripon, CA 95366
(209) 599-2216

Claude A. Valenti, O.D.
8950 Villa La Jolla Drive, #1114
La Jolla, CA 92037
(619) 453-0442

Irving S. Werksman, O.D., F.C.O.V.D.
372 N. Moorpark Road, #1465
Thousand Oaks, CA 91360
(805) 495-0446

Paul Yamashita, O.D.
1611 Lewis Street, #367
Kingsburg, CA 93631
(209) 897-2464

Shaw Yorizane, O.D.
Shaw 6 Square
5150 N. 6th, #100
Fresno, CA 93710
(209) 222-6576

COLORADO

John Denhof, O.D.
2500 S. Broadway
Denver, CO 80210
(303) 777-6633

Roger T. Dowis, O.D.
1645 28th Street
Boulder, CO 80301-1001
(303) 443-4545

Mr. Michael Ebeling
918 Pleasant Street
Boulder, CO 80302
(303) 444-1437

Lynn F. Hellerstein
6979 S. Holly Circle, #105
Englewood, CO 80112
(303) 850-9499

Jay E. Highland, O.D.
49 West Mill Street, P.O. Box 560
Bayfield, CO 81122
(303) 884-9559

Rebecca Hutchins, O.D.
3065 Center Green Drive, #120
Boulder, CO 80301-5407
(303) 443 7312

Lewis E. Mock, O.D.
330 N. Limit Street
Colorado Springs, CO
(316) 227-8658

John H. Philip, D.C.
711 Main Street
Carbondale, CO 81623
(303) 963-1575

Stuart M. Tessler, O.D.
6979 S. Holly Circle, #105
Englewood, CO 80112
(303) 850-9499

Gary Trexler, Ph.D.
831-17th Avenue, #27
Longmont, CO 80501
(303) 651-3173

CONNECTICUT

Kenneth L. Burke, O.D.
175 Main Street South, P.O. Box 384
Woodbury, CT 06798
(203) 263-3391

Marc Denigris, O.D.
36 Summer
Stratford, CT 06497

Sheila W. Doyle, O.D.
281 Connecticut Avenue
Norwalk, CT 06854
(203) 866-5227

Constantine J. Forkiotis, O.D.
437 Tunxis Hill Road, P.O. Box 741
Fairfield, CT 06430
(203) 333-2772

William M. Goldberg, O.D.
149 Hazard Avenue
Enfield, CT 06082

Phyllis A. Liu, O.D.
1266 Ella Grasso Boulevard
New Haven, CT 06511
(203) 865-2948

Andrew Parker, M.D.
85 Seymour Street, #522
Hartford, CT 06106

John J. Pulaski, O.D.
53 Central Avenue
Waterbury, CT 06702

Christine Semenza, O.D.
562 Chapel Street
New Haven, CT 06511

Roy A. Shankman
45 Liberty Avenue
Danbury, CT 06810
(203) 730-2147

Andrew Stack, O.D.
18 Wepawaug Road
Woodbridge, CT 06525-2423

Harvey M. Tuckman, O.D.
Duck Pond Road
Norwalk, CT 06855

Benjamin Zeldes, O.D.
1268 Main Street
Newington, CT 06111
(203) 666-5431

DELAWARE

Gregory E. Colalillo
3217 Brookline Drive
Fairway Falls
Wilmington, DE 19808-2612
(302) 737-4363

FLORIDA

James B. Adair, D.C.
7203 East Aloma Avenue
Winter Park, FL 32792
(407) 679-8875

Melvin J. Apple, O.D.
784 Glouchester Street
Boca Raton, FL 33487
(407) 998-9846

Walter J. Chao, O.D.
7867 Pines Boulevard
Pembroke Pines, FL 33024
(305) 966-4335

William A. Clement, O.D.
123 W. Oak Street, P.O. Box 1099
Arcadia, FL 33821
(813) 494-2662

Syntonic Optometry Membership—Continued

Philip Czyz, O.D.
21178 Olean Boulevard, #A
Port Charlotte, FL 33952
(813) 629-1090

Salvatore M. De Canio, Jr., O.D.
900 N.W. 13th Street, #101
Boca Raton, FL 33486-2350
(407) 392-0660

Joseph Devine, O.D.
948 Pine Hills Road
Orlando, FL 32808

Mr. & Mrs. Robert DiTosti
4751 Gulf Shore Blvd. North, #1805
Naples, FL 33940

Mark B. Frank, D.C.
4900 Allen Road
Zephyr Hills, FL 33541
(813) 788-0496

Gayle H. Fuqua, O.D.
1635 S. Ridgewood #107
Daytona Beach, FL 32119
(904) 760-7799

George L. Haffner, O.D.
408 Lakewood Avenue
Tampa, FL 33611
(813) 961-6168

Kirby R. Hotchner, D.O.
185 N. E. 84th Street
Miami, FL 33138
(305) 751-5155

W. L. Howard, O.D.
P.O. Box 776
Wauchula, FL 33873
(813) 773-6459

George Kaplan, O.D.
431 W. Vine Street
Kissimmer, FL 32741
(305) 846-0728

Robert Lebwohl, O.D.
4146 Marina Court
Coriez, FL 34215
(516) 785-2374

Mr. Robert Lydic
3923 Coconut Palm Drive, #101
Tampa, FL 33619
1-800-842-8848

Casey McCreery, R.N.
P.O. Box 929
Windermere, FL 34786
(407) 876-6352

Ralph F. Mead, O.D., F.A.A.O.
1225 E. Mt. Vernon
Orlando, FL 32803
(305) 896-4511

Rick Morris, O.D.
3288 N.W. 27th Avenue
Boca Raton, Fl 33434-3436

Dr. John Ott, Ph.D. (hon)
8118 Sanderling Road
Sarasota, FL 33581
(813) 349-4514

Jane Pedrick
P.O. Box 929
Windermere, FL 34786
(407) 876-6352

Martha Peterson, O.D.
P.O. Box 40
Pineland, FL 33945
(813) 283-0838

Wayne M. Pharr, O.D., F.A.A.O.
1504 S.E. 8th Drive
Okeechobee, FL 34974

Albert A. Sutton, O.D.
820 Lakeview Drive
Miami Beach, FL 33140

Hanoch Talmor, M.D.
1011 N.W. 39th Street
Gainesville, FL 32605
(904) 376-5103

Syntonic Optometry Membership—Continued

Jack R. Walesby, O.D.
7110 Nebr Avenue
Tampa, FL 33604
(813) 238-6471

GEORGIA

Bruce K. Bell, O.D.
225 South Marble
Rockmart, GA 30153

R. H. Pinckney, O.D.
PO Drawer 3860
Jackson, GA 30233

Edward B. Quinton, O.D.
218 E. Gordon Avenue
Rossville, GA 30741
(404) 866-7066

Robert Searfoss
American International Instruments
1370-3 Chalmette Drive N.E.
Atlanta, GA 30306

John Stephens
300 Miller Court West
Norcross, GA 30071
(404) 242-9087

James E. Tillman, O.D.
P.O. Box 927
Americus, GA 31709

HAWAII

Clayton Gushiken, O.D.
2353 South Beretania, #101
Honolulu, HI 96826-1413
(808) 941-3811

Glen Swartwout, O.D.
311 Kalanianaole Avenue
Hilo, HI 96720
(808) 934-3235

IOWA

Don H. Hansen, O.D.
1923 Main Street
Davenport, IA 52803
(319) 324-3241

Kenneth R. Hanson, O.D.
301 N. Ankeny Boulevard, #210
Ankeny, IA 50021

L. D. Peck, O.D.
1813 Main Street
Keokuk, IA 52632

ILLINOIS

Jackie M. Calamos
412 Bonnie Brae Road
Hinsdale, IL 60521
(708) 986-8412

Ronald A. Deyo, D.C.
Route 88 South, #147
Mt. Carroll, IL 61053
(815) 244-2091

Sharon M. Luckhardt, O.D.
136 North Cass
Westmont IL, 60559-1687
(708) 969-2807

Gary D. Meier, O.D.
1318 Mercantile Drive
Woodcrest Plaza
Highland, IL 62249
(618) 654-7774

Edward L. Montwill, O.D.
5450 S. Archer Avenue
Chicago, IL 60638

Chester J. Nowak, O.D.
8150 Milwaukee Avenue
Niles, IL 60648-2866
(708) 823-5988

Irving J. Peiser, O.D.
7851 W. Ogden Avenue
Lyons IL 60534
(708) 447-1515

Warren Shore
3412 Arcadia Street
Evanston, IL 60203
(708) 831-1592

Mark A. Yates, O.D.
1318 Mercantile Drive
Woodcrest Plaza
Highland, IL 62249
(618) 654-7774

INDIANA

William J. Kokenge, D.C.
105 N. State Street, #A
W. Harrison, IN 47060
(812) 637-3400

Robert Martindale, O.D.
510 E. Highway #131
Clarksville, IN 47130
(812) 232-8269

Pat McMillen, O.D.
319 Vigo Street, P.O. Box 138
Vincennes, IN 47591
(812) 882-0738

James L. Wessar, O.D.
525 W. 38th Street, P.O. Box 1578
Anderson, IN 46014
(317) 649-2278

Edmund P. Zaranka, O.D.
6717 Kennedy Avenue, P.O. Box 2520
Hammond, (Hessvl), IN 46323

KANSAS

Ralph F. Alexander, O.D.
7505 Quivira Road
Shawnee Mission, KS 66216
(913) 631-0090

Robert J. Falta, O.D.
534 S. Santa Fe Avenue
Salina, KS 67401-4146
(913) 827-8012

Lowell Goodwin, O.D.
704 N. Main Street, P.O. Box 638
Garden City, KS 67846-5433
(316) 276-2261

Roger Grant, O.D.
900 N. Poplar
Newton, KS 67114
(316) 283-4735

Ron Huffman, O.D.
214 W. Commercial
Lyons, KS 67554

L. L. McCormick, O.D.
1001 N. Main
Hutchinson, KS 67501
(316) 663-5417

Lewis Mogel, O.D.
1001 N. Main
Hutchinson, KS 67501
(316) 663-5417

Jim Morrison, O.D.
Box 34, 180 W. 6th
Colby, KS 67701

M. J. Philbrook, O.D.
7161 State Avenue
Kansas City, KS 66112
(913) 299-3548

Robert Shoof, O.D.
1206 Frontview Street, #206 Ex. Sq.
Dodge City, KS 67801
(316) 227-8658

Larry Young, O.D.
1001 N. Main
Hutchinson, KS 67501
(316) 663-5417

KENTUCKY

Pauline Cox Johnson, M.Ed., L.H.D.
R.E.A.D. Johnson
7133 Johnson Road,
London, KY 40741-9515
(606) 878-1907

William E. Leadingham, O.D.
1330 Carter Avenue, P.O. Box 2005
Ashland, KY 41105-2005
(606) 329-8672

LOUISIANA

Cecil Henry, O.D.
2041 S. Kirkwood Drive
Shreveport, LA 71108

MAINE

Arnie Hoffman
141 Main Street, P.O. Box 2777
South Portland, ME 04106
(207) 799-2371

Bradford D. Smith, O.D.
15 Western Avenue
Augusta, ME 04330
(207) 623-3911

MARYLAND

Stanley A. Appelbaum, O.D.
6509 Democracy Boulevard
Bethesda, MD 20817
(301) 897-8484

Sanford R. Cohen, O.D.
3933 Ferrara Drive
Wheaton, MD 20906
(301) 946-2550

Paul Harris, O.D.
16 Greenmeadow Drive, #103
Timonium, MD 21093
(301) 252-5777

Walter J. Kaplan, O.D.
20 South Summit Avenue
Gaithersburg, MD 20877
(301) 977-7879

Timothy Madgar, O.D.
7952 Harford Road
Ba Ho, MD 21234

Gordon D. Wallace
7315 Wisconsin Avenue, #900E
Bethesda, MD 20814-3202
(301) 961-8557

MASSACHUSETTS

Sol Aisenberg, Ph.D.
36 Bradford Road
Natick, MA 01760
(508) 651-0140

Martin J. Baer, O.D.
65 Pleasant Street
Woburn, MA 01801
(617) 935-1025

Leo DeCatzo, O.D.
204 Mallard Way
Waltham, MA 02154
(617) 484-1644

Celia Hinrichs, O.D.
169 Powers Road
Sudbury, MA 01776
(508) 668-0910

Joan Jordan, RN
34 Glad Valley Drive
Billerica, MA 01821

Syntonic Optometry Membership—Continued

Catherine A. Kennedy, O.D.
2 Richardson Road
Burlington, MA 01803
(617) 229-2041

Isabelle B. King, Ph.D
70 Run Hill Road
Brewster, MA 02631
(508) 896-3858

Barbara Lawrence
176 Main Street, P.O. Box 711
Easthampton, MA 01027
(413) 527-4881

Wilbert E. Libbey, O.D.
66 Eastern Avenue
Dedham, MA 02026

Earl Lizotte, O.D.
176 Main Street, P.O. Box 711
Easthampton, MA 01027
(413) 527-4881

Ernest V. Loewenstein, O.D.
471 Washington Street
Newton, MA 02158
(617) 244-6454

M.L. Mathias, O.D.
391 Broadway, P.O. Box 226
Everett, MA 02149
(617) 387-5665

Antonia Orfield, O.D.
129 Inman Street
Cambridge, MA 02139

Myron Rubinstein, O.D.
2211 Pleasant Street
Fall River, MA 02723
(508) 673-4656

Harvey G. Schneider, O.D.
336 Baker Avenue
Concord, MA 01742
(508) 369-4453

Cora Scott, Ph.D.
12 Pamela Lane
Amesbury, MA 01913
(508) 462-3286

Solomon K. Slobins, O.D.
1200 Robeson Street
Fall River, MA 02720
(508) 673-1251

Michael Smookler, O.D.
19 Englewood Avenue, #5
Brookline, MA 02146
(617) 232-3392

Cathy Stern, O.D.
27 Harvard Street
Brookline, MA 02146
(617) 277-7754

Theodore S. Thamel, O.D.
52 Fruit Street
Worcester, MA 01609
(508) 754-8872

Maryellen Visconti
8 East Indian Road, #19H
Boston, MA 02110
(617) 367-0101

Gerald Matthew Webb, O.D.
321 Maple Street
Danvers, MA 01923
(508) 777-5732

MICHIGAN

Richard Bratt, O.D.
5364 Franklin Ridge Circle
West Bloomfield, MI 48322
(313) 851-4086

Robert A. Hohendorf, O.D.
4364 S. Division
Grand Rapids, MI 49548

Robert Kocembo, O.D.
666 Chene (at Lafayette)
Detroit, MI 48207
(313) 259-6006

Syntonic Optometry Membership—Continued

Ronald L. Mead, O.D.
829 West Main, Alpine Plaza
Gaylord, MI 49735
(517) 732-6261

Dale Peterson
North Saginaw Street, #300
Flint, MI 48502
(313) 234-3658

Dirk Schrotenboer, O.D.
285 James Street
Holland, MI 49423
(616) 399-3585

Myron Spalter, O.D.
20512 Dequindre
Detroit, MI 48234
(313) 891-6200

Marv Weston, O.D.
202 W. 4th
Royal Oak, MI 48067

Elliott D. Yush
2627 Braeburn Circle, P.O. Box 1064
Ann Arbor, MI 48106-1064
(313) 973-8554

MINNESOTA

Patrick J. Flanagan, O.D.
4473 Olson Lake Tr. N.
Lake Elmo, MN 55042
(612) 779-8887

Keith P. Winter, O.D.
P.O. Box 178
Slayton, MN 56172

Robert E. Zwicky, O.D.
2550 W. University Avenue, #163 South
St. Paul, MN 55114
(612) 645-8124

MISSISSIPPI

Logan G. Eaton, O.D.
127 Washington Street, Route 53
Norwell, MS 02061

MISSOURI

Al Breitenstein, O.D.
7611 State Line
Kansas City, MO 64113
(816) 252-9222

Charles Butts, O.D.
Route 1 Box 195A
Sunrise Beach, MO 65079
(314) 374-6326

David B. Clark, D.C.
106 East 12th Street, P.O. Box 126
Oak Grove, MO 64075
(816) 625-4497

David J. Luke, O.D.
121 N. Allen, P.O. Box 82
Centralia, MO 65240
(314) 581-3848

Donald Miller, O.D.
549 E. Camino Street
Springfield, MO 65810
(417) 887-8036

John N. Searfoss, O.D.
70 E. Arrow Street, P.O. Box 70
Marshall, MO 65340
(816) 886-3755

Linda K. Turner, O.D.
University of Missouri Eye Center
8001 Natural Bridge Road
St. Louis, MO 63121-4499
(314) 553-5131

Michael Wiejaczka, O.D.
314 N. Broadway, #825
St. Louis, MO 63102

Kent R. Wolber
413 Broadway
Hannibal, MO 63401
(314) 221-0040

Richard Wolken, O.D.
401 Locust Street
Columbia, MO 65201
(314) 449-4356

NORTH CAROLINA

Robert Driggers
302 Covewood Trail
Ashville, NC 28805
(704) 253-5336

James C. Herring, O.D.
2409 N. Elm Street
Lumberton, NC 28358
(919) 730-8141

C. Patrick Patton, D.C.
346 Merrimon Avenue
Ashville, NC 28801
(704) 258-2051

NORTH DAKOTA

Steve M. Agnus, O.D.
Agnus Vision Center
118 3rd Street N.E., P.O. Box 841
Rolla, ND 58367
(701) 477-3640

J. Gregory Dye, O.D.
1207 Prairie Parkway
West Fargo, ND 58078
(701) 282-2020

NEBRASKA

Rex Cross
C & J Instruments
2620 Pawnee
North Platte, NE 69101-0824
(308) 534-2537

J. O. Jenkins, O.D.
209 W. Circle Drive
N. Platte, NE 69101
(308) 532-3799

R.A. Manthey, O.D.
237 So. 70th Street, Esq. Plaza #101
Lincoln, NE 68510
(402) 483-0042

Kerri Pillen, O.D.
1227 St. Andrews
Bellview, NE 68005

James Plouzek
424 Village View
Hickman, NE 68372

NEW HAMPSHIRE

Wayne Flewelling
41 Manchester Street
Nashua, NH 03060
(603) 595-4450

Shirley S. Snow
755 Straw Hill
Manchester, NH 03104
(603) 644-4525

NEW JERSEY

Herman Cohn, O.D.
217 Glenridge Avenue
Montclair, NJ 07042

Darius Dinshah, S.C.N.
1399 N. Orchard Road
Vineland, NJ 08360
(609) 692-4686

Syntonic Optometry Membership—Continued

Rudolph S. Domino, O.D.
228 Plainfield Avenue
Edison, NJ 08817
(201) 985-5009

Peter L. Ehrhardt, O.D.
111 Murray Street
Elizabeth, NJ 07202
(201) 352-4842

Norman Phil Einhorn, O.D.
613 10th Avenue
Belmar, NJ 07719
(908) 681-2320

Jay Feder, O.D.
17 Icemeadow
Matawan, NJ 07747
(201) 583-9192

Ray Gottlieb, O.D., Ph.D.
10 West Lane
Madison, NJ 07940
(201) 377-6556

Gabriel Gregory, O.D.
217 Washington Street
Tom's River, NJ 08753

Irving Grossman, O.D.
525 Belford Road
Cranbury, NJ 08512
(201) 655-1531

David E. Kraus, O.D.
9226 Kennedy Boulevard
North Bergen, NJ 07047
(201) 861-7202

Ben Lane, O.D.
16 N. Beverwyck Road
Lake Hiawatha, NJ 07034

Stanley H. Levine, O.D.
240 Amboy Avenue
Metuchen, NJ 08840
(201) 548-3636

Joseph R. Miele, O.D.
36 Cherry Tree Farm Road
Middletown, NJ 07748
(201) 763-3511

Raksha Naik, O.D.
146 Abbot Court
Piscataway, NJ 08854
(201) 463-7547

Stephen R. Niemiera, O.D.
474 Amboy Avenue
Perth Amboy, NJ 08861
(201) 826-9330

Dr. Andrew Pritchard
702 Stillholse Lane
Marlton, NJ
(609) 596-9126

Bruce Rosenfeld, O.D., F.C.S.O.
112 W. Franklin Avenue #I-7
Pennington, NJ 08534
(609) 737-7147

Russell Sinoway, O.D.
309 South Orange Avenue
South Orange, NJ 07079
(201) 763-3511

Roy Soloff, O.D.
2020 New Road
Linwood, NJ 08221

Charles Sosis, O.D.
Oak Ridge Pkwy & Cardinal Drive
P.O. Box 383
Toms River, NJ 08754
(201) 240-0020

Richard Stein, O.D.
53 Sunset Terrace
Wayne, NJ 07470
(201) 696-7089

Raymond P. Taub, O.D.
#1 W. Cliff Street
Somerville, NJ 08876
(201) 725-2915

Syntonic Optometry Membership—Continued

Mr. William Turon, CBT Enterprises
1655-300 Oak Tree Road
Edison, NJ 08820
(908) 603-0060

Norman L. Tursh, O.D.
701 Valley Road
Wayne, NJ 07470
(201) 633-9060

A.R. Van Beveren, Ph.D.
952 Route 518
Skillman, NJ 08558
(609) 924-7337

Vincent R. Vicci Jr., O.D.
123 North Union Avenue
Cranford, NJ 07016
(201) 272-1133

James Washington, O.D.
104 South Munn Avenue
East Orange, NJ 07018
(201) 675-5392

Harold & Marc Wiener, O.D.
64 Ridge Road
N. Arlington, NJ 07032
(201) 991-2211

Herbert L. Zussman, O.D.
P.O. Box 277
Tennent, NJ 07763-0277
(609) 448-0250

NEW MEXICO

Jay Allen Dillon
1020 Canyon Road, P.O. Box 16055
Santa Fe, NM 87501
(505) 989-8094

Robert B. Pomeranz, O.D.
651 Campfire Road, SE
Rio Rancho, NM 87124
(505) 892-1437

NEVADA

Stanley Abelman, O.D.
4520 Red Cider Lane
Las Vegas, NV 89130-5152

Mary C. Carrol, O.D.
2225 E. Flamingo Road, #100
Las Vegas, NV 89119
(702) 369-0225

Darrell Grise, O.D.
3952 Wingedfoot Avenue
Las Vegas, NV 89110
(702) 459-9565

NEW YORK

Alison Bentley, O.D.
91 Bushwick Road
Poughkeepsie, NY 12603

Michele R. Bessler, O.D.
140 Cadman Plaza West, #76
Brooklyn, NY 11201
(212) 420-4972

Ellen Brand, O.D.
645 E. 14th Street
New York, NY 10010

Jay M. Cohen, O.D.
802 Dorian Court
Far Rockaway, NY 11601
(212) 989-4238

Bonnie Farese
18 Heather Hill Lane
Suffern, NY 10901
(914) 353-3311

Nancy Gahles, D.C.
231 E. 58th Street, 1st Floor
New York City, NY 10022-1224
(212) 989-0211

Steven Greenstein, O.D.
281 Avenue #C
New York, NY 10009

Syntonic Optometry Membership—Continued

Mark R. Grossman, O.D.
20 Chestnut Street
Rye, NY 10580
(914) 967-1740

William Gruen
731 Saw Mill River Road, P.O. Box 609A
Ardsley, NY 10502
(914) 693-9240

George Hellinger, O.D.
10 Barkswood Lane
Lawrence, NY 11559

Barbara Higgins, O.D.
Oakhill Terrace
Ossining, NY 10562

Carole Hong, O.D.
20 West 64th Station
New York, NY 10023

Ronald A. Horst, O.D.
2135 Cornwall Road, #210
Southwales, NY 14139

Robert Krall, O.D.
P.O. Box 570, Washington Plaza
Millbrook, NY 12545
(914) 677-5012

Stuart M. Lazarus, O.D.
400 Troy-Schenectady Road
Latham, NY 12110
(518) 785-7891

Mark J. Licht, O.D.
2717 East 28th Street
Brooklyn, NY 11235
(718) 646-4000

Stephen Morgenstern, O.D.
554 Larkfield Road
East Northport, NY 11731

Richard D. O'Connor, O.D.
411 Main Street
East Aurora, NY 14052
(716) 652-0870

Stephen Rozenberg, O.D.
1010 2nd Avenue
New York, NY 10022
(212) 753-7733

Jean Rudy
Orange County AHRC
Mt. Hope Road
Middletown, NY 18504

Salvatore Shakir, O.D.
2048 Flatbush Avenue
Brooklyn, NY 11234

Joseph Shapiro, O.D.
80 Fifth Avenue #1105
New York, NY 10011
(212) 255-2240

Howard Sherman, O.D.
1474 Ocean Avenue
Brooklyn, NY 11230
(718) 252-0241

Lorraine Tomasi
302 Quickway Plaza
Chester, NY 10918

Jesse Vics, O.D., M.P.A.
264 Osborn Road
Loudonville, NY 12211
(518) 459-7337

Larry B. Wallace, O.D.
322 North Aurora Street
Ithaca, NY 14850
(607) 277-4749

Kenneth Weiner, O.D.
Lenscrafters
2000 Walden Avenue
Cheektowaga, NY 14225

Syntonic Optometry Membership—Continued

Gerald Wintrob, O.D.
380 Marlborough Road
Brooklyn, NY 11226
(718) 856-2020

Aaron Zinney, O.D.
175 Main Street, P.O. Box 494
Fish Kill, NY 12525
(914) 896-6700

OHIO

Dru Grant, O.D.
1520 Portage Trail
Cuyanoga Falls, OH 44223

Richard Horn, O.D.
6580 North Main Street
Dayton, OH 45415

Joseph A. Miller, O.D.
2620 Lorain Avenue
Cleveland, OH 44113
(216) 621-1822

Paul Newman, O.D.
279 South Main Street
Akron, OH 44308
(216) 253-1627

OKLAHOMA

Carl Mahaney, O.D.
908 Callie Avenue
Tahlequah, OK 74464
(918) 456-3504

OREGON

Joseph C. Beattie, O.D.
7826 S.W. Capitol Highway
Portland, OR 97219

Larry K. Burr, O.D., F.C.O.V.D.
1631 Oak Street
Eugene, OR 97401
(503) 342-4243

Thomas H. Emerson
1134 S.E. Lexington
Portland, OR 97202
(503) 234-6835

Eric Halperin, O.D.
102 Stillwell
Tillamook, OR 97141
(503) 942-5568

Brian L. Hill, O.D.
2736 Main Street, #72
Forest Grove, OR 97116
(503) 357-2273

Todd H. Hnatko
2636 26th Avenue
Forest Grove, OR 97116-1525
(503) 357-1752

Marlene Hunt, O.D.
24440 Wilson River Highway
Tillamook, OR 97141
(503) 356-5584

Dean W. Kyle, O.D.
1351 Main, P.O. Box 585
Sweet Home, OR 97386

Sandra K. Landis, O.D.
14385 S.W. Allen Boulevard, #102
Beaverton, OR 97005
(503) 646-8592

Susan Morse
25911 Fleck Road
Veneta, OR 97487
(503) 935-5141

Thomas A. Neal, O.D.
2701 N. Main Street, #41
Forest Grove, OR 97116
(503) 359-4937

Syntonic Optometry Membership—Continued

Robert M. Paluska, O.D.
Pacific University
Forest Grove, OR 97116
(503) 357-3619

Alan P. Pearson
2528-21st Avenue, #8
Forest Grove, OR 97116

Paul S. Preston, O.D.
2602-21st Avenue
Forest Grove, OR 97116
(503) 357-2379

Joseph J. Raffa, O.D.
3002 19th Avenue, #10
Forest Grove, OR 97116
(503) 359-9399

Bruce Winters, O.D.
1607 William Highway, #3
Grants Pass, OR 97527
(503) 479-4033

Bruce R. Wojciechowski
7831 Lake Road
Milwaukee, OR 97267

PENNSYLVANIA

Stephen Blaschak, O.D.
733 North 7th Street
Allentown, PA 18102

Arta Marie Buclay, O.D.
445 Shirley Street
Mount Union, PA 17066

Stuart M. Clark, O.D.
714 N. 5th Street
Reading, PA 19601
(215) 489-0870

Janine Davis, O.D.
601 Ridge Avenue
Pottsville, PA 17901
(717) 628-2932

Ellis S. Edelman, O.D.
313 N. Newtown Street, #107
Newtown Square, PA 19073
(215) 356-1889

Stan Finkelstein, D.C.
638 South Street
Philadelphia, PA 19147
(215) 440-9600

Jonathan French, D.C.
727 Chestnut Street
Emmaus, PA 18049
(215) 967-5543

Steven J. Gallop, O.D.
313 N. Newtown Street, #107
Newtown Square, PA 19073
(215) 356-1889

Richard N. Gross, O.D.
210 Fairfield Avenue
Johnstown, PA 15906

Robert B. Halberstadt, O.D.
116 South Broad Street
Nazareth, PA 18064

Jillian Hollands, O.D.
3 Rosewood Court
Danville, PA 17821

Stanley T. Hozempa, O.D.
215 Ferguson Avenue
Shavertown, PA 18708

Leonard B. Krachman, O.D.
403 Avenue Of The States, P.O. Box 466
Chester, PA 19013
(215) 874-9404

Mark Landau, O.D.
555 Van Reed Road
Wyomissing, PA 19610

Jacob Parker, O.D.
8595 Bustleton Avenue
Philadelphia, PA 19152
(215) 722-1133

Syntonic Optometry Membership—Continued

Talitha Robinson, O.D.
2928 Linda Lane
Sinking Spring, PA 19608
(215) 678-4829

Christa Roser, O.D.
882 Indian Springs Drive
Lancaster, PA 17601
(717) 741-5531

Ronald Shane, O.D.
826 N. 4th Street
Sunbury, PA 17801
(717) 286-5401

Gail Wetzel, O.T.
#1 Winding Way
Philadelphia, PA 19131
(215) 879-3430

Kenneth Weyback, O.D.
1002 Roundhouse Court
Westchester, PA 19380-1704
(201) 751-4321

PUERTO RICO

Maria H. Gorbea, O.D.
Hato Rey Plaza, #3-C
Hato Rey Plaza, PR 00918
(809)780-0677

Ana M. Pico, O.D.
Calle 2 J-12A Hnas Davila
Bayamon, PR 00619
(809) 780-0677

Edgar R. Saez, AT
Paseo Morell Campos Y-5
Punto Oro Ponce, PR 00731
(809) 878-8275

Wanda M. Tort, O.D.
Calle 2 #J-12A, Vrb. Hnas Davila
Bayamon, PR 00619
(809) 780-0677

RHODE ISLAND

Howard M. Coleman, O.D.
428 Pawtucket Avenue
Rumford, RI 02916
(401) 434-2700

Edward I. Lyons, O.D.
989 Reservoir Avenue
Cranston, RI 02910
(401) 943-1122

George S. Shola, O.D.
180 A. Danielson Pike, P.O. Box 243
North Scituate, RI 02857
(401) 647-3106

SOUTH CAROLINA

John L. Brinkley, O.D.
426 Bush River Road
Columbia, SC 29210
(803) 772-9040

Alva Pack, O.D.
399 E. Henry Street, P.O. Box 851
Spartanburg, SC 29302
(803) 585-0208

Brant Sweet, O.D.
P.O. Box 8009
Greenwood, SC 29646
(803) 223-8226

SOUTH DAKOTA

Charles Howlin, O.D.
3712 S. Western Avenue
Sioux Falls, SD 57105-6171
(605) 332-2231

TENNESSEE

Edward E. Cho, O.D.
699 S. Mendenhall Road
Memphis, TN 38117
(901) 767-1255

TEXAS

Russ Arnold
17502 Bamwood
Houston, TX 77090
(713) 586-6070

Robert M. Batte, M.D.
20725 Hollandale Drive
Houston, TX 77082
(713) 932-0552

Dhavid Cooper, O.D.
2055 Westheimir, #115
Houston, TX 77098
(713) 520-6600

Martha C. Frede, Ph.D.
2703 Maria Anna Road
Austin, TX 78703-1628
(512) 458-8090
(512) 452-6828

Gloria Keraga, M.D.
17215 Red Oak Drive, #105
Houston, TX 77090
(713) 580-0046

David Saul Mora, O.D.
1601 Corpus Christi
Laredo, TX 78043
(512) 726-1007

Teresa Peck, O.D.
1012 Robinhood
Angleton, TX 77515
(409) 849-7321

Eleanor A. Reckrey, O.D.
308 E. Irving Boulevard
Irving, TX 75060
(214) 579-1747

Russel Reiter, Ph.D.
University of Texas
Health & Science Center
7703 Floyd Curl Drive
San Antonio, TX 78284-7762

Linda K. Rogers
800C Forest Oaks Lane
Hurst, TX 76053
(817) 268-4221

Nick Soto, O.D.
P.O. Box 887
Brownsville, TX 78522

Elliot Stendig, O.D.
1821 Old Mill Run
Garland, TX 75042
(214) 494-2020

Marie Thome
14815 Cindywood Drive
Houston, TX 77079

Ted Vorster, O.D.
2905 S. Shepherd
Houston, TX 77098
(713) 522-3183

Ann Voss, O.D.
7324 SW Freeway, #985
Houston, TX 77074
(713) 771-8204

Catherine West, O.D.
800 W. Sam Houston Pkwy N. #E305
Houston, TX 77024
(713) 465-2516

Leonard R. White, O.D.
4747 S. Hulen Street, #110
Ft. Worth, TX 76132-1413
(817) 370-2600

UTAH

L.D. Hansen, D.C.
150 South State Street
Orem, UT 84058
(801) 224-7246

VIRGINIA

Anthony W. Anneski, O.D.
P.O. Box 1531
Pulaski, VA 24301
(703) 980-3705

Dennis R. Cantwell, O.D.
7409 E. Little River TPK
Annandale, VA 22003
(703) 941-3937

Craig S. Dacales, O.D.
13950 Lee Jackson Highway
Chantilly, VA 22021
(703) 830-6379

Genevieve M. Haller, D.C.
P.O. Box 1097
Virginia Beach, VA 23451-1097
(804) 486-3943

Janet E. Kemmerer, O.D.
1208 Hatteras Road
Sandston, VA 23150
(714) 447-8161

WASHINGTON

George N. Dever, O.D.
1511 3rd Avenue, #411
Seattle, WA 98101
(206) 624-0737

John Ellson, O.D.
P.O. Box 589
Pasco, WA 99301

Agnes J. Forras
10756 Exeter Avenue NE
Seattle, WA 98125
(206) 364-4489

Sidney Hays, O.D.
7902 W. 27th
Tacoma, WA 98466
(206) 564-9262

Tracy J. Knight, O.D.
800 Sixth Street
Clarkston, WA 99403
(509) 758-3788

Jennifer E. Nelson, O.D.
644 Lovejoy Court NE
Olympia, WA 98506-9619

William C. Nielsen
619 NW 116th
Seattle, WA 98177
(206) 362-6624

Wm. C. Nielsen, O.D.
P.O. Box 85147
Seattle, WA 98105

Lawrence R. Weathers, Ph.D.
West 1525 8th Avenue
Spokane, WA 99204
(509) 838-8473

Gerald Wodtli, O.D.
P.O. Box 2278
Pasco, WA 99302
(509) 542-8409

Jonathan Wright, M.D.
24030 132nd SE
Kent, WA 98042
(203) 631-8920

Pamela Ziobro
3404 W. 46th Avenue
Kennewick, WA 99337

WASHINGTON, D.C.

Barbara S. Anan, O.D.
1901 Pennsylvania Avenue NW #200
Washington, DC 20006
(202) 466-7830

Jeffrey Kraskin, O.D.
4600 Massachusetts Avenue NW
Washington, DC 20016
(202) 363-4450

WISCONSIN

Robert B. Bower, O.D.
2301-75th Street
Kenosha, WI 53140
(414) 654-6005

James Reedstrom, O.D.
1325 Tower Avenue
Superior, WI 54880

WEST VIRGINIA

Michael Lebowitz, D.C.
P.O. Box 25
Mount Zion, WV 26151
(304) 354-6141

WYOMING

Sue E. Lowe, O.D.
P.O. Box 927
Laramie, WY 82070
(307) 742-8159

INTERNATIONAL

For International dialing: dial "00" for international operator assistance. In the white pages of phone books there are listings for international calling. Allow 45 seconds for ringing to begin after dialing.

AUSTRALIA

Hans-Peter Abel, AOM
18 Starkey Street
Forestville, NSW
Australia 2087
011-61-2-452-1085

Claire Alexander, O.D.
357 Gympie Road
Strathpine, Queensland
Australia 4500
011-61-7-205-1593

Robert J. Alexander, O.D.
2/288 Dawson Pde
Arana Hills,
Australia 4551
011-61-7-351-5762

Margaret Banks, O.D.
30 Rubens Grove
Canterbury,
Australia 3126
011-61-2-383-64987

Adrian J. Bell, O.D.
67 Bulcock Street
Caoundra,
Australia 4551
011-61-7-491-1288

Chris Chong, O.D.
P.O. Box 3527
Darwin, North Territory
Australia 0801
011-61-8-981-8130

Stephen J. Daly, O.D.
514 Princes Highway
Rockdale, NSW
Australia 2216
011-61-2-597-6413

Simon Grbevski, O.D.
458 Princes Highway, 1st Floor
Rockdale, Australia 2216
P.O. Box 697, 107 Barker Street
Casino, NSW
Australia 2470
011-61-6-662-1416

Dominic J. Kelly, O.D.
357 Gympie Road
Strathpine, Queensland,
Australia 4500
011-61-7-205-1593

Susan C. Larter, O.D.
374 Pennant Hills Road
Pennant Hills,
Australia 2120
011-61-2 481-0449

Graham T. Peachy, O.D.
8 Nilmar Avenue
Wodonga,
Australia 3690
011-61-6-024-2522

Beverley A. Roberts, O.D.
357 Gympie Road
Strathpine, Queensland
Australia 4500
011-61-7-285-5883

Michael JW Smith, O.D.
P.O. Box 381D
Hobart, Tasmania
Australia 7001
011-61-2-024-0077

Graeme H. Thompson, O.D.
374 Pennant Hills Road
Pennant Hills, NSW
Australia 2120
011-61-2-481-0449

Peter J. Woolf, O.D.
P.O. Box 102
Kotara Fair, NSW
Australia 2289
011-61-4-969-5500

BELGIUM

Bernard Cassiers, O.D.
Lange Leemstraat 142 B2018
Antwerpen 7, Belgium
011-32-3-230-9799

CANADA

Steve G. Briggs, O.D.
823 2nd Avenue East, Box 69
Owen Sound, Ontario
Canada N4K 5P1
1-(519) 376-0936

George Edworthy, O.D.
443 Wildwood Drive SW
Calgary, Alberta
Canada T3C 3E4
1-(403) 242-2731

Sonja G. Hagemann, O.D.
#3 1836-29 Avenue SW
Calgary, Alberta
Canada T2T 1M8
1-(403) 228-5915

John Heisler M.D.
P.O. Box 149
Shubenacadie Nova Scotia
Canada B0N 2H0
1-(902) 758-2213

Doug Holroyd, O.D.
39 Royal Road, North Portage
La Prairie Manitoba
Canada RIN 1W8
1-(214) 857-8559

Stewart McLeod, O.D.
471 Ellis Street
Penticton, BC
Canada V2A 4M1
1-(604) 492-5741

Gerard G. Murray, O.D.
39 Royal Road North, P.O. Box 97
Portage La Prairie, Manitoba,
Canada RIN 1W8
1-(214) 857-4760

June G. Robertson, O.D.
1515 Rebecca Street, #208
Hopedale Mall
Oakville, Ontario,
Canada L6L 5G8
1-(416) 827-4711

Edward L. Robock, O.D.
690 Charlotte Street
Peterborough, Ontario,
Canada K9J 2X4
1-(705) 742-5081

Howard C. Thompson, O.D.
4 Algonquin Boulevard
Bramalea, Ontario,
Canada L6T 1R8
1-(416) 793-2020

Rick H. Thompson, O.D.
25 Kingscross Road, #2
Bramalea, Ontario,
Canada L6T 3V5
1-(416) 793-2020

James C. Thompson, O.D.
3-3260 Edgemont Boulevard N
Vancouver, B.C.
Canada V7R 2P2
1-(604) 987-4224

Harry Wohlfarth
1101, 11025-82 Avenue
Edmunton, Alberta,
Canada T6G OT1

NETHERLANDS

Hans V. Brink, M.D.
Weegbreestraat 44 3765 XW
Soest, Netherlands
011-31-2155-17255

Jan W. Dijkhof, O.D.
DiJK 46, 1811 MC
Alkmaar, Netherlands
011-31-72-117-235

Will Kock, O.D.
Herenstraat 31, 1211 BZ
Hilversum, Netherlands
011-31-35-233-541

Robert Werrelman, O.D.
150 Kruisstaraat 5612 CM
Eindhoven, Netherlands
011-31-40-437-619

NEW ZEALAND

Adrian Young, O.D.
P.O. Box 13863
Onehunga Aukland
New Zealand
011-64-9-634-3852

TRINIDAD

Chabinath H. Ramnarine, M.D.
Esmeralda Road, Cunupia
Trinidad, West Indies
1-(809) 665-1234

VIRGIN ISLANDS

Donald E. Young, O.D.
Upper Haven Sight Mall, P.O. Box 7939
St. Thomas, VI 00801
1-(809) 774-6315
1-(809) 774-8041

5. COLORPUNCTURE PRACTITIONERS & TRAINERS

Manohar Croke, B.A.
Colorpuncture & Kirlian Photography
Institute for Esogetic Colorpuncture
1705 14th Street, #198
Boulder, CO 80302
(303) 443-1666
(303) 938-9189
Certified colorpuncture and kirlian photography practitioner and trainer specializing in the use of colorpuncture and other energetic subtle vibration therapies.

Akhila Dass, O.M.D., L.Ac.
Licensed & Certified Acupuncturist
P.O. Box 3013
San Anselmo, CA 94979
(415) 461-6641
Teaches and practices acupuncture and colorpuncture internationally. Call for sessions, equipment, information, and training. Distributor of Esogetic oils and sound tapes based on the teachings of Peter Mandel.

MANDEL INSTITUT
Hildestrasse 89
D-76646 Bruchsal, Germany
011-49-7251-800140
FAX: 011-49-07251-800155
For session bookings at the Institute with Peter Mandel.

MANDEL INSTITUT FÜR ESOGETISCHE MEDIUN
KAMLA AG
Ch-6006 Luzern, Switzerland
(041) 36-58-36
FAX: (041) 36-59-36

Helge Prosak, Ph.D., L.Ac.
Acupuncture & Colorpuncture
P.O. Box 816
Mill Valley, CA 94941
(415) 435-1578
(415) 721-4383 Voice Mail
For the last ten years she has successfully used light therapy in conjunction with acupuncture in her private practice. Dr. Prosak conducts Acu-Light seminars worldwide, based on the colorpuncture techniques. She received a B.A. degree from U.C.L.A. and attended the American College of Traditional Chinese Medicine in San Francisco. She received her doctorate on the effect of colorpuncture on the human body as measured by Kirlian Photography. She is a former teacher of Traditional Chinese Medicine at the Oriental Medical Institute located in Honolulu.

Helge has joined forces with Light Years Ahead, located at Tiburon, California and is currently teaching Acu-Light workshops for both health professionals and lay people. Dr. Prosak has studied extensively in Germany with Peter Mandel for many years.

Neera Hunton
770 Mountain Meadows
Boulder, CO 80302
303-449-2532

Roberto Borrebach
Apartado de Correos 1.100
ES–07800, Ibiza, Baleares, Spain
011-34-71-312656

Christine King
P.O. Box 12
Calistoga, CA 94515
(707) 967-9031
Certified in massage, Neurolink and Reiki. "Christine finds colorpuncture to be a tremendous tool in moving blocks and balancing the body, especially the endocrine system and the emotional body."

Jaldhara Kristen
Gehrstrasse 13
CH–8908
Hedingen, Switzerland
011-41-1-761-830

Patrick Matthews
800 East Fairview Road
Asheville, North Carolina 28803
(704) 683-4885
Massage therapist; teaches classes and sells colorpuncture instruments.

Colorpuncture Practitioners—Continued

Antonio Micalvez
Via Liruti 12
I-33100, Udine, Italy
011-39-432-510046

OSHO ESOGETIC VERTRIEB
Gertrud Cordez
Am Steinberg 11
D-21271 Hanstedt, Germany
011-49-4184-7089
FAX: 011-49-4184-1866
Information on equipment and training.

ME TE PRO
Medizisch–Techische
Produbte Vertrieb Gmbh
Hildestrasse 8, Germany
011-49-7-251-800102
FAX: 011-49-7-251-800155
Colorpuncture equipment.

Reinhard Stubenreich
Berg 69, AU
5023 Salzburg, Austria
011-43-662-660473

SYNERGY
3-21-4 Kichijohji–Minami–cho
Musashino–shi
Tokyo 180, Japan
011-81-481-481-221 (Telephone & Fax)

Praveeta Timmermann
Oude Yselstraat 9 III,
NL-1078 CL, Amsterdam, Holland
011-31-20-676-4670

YASUHIDE, IS CO., LTD.
Jiyugaoka Townhouse 102
2-12-5 Okusawa, Setagya
Tokyo 158, Japan
011-81-3-371-87613 (Telephone & Fax)

PRODUCTS USED IN THERAPY

6. COLORED LIGHT THERAPY INSTRUMENTS

SENSORY LEARNING
Mary L. Bolles, B.A.
1705-14th Street, Suite 344
Boulder, CO 80302
(303) 530-4911

Developer of Light, Sound and Motion Instrumentation', portable, computerized light therapy instruments appropriate for home or office use, consisting of six colors, and the ability to change flash rate, light intensity, as well as computerized programs that can sequence a variety of colors.

APPLIED LIGHT TECHNOLOGY
Ernest Baker, Jr., CEO
79 Belvedere Street, Suite 11
San Rafael, CA 94901
(415) 456-5046
FAX: (415) 456-4708

The Lumatron Ocular Light Stimulator' is the first significant breakthrough in clinical optometric light therapy equipment since the 1940s. State-of-the-art light therapy instrument uses eleven colors and has adjustable strobe flicker rates from .1 to 60 hertz. Several models are available that are appropriate for home or office use. The new portable model, Photron is currently available.

UNIVERSAL LIGHT TECHNOLOGY
Jacob Liberman, O.D., Ph.D.
P.O. Box 520
Carbondale, CO 81623
(303) 927-0100
FAX: (303) 927-0101
1-800-81-LIGHT

Dr. Liberman has developed the Color Receptivity Trainer', a non-medical device designed to enhance receptivity to the entire visible spectrum. The Trainer offers the unique advantage of being able to shine light either directly on the body or in the eyes. This instrument offers many advantages in terms of size, price, and design, as well as having a color wheel with 13 color gels. Newsletter available.

7. GELS AND COLOR FILTERS

EDMUND SCIENTIFIC COMPANY CATALOG
101 Gloucester Pike
Barrington, NJ 08007
(609) 573-6250

Order item number F7068 to receive a book of 44 Roscolene' filters, 8 x 10 inch, a good size to use in projectors.

These colors and formulas are:
Red 818, 828
Orange 809, 828
Yellow 809
Lemon 809, 871
Green 871
Turquoise 861, 871
Blue 866
Indigo 818, 859, 861
Violet 832, 859, 866
Purple 832, 866
Magenta 818, 828, 866
Scarlet 810, 818, 861

The above combinations give the closest available for Spectrochrome Tonations; some numbers are different from previous listings because the Edmund Catalog does not contain a certain color filter due to manufacturing changes.

On page 22, of *Let There Be Light*, Dinshah Ghadiali mentions six additional colors, giving a more "flexible" Spectrochrome. For example, if a particular tonation color was too strong or powerful, then the practitioner could switch to a different gradation within a similar range of the color (*if Yellow was too strong, the practitioner could switch to a Yellow-Lemon gel*).

These colors and the formulas include:
Red-Orange 809, 818
Orange-Yellow 809, 826
Yellow-Lemon 809, 878
Lemon-Green 810, 871
Green-Turquoise 871, 877
Turquoise-Blue 871, 866

Gels and Color Filters—Continued

LEE FILTERS LIMITED
Central Way, Walworth Ind. Estate,
Andover, Hampshire SP10, 5 AN
England

U.S.A. East Coast Distributor:
Lee Colortran Inc.
40-B Commerce Way
Totowa, NJ 07512
(201) 256-7666

U.S.A. West Coast Distributor:
Lee Colortran Inc.
1015 Chestnut St.
Burbank, CA 91506
(818) 843-1200

Both U.S. distributors have many local dealers. Check your phone book YELLOW PAGES under "Theatrical Supplies."

ROSCO LABORATORIES
36 Bush Avenue
Port Chester, NY 10573
(914) 937-1300
The twelve original Spectrochrome colors by Dinshah Ghadiali can be made by combining a series of plastic filters with certain color formulas of eleven Roscolene filters:
809, 810, 818, 819, 832, 839, 858, 861, 863, 866, 871.

Red, 818 and 832
Orange, 809 and 839
Yellow, 809
Lemon 809 and 871
Green 871
Turquoise 861 and 871
Blue 866
Indigo 832 and 858 and 866
Violet 832 and 863 and 866
Purple 810 and 832 and 866
Magenta 818 and 819 and 866
Scarlet 810 and 818 and 861
Roscolene™, Roscolux™ and Super Gel filters™ (all made by Rosco Laboratories).

8. FULL SPECTRUM LIGHT PRODUCTS

APOLLO LIGHT SYSTEMS, INC.
352 West 1060 South
Orem, UT 84058
1-800-545-9667

BIO-BRITE INC.
Bio-Brite Light Visor™
Gordon Wallace, DVM, MPH
President and Scientific Director
7315 Wisconsin Avenue, #900E
Bethesda, MD 20814
1-800-621-LITE
(301) 961-8557
Bio-Brite Light Visor™, is the world's first head-mounted device for treating *seasonal affective disorder (SAD)*. The product of over three years of extensive clinical trials, the visor was developed with leading researchers from the Thomas Jefferson Medical Center and the National Institute of Mental Health. Bio Brite's portable, light-weight visor offers significant advantages over other products used by SAD sufferers. Because it is worn on the head, the Light Visor delivers constant, consistent illumination to the eyes. This approach means users no longer need to sit directly in front of a light source; they can watch television, read a book or even do office or housework. Battery power is supplied by rechargeable nicad batteries. Light intensity is adjustable between approximately 500 and 3,000 lux at a distance of two inches from the lens. The Visor uses a full spectrum white light source with the ultraviolet range filtered out.

DURO-TEST CORPORATION
9 Law Drive
Fairfield, NJ 07007
1-800-289-3876
Producers of VITA-LITE™ full spectrum fluorescent light tubes.

Full Spectrum Light Products—Continued

ENVIRONMENTAL OFFICE SYSTEMS
6 Victoria House
121 Longacre
Covent Garden
London WC2, England
(44-71) 379-7940

FSL (FULL SPECTRUM LIGHTING)
Unit 5, Wye Trading Estate
London Road
High Wyciombe
Bucks HP11 1LH
England
(0494) 4 448-7272

G.E. LIGHTING
Product Service
Nela Park
Cleveland, OH 44112
1-800-626-2000
Product: CHROMA 50

GTE PRODUCTS CORPORATION
U.S. Lighting Division
Danvers, MA 01923
1-800-225-5483
Product: Design 50

LIGHT ENERGY COMPANY FULL SPECTRUM LIGHTS
David Olzewski, E.E., I.E.
Pam Baker, R.N.
1056 NW 179th Place
Seattle, WA 98177
1-800 LIGHT-CO
1-800-544-4826

National distributor for all John Ott full spectrum fluorescent *Ott-Lite™* products, including all sizes and shapes of fluorescent tubes, Task Lamps, Ergo Lamps, Screw-in Capsule Bulbs, and Light Boxes. Full spectrum sunglasses, Sun-up Dawn Simulator, and LED phototherapy units are also available.

WEST COAST DISTRIBUTOR FOR OTT-LITE™ SYSTEMS
Ott-Lite® Systems Inc.
Ken Cedar
28 Parker Way
Santa Barbara, CA 93101
(808) 564-3467
1-800-234-3724

John Nash Ott, a pioneer in the development of time lapse photography for Disney Studios, was the first to develop full spectrum fluorescent light tubes yielding a color that more closely approximates natural sunlight. The Ott Lite® full spectrum light panels have an additional ultraviolet, black light tube and have the advantage of being electromagnetically shielded and grounded. The Ott safety light is the only patented radiation shielded lighting system. Also available from this company are Ott-Lite® full spectrum compact fluorescent bulbs that fits into incandescent fixtures.

EAST COAST DISTRIBUTOR FOR OTT-LITE® SYSTEMS
Environmental Lighting Concepts, Inc.
3923 Coconut Palm Drive, #101
Tampa, FL 33619
(813) 621-0058
FAX: (813) 626-8790
1-800-842-8848

INTERLIGHT TRU-LITE
Australia Pty Ltd.
3121 Eileen Road, Clayton South
Victoria 3169
Australia
03-5623466

MEDIC-LIGHT INC.
Yacht Club Drive,
Lake Hopatcong, NJ 07849
1-800-LIGHT-25

NORTH AMERICAN PHILIPS
200 Franklin Square Drive
Somerset, NJ 08873
1-800-752-2852
Product: COLORTONE 50

Full Spectrum Light Products—Continued

THE SUNBOX COMPANY
Neil Owens
19217 Orbit Drive
Gaithersburg, MD 20879
1-800-LITE-YOU
(301) 762-1-SUN
(301) 762-1-786

This group is the manufacturer of the full spectrum light panels that were originally used in the initial *seasonal affective disorder* research by Norman Rosenthal, M.D., at the National Institute of Mental Health (NIMH) in Bethesda, MD. Several powerful models of full spectrum light panels are available and include: The Sunsquare™, the Sunray™, and the Sunbox™. Quarterly newsletter available.

SUNBOX DESIGNS, LTD.
34 Kings Avenue
London N10 1PB
England
(44-81) 444-9504

VERILUX INC.
Nicholas Harmon
P.O. Box 7633
Vallejo, CA 94590
1-800-786-6850
FAX: (707) 554-8370

Manufacturer of balanced full spectrum UV-filtered fluorescent light, "The True Color Light," since 1956. Lights tubes with the highest color rendering index of any tubes available. Direct sales and distribution of lights for home and commercial use. In addition to the health benefits of full spectrum lights, these lights offer the truest color available and are widely used by artists, horticulturists, and those in animal husbandry, photographers, libraries, museums, jewelers, medical centers, laboratories, and schools. This company offers the smallest compact fluorescent light that fits into regular incandescent lamps. Also available is a line of color corrected incandescent bulbs known as "Neodymium."

WINTERLITES
667-810 West Broadway
Vancouver, British Columbia,
Canada V5Z4C9
(604) 926-4287

9. OTHER PHOTOTHERAPY INSTRUMENTS

LIGHT EMITTING DIODE (LED) UNITS
Light Energy Co.
David Olszewski, E.E., I.E.
Pam Baker, R.N.
1056 N.W. 179th Place
Seattle, WA 98117
1-800-LIGHT CO
1-800-544-4826

Manufacturer and distributor of safe and inexpensive monochromatic Light Emitting Diode (LED) light therapy units, which replace low power laser devices for use in acupuncture, pain relief, and tissue regeneration. Products include: Light Shaker™, Tri-Light™, Tri-Light Mod II™, and the Light-Disc™.

LIGHT PEN FOR ACUPUNCTURE–COLORPUNCTURE/ACULIGHT
Perlux Model B-111
KAMLA AG
Ch-6006 Luzern, Switzerland
(041) 36-58-36
FAX: (041) 36-59-36

U.S.A. DISTRIBUTORS:

Manohar Croke, B.A.
1705 14th Street, #198
Boulder, CO 80302
(303) 443-1666

Helge Prosak, Ph.D., L.Ac.
Acupuncture & Colorpuncture
21 Main Street, PO Box 174
Tiburon, CA 94920
(415) 435-1578

Kamla makes products for light and color therapies according to the theories of Dr. Peter Mandel. The Perlux Model B 111 unit consists of a battery-powered, illuminating pen with a series of seven glass rods of different colors. This instrument can be used to either tonify or sedate different acupuncture points or brain and nervous system points or Transmitter Relay Points. See *Resource List: Section Five, page 371, for Colorpuncture Practitioners and Trainers.*

Other Phototherapy Instruments—Continued

THE SUN-UP DAWN SIMULATOR™

PI Square Incorporated
12305-9th Avenue S.W.
Seattle, WA 98146
1-800-786-3296
also available from:
Tools for Exploration Catalog
4460 Redwood Highway, #2
San Rafael, CA 94903
(415) 499-9050
1-800-456-9887

Sun-Up is the brainchild of Seattle professor Blaine Shaffer, who wanted to create **an alarm clock using gentle light** for people who hate to get jolted out of their sleep in the dark. Shaffer has developed a compact, automatically timed device that can control any plug-in lamp or light source. Just plug the lamp into Sun-Up, set the timer to a chosen interval, and the room will gradually brighten at the time you set.

BIOPTRON™ LAMP

Tools for Exploration
4460 Redwood Highway, #2
San Rafael, CA 94903
(415) 499-9050
1-800-456-9887

The Swiss-made Bioptron Lamp uses polarized infrared light with no ultraviolet and is the product of over ten years of research and development. The Bioptron has been successfully used throughout Europe since 1992, with excellent results reported for temporary relief of minor pain due to *arthritis, bursitis, muscle spasm, pinched nerves, neuralgia, back and muscle strains and sinusitis.*

THE SHEALY RELAXMATE™ SYSTEM

Available through Health & Wealth Inc.
2432 Ellsworth St.
Berkeley, CA 94704
1-800-642-WELL

A portable light and sound self treatment system ideal for home or office use that was developed by holistic physician, author, and educator, Norman Shealy, M.D., Ph.D. The Shealy Relaxmate guides the mindbody into a state of deep relaxation. This system has benefitted thousands of people suffering from *jet lag, pain, insomnia, anxiety and depression.*

10. OTHER INSTRUMENTS MENTIONED IN THIS BOOK

BGC ENTERPRISES INC.

D.A. George
4721 Murat Place
San Diego, CA 92117
(619) 273-2868
FAX: (619) 273-0416

This is the manufacturer of the Audio Effects Generator Model AEG 102-1, used by the *sensory impaired.* This is a safe, technically superior audio trainer with high accuracy filters and excellent capabilities. This machine provides the audio filtration component of Mary Bolles' light, sound and motion treatment of *learning disabled and developmentally delayed children.* This trainer has been successfully used to modify the behavior and cognitive functioning of *autistic children.*

CRANIAL ELECTRIC STIMULATOR THE CES 100HZ™

Available with Physician's Prescription from:
Tools for Exploration
4460 Redwood Highway, #2
San Rafael, CA 94903
(415) 499-9050
1-800-456-9887

As described in Dr. Norman Shealy's chapters, the Cranial Electric Stimulator has been shown to be effective in the treatment of *depression.* This product is based upon over 20 years of research and refinement in Europe, Asia, and America. It is also prescribed by physicians in the treatment of *anxiety, insomnia, and substance abuse recovery, pain management, and attention deficit disorders.* The CES 100Hz fits in the palm of your hand and delivers a barely perceptible electrical current via electrodes placed behind the ears to induce a feeling of relaxation and well-being after only a half hour of use.

THE GRAHAM POTENTIALIZER™
Bruce Lloyd
P.O. Box 637
Orillia, Ontario L3V 6K5
Canada
(705) 326-7728
The Graham Potentializer is a motion table used by Mary Bolles to provide vestibular stimulation as part of her light, sound, and motion treatment of *learning disabled or developmentally delayed children*. Bruce Lloyd was the chief engineer for David Graham, who originally designed this motion table.

---

11. HEALING EYEWEAR

COLOR THERAPY EYEWEAR
Terri Perrigoue-Messer
P.O. Box 3114
Diamond Springs, CA 95619
(916) 622-4474
Color Therapy eyewear is attractive, non-prescription color glasses designed to incorporate the use of color therapy into our daily lives. These lightweight plastic frames with acrylic lenses, meet current FDA standards blocking out 95% of ultraviolet B and 60% of ultraviolet rays. There are eight different colored specs available that correspond to the seven Chakras. These colored glasses are quite powerful.

DR. JOHN OTT'S TOTAL SPECTRUM SUNGLASSES
Environmental Lighting Concepts
3923 Coconut Palm Drive, #101
Tampa, FL 33619
(819) 621-0058
1-800-842-8848
FAX: (813) 626-8790
Ott Total Spectrum Sunglasses are gray-tinted to allow the eyes to take in the full spectrum of natural sunlight, while protecting them from the harmful effects of ultraviolet light. Dr. Ott believes that green, red, yellow, and orange sunglasses distort the spectrum of light intake. Whereas gray tinted sunglasses allow the eye to take in a more balanced spectrum of light energy and may have positive health benefits (such as decreased eye muscle fatigue).

MINDLABS LIGHT/SOUND AUDIO/VISUAL SYSTEM
Synetic Systems, Inc.
P.O. Box 95530
Seattle, WA 98145
Information: (206) 632-1722
Orders: 1-800-388-6345
Manufacturers of light/sound technology that downloads cassette software and syncs with audio tape. Unit includes manual, recharger, free sample cassette, and a one-year warranty.

---

12. FUTURE LIGHT TOOLS

LIGHTFIELD SYSTEMS
William Croft
327 Waverly Street
Menlo Park, CA 94025
(415) 322-8306
Internet: croft@igc.org
Inventor of a prototype variable frequency or "tuneable" light source to balance the human energy field through the eyes and body to affect the chakras. This technology involves shining very pure colors of variable frequency light into the chakras to balance and help clear distorted energy patterns. By applying pure color of the appropriate frequency, the chakra entrains with the applied frequency or a harmonic of that frequency and hence, strengthens its native frequency. The light produces a resonant phenomenon similar to striking a tuning fork next to a piano. After balancing the body, light is then applied through the eyes. In this way a resonant process happens throughout the brain and nervous system.

13. CATALOGS

EARTH OPTIONS™
P.O. Box 1542
Sebastopol, CA 95473
1-800-269-1300
Solar power and full spectrum energy efficient lighting gear for a better environment.

PACIFIC SPIRIT
WHOLE LIFE PRODUCTS
1334 Pacific Avenue
Forest Grove, OR 97116
1-800-634-9057
The latest in subtle energy tools: color, sound, and fragrance kits. Also available are full spectrum light bulbs, Vita-Lite fluorescent, and the OTT Lite™.

REAL GOODS
966 Mazzoni Street
Ukiah, CA 95482-3471
1-800-762-7325
FAX: (707) 468-9486
International: (707) 468-9214
Products and ideas that complement nature and sustain life, include: 528-page *Alternative Energy Sourcebook,* featuring renewable energy; *The Real Goods News,* a tri-annual newsletter *(call for free copy); The Book of Light,* the 48-page definitive source for state-of-the-art lighting. **"Anything's possible when you plug into the sun!"**

HEALTH HARVEST UNLTD, INC.
25 Mitchell Blvd., #8
San Rafael, CA 94903
(415) 472-2343 or 415-455-4656
FAX: (415) 472-7636 or (415) 381-3141
Products including Chakra T-shirt and decal as well as other consciousness fashions, including Sole-Sox with Reflexology Chart and Anatomy for the foot and lower leg. Specializing in "Consciousness Fashions and Living Books."

THE SHARPER IMAGE CATALOG
650 Davis Street
San Francisco, CA 94111
(415) 445-6000
1-800-344-4444 for Orders
ELF monitor under $100 measures radiation. Ten LEDs indicate from 1-24 miligauss. Detects frequencies 30-1000 Hz over a range of 1,000 yards. Runs on 9V battery.

TOOLS FOR EXPLORATION
Terry Patten
4460 Redwood Highway, Suite 2
San Rafael, CA 94903
Inquiries: (415) 499-9050
To Order: 1-800-456-9887
An amazingly complete color catalog, advertised as the world's most complete source of the latest information on light therapy instruments, mind machines, audiotapes, books, videos, software, and subtle energy devices. A unique product selection and low price guarantee.

EDUCATIONAL AND RESEARCH ORGANIZATIONS

14. REFERRALS AND EDUCATIONAL INFORMATION

THE SCHOOL OF SYNTONIC OPTOMETRY

A non-profit corporation dedicated to research in photoretinology, the therapeutic application of light to the visual system.

For membership and journal subscriptions contact:

Dr. Samuel Pesner, Journal Editor
133 Second Street
Los Altos, CA 94002
(415) 948-3700

Dr. Harry Riley Spitler developed the clinical science which he called Syntonics *(from 'syntony' which means — "bring into balance")* in the 1920s. His research and clinical studies validated the profound effect that light has on human function and health. For the last sixty years this organization of optometrists has pioneered the research and clinical applications of colored light applied through the eyes. Associate membership by other professionals and lay people is currently available. A yearly conference and continuing professional education address both the historical and leading edge advances in phototherapy. The proceedings of the conferences are available in *The Journal of Optometric Phototherapy.*

Betsy Hancock, D.O.
21 East Fifth Street
Bloomberg, PA 17815
(717) 784-2131
Librarian for the historical archives of The Syntonic School of Optometry

SOCIETY FOR LIGHT TREATMENT AND BIOLOGICAL RHYTHMS (SLTBR)
For U.S.A. membership contact:
P.O. Box 478
Wilsonville, OR 97070
(503) 694-2404

For European membership contact:
Dr. Anna Wirz-Justice
Psychiatrische Universitaets Klinik
University of Basel
Wilhelm Klein-Strasse 27
Ch 4025 Basel
Switzerland
While the primary members of this organization are physicians, limited membership is also available to the general public, researchers, and graduate students in the fields related to *phototherapy or chronobiology,* as well as professional corporations, such as, light panel manufacturers, publishers, and pharmaceutical companies. Quarterly newsletter available describing the latest advances in medical research in the use of full spectrum and colored light. This is a quality publication.

LIGHT THERAPY INFORMATION SERVICE
New York Psychiatric Institute
(212) 960-5714
A referral source for information on light therapy for *seasonal affective disorder, sleep disorders, jet lag, shift work adjustment, chronobiology, and biological rhythms.* Callers are connected to research programs or health practitioners in the U.S. or Europe. Information is also available on full spectrum or other phototherapeutic lights, safety recommendations, and insurance reimbursement.

Referrals and Educational Information—Continued

NOSAD
National Organization of
Seasonal Affective Disorder
P.O. Box 4013
Washington, DC 20016
Organizes support groups for those suffering from *seasonal affective disorder* (SAD). A quarterly newsletter provides education on the latest research findings on SAD, as well as a national SAD support group referral and network suggestions for forming new groups.

SAD ASSOCIATION
Jennifer Eastwood
51 Bracewell Road
London, W10 6AF
England
(011-081) 969-7028
SAD is a registered charity which was set up in 1987, to support SAD sufferers, their families and friends. The Association provides a listing of SAD sufferers who can be contacted for advice or support. A quarterly newsletter is published that addresses the latest research on SAD and its treatment as well as a list of light therapy products. SAD holds an annual meeting to discuss the latest issues concerning SAD sufferers.

THE DINSHAH HEALTH SOCIETY
President, Darius Dinshah
100 Dinshah Drive
Malaga, New Jersey 08328
(609) 692-4686
Darius continues to disseminate literature on Spectrochrome, a therapeutic approach that uses colored light directly on the body which was pioneered by his father Dinshah Ghadiali. There is a monthly newsletter as well as a holistic health network dedicated to the principles of his father's book, *Let There Be Light*.

THE INTERNATIONAL SOCIETY FOR THE STUDY OF SUBTLE ENERGIES AND ENERGY MEDICINE
5800 West 6th
Topeka, KS 66606
(913) 273-7500
FAX: (913) 273-8625
The Society produces an interdisciplinary journal of energetic and informational interactions

called subtle energies. Membership is available to professionals in a variety of healing arts as well as lay people. An annual conference brings together the leading edge physicists, healers, and other health professionals.

THE FETZER INSTITUTE
Dr. Arthur Zajonc, President
Kalamazoo, MI 49009
(616) 345-8387
The Fetzer Institute is non-profit and is the largest independent source of funding for research and education. The Fetzer Institute is dedicated to mindbody approaches to health and healing. They are particularly interested in supporting research that emphasizes the bio-electromagnetic and subtle energetic nature of the human body. The Institute seeks to promote health care innovation and seeks projects that recognize the importance of healing the whole person – the body, mind, and spirit. They believe that health and the well-being of humanity will be greatly enhanced as both scientific and spiritual knowledge and techniques are incorporated into the health care delivery systems.

John Fetzer was trained as an electrical engineer shortly after World War I. He frequently encountered phenomena which suggested a link between engineering and spiritual philosophies. When he studied the works of Nicola Tesla, he recognized there are energy wave forms in the physical world and he began to speculate about the existence of other, more subtle wave forms.

THE QI GONG INSTITUTE
EAST-WEST ACADEMY OF
HEALING ARTS
Kenneth M. Sancier, Ph.D.
Co-president of Research
450 Sutter Street, #2104
San Francisco, CA 94108
(415) 788-2227 or (415) 3123-1221
Membership and *Qi gong Magazine* are available. The Institute promotes both the research and education of a variety of Qi gong practices.

THE NATIONAL DEPRESSION AND MANIC DEPRESSION ASSN.
Merchandise Mart #3395
Chicago, IL 60654
A support group for patients with all types of *mood disorders.*

CFIDS BUYERS CLUB
1187 Coast Village Road #I-280
Santa Barbara, CA 93108-2794
(805) 963-5404 for orders only
1-800-366-6056 for catalog orders only.
Nutritional supplements and health resources dedicated to serving the patient community. Newsletter sent free to members.

THE WORLD RESEARCH FOUNDATION
Julianne Balistreri,
Information Services
15300 Ventura Blvd., #405
Sherman Oaks, CA 91403
(818) 907-5483
FAX (818) 907-6044
This organization provides the latest information on alternative and traditional therapeutics for a large number of diseases. For a nominal fee, clients are sent literally boxloads of self-care information extracted from medical literature around the world.

THE UNITED STATES FOOD AND DRUG ADMINISTRATION (FDA)
Consumer H-E-L-P
716 20th St. N.W.
Washington, DC 20052
Publication Information
(301) 443-3220
Publications and direct information are available regarding classification of medical devices and procedures necessary for FDA clearance and approval, which may be appropriate in developing phototherapeutic instruments.

15. PHOTOTHERAPY FOR CANCER WITH PHOTOFRIN

Dr. Oscar J. Balchum
St. Francis Medical Center
3630 E. Imperial Highway #253
Lynwood, CA 90262
(213) 226-7906

Dr. George Fisher
Clinical Professor of Medicine
University of Southern California
Goleta Valley Community Hospital
601 East Arrellaga Street #101
Santa Barbara, CA 93103
(805) 963-2029

Dr. Warren Grundfest
Cedars-Sinai Medical Center
8700 Beverly Boulevard #8215
Los Angeles, CA 90048
(213) 855-4685

Dr. Stephen Heier
Director, Edoscopy Unit
New York Medical College
Westchester County Medical Center
Department of Gastroenterology
Valhalla, NY 10595
(914) 285-7337

Dr. Steven Lam
Vancouver General Hospital
Department of Medicine
#102-2775 Heather Street
Vancouver, B.C. V5Z 3J5
(604) 875-4122

Dr. Norman Marcon
Chief, Division of Gastroenterology
Wellesley Hospital
#121 Elsie K. Jones Bldg.
160 Wellesley Street East
Toronto, Ontario, Canada M4Y IJ3
(416) 926-7039

Phototherapy for Cancer with Photofrin—Continued

Dr. James McCaughan
Grant Laser Center
Laser Medical Research Foundation
323 East Towne Street
Columbus, OH 43215
(614) 221-2643

Dr. Unyime Nseyo
VA Medical Center
150 Muir Road
Martinez, CA 94553
(510) 228-6800

Dr. Anne-Marie Regal
Roswell Park Memorial Institute
666 Elm Street
Buffalo, NY 14263
(716) 845-8577

Dr. Bryan Shumaker
North Woodward Urologic Association
909 Woodward Avenue
Pontiac, MI 48053
(313) 338-4038

16. LUMINARIES

Dorothy Fadiman
Concentric Media
1070 Colby Avenue
Menlo Park, CA 95025
(415) 321-1533
Writer, filmmaker, and director. Creates media to deepen the connection between human understanding and pure consciousness. Response to her work includes an Academy Award nomination, screenings in both Houses of Congress, and nationwide Public Television screenings. Her films include *RADIANCE: The Experience of Light* and *Why Do These Kids Love School?*, audio tapes include *Open Secret — the Poetry of Rumi* (with Coleman Barks) and *Bringing Visions into Form* (with New Dimensions Radio).

SPECTRUM SPORTS RESEARCH INSTITUTE
Irene Lamberti, D.C.
21 Tamal Vista Blvd., Suite 155
Corte Madera, CA 94925
(415) 924-7277
1-800-488-BACK
These products are of exceptional quality and very reasonably priced. The exercise video entitled *Relief From Back Pain;* the audio cassette *Stress Reduction and Pain Control;* and her fully illustrated book, *Pearls of Sweat: Aerobic Injury Preventions.* Dr. Lamberti is also available for seminars. Call or write for a brochure.

QUANTUM BIOLOGY RESEARCH LAB
(Subtle Energy Medical Research)
Biochemistry and Neurophysics
Glen Rein, Ph.D
P.O. Box 60653
Palo Alto, CA 94306
(415) 324-9054
Coined the term "bioelectromagnetics," how electromagnetic energy affects the body's healing. Electromagnetics is the next level up from the physical. Dr. Rein's research suggests that subtle energy generated by machines affect tissue cultures similarly to drugs.

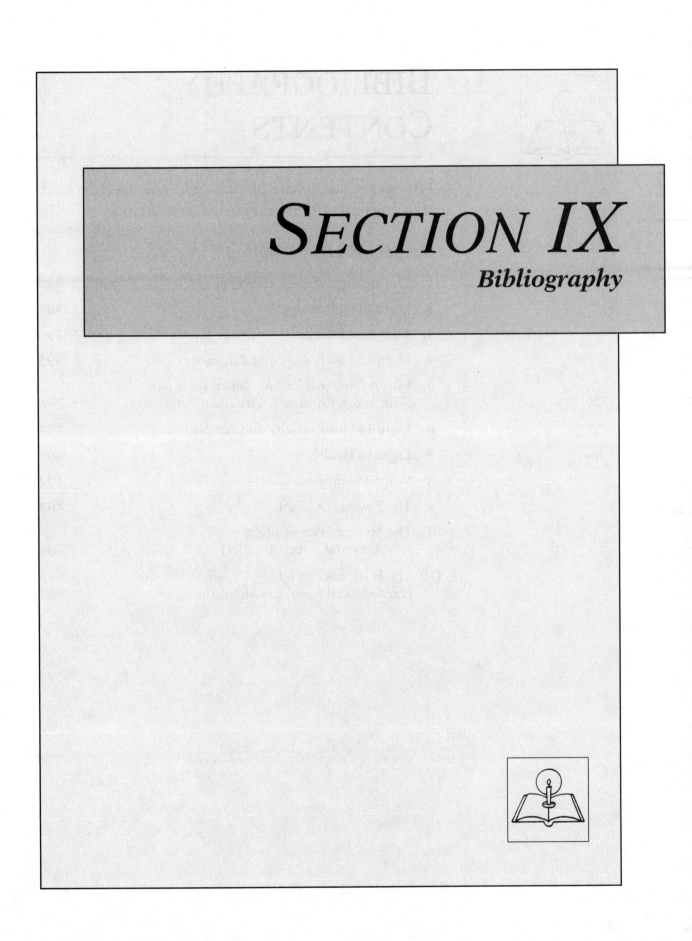

SECTION IX

Bibliography

BIBLIOGRAPHY
CONTENTS

For ease of access the *Bibliography* has been divided into eleven content categories that include:

Suggested Light Reading

BIBLIOGRAPHY:
RECOMMENDED "LIGHT READING"

1. THE HISTORY OF PHOTOTHERAPY

Babbitt, Edwin D. *The Principles of Light and Color.* New York, NY: Babbitt & Co., 1878. An extensive volume which influenced the work of Spitler, Dinshah, and all who followed. Currently out of print. Reproduced in part in *Color Healing: An Exhaustive Survey,* compiled by Health Research from the 21 works of the leading practitioners of chromotherapy. Mokelumne Hills, CA: Health Research, 1956.

Bach, Hugo. *Ultra-Violet Light by Means of the Alpine Sun Lamp: Treatment and Indications.* New York, NY: P.B. Hoeber, 1916.

Bloch, H. *"Solartheology, Heliotherapy, Phototherapy, and Biologic Effects: a Historical Overview."* Journal of the National Medical Association, 1990, 82(7): 517-21.

Burnie, David. *Light, Eyewitness Science.* New York, NY: Dorling Kindersley, Inc., 1992. Tantalizing, full color illustrations, from von Leeuwenhoek's microscope to advanced lasers and fiberoptics. Accessible information about inventions, scientific theories, personalities, and the history of light.

Cleaves, Margaret Abigail. *Light Energy, It's Physics, Physiological Action and Therapeutic Applications.* New York, NY: Rebman Company, 1904.

Daniell, M.D. and J.S. Hill. *"A History of Photodynamic Therapy."* Australian and New Zealand Journal of Surgery, 1991, 61(5): 340-8.

Deutsch, Felix. *"Psycho-physical Reactions of the Vascular System to Influence of Light and to Impression Gained Through Light."* Folia Clinica Orientalia, 1937, Vol. 1.

Dinshah, Darius. *Let There Be Light.* Malaga, NJ: Dinshah Health Society, 1985. A concise history and description of Dinshah Ghadiali's work written by his son.

Eaves, A. Osborne. *The Colour Cure.* London: Philip Wellby, 1901.

Ghadiali, Dinshah P. *Spectro-Chrome-Metry Encyclopedia, Measurement and Restoration of the Human Radioactive and Radio-Emanative Equilibrium by Attuned Color Waves.* Malaga, NJ: Spectro-Chrome Institute, 1939. (1st Published in 1933.) A three-volume treatise on the systematic application of light to the body for healing and restorative purposes.

Goethe, Johann Wolfgang von. *Theory of Colors.* Translated by Charles Lock Eastlake, Cambridge, MA: The MIT Press, 1970 (1st published in London: 1840).

Hall, Percy. *Ultra-Violet Rays in the Treatment and Cure of Disease.* St. Louis: The C.V. Mosby Company, 1928.

Hanoka, N.S. *The Advantages of Healing by Visible Spectrum Therapy.* Health Booklet Series 1. India: Bharti Association Publications, 1957.

Jones, David Arthur. *Actinotherapy Technique: An Outline of Indications and Methods for the Use of Modern Light Therapy.* With a foreword by Sir Henry Gauvain. 5th edition, revised. Newark, NJ: J.J. Alpine Press, 1940.

Kern, H.E., and R.J. Lewy. *"Corrections and Additions to the History of Light Therapy and Seasonal Affective Disorder."* Archives of General Psychiatry, 1990, 47(1): 90-1.

Kovacs, Richard. *Light Therapy.* Springfield, IL: C.C. Thomas, 1950.

Kovacs, Richard. *Electrotherapy and Light Therapy.* Philadelphia, PA: Lea & Febiger, 1935.

Lavie. P. *"Two 19th Century Chronobiologists: Thomas Leycock and Edward Smith."* Chronobiology International, 1992, 9(2): 83-96 and 97-101.

Lorand, Arnold. *The Ultra-Violet Rays, Their Action on Internal and Nervous Diseases and Use in Preventing Loss of Color and Falling of the Hair.* Philadelphia, PA: F.A. Davis Company, 1928.

Mayer, Edgar. *The Clinical Application of Sunlight and Artificial Radiation: Including the Physical Effect.* 1889.

Mayer, Edgar. *The Curative Value of Light; Sunlight and Sun-Lamp in Health and Disease.* New York, NY: and London: D. Appleton & Company, 1932.

Meffert, H., and I. Bahr. *"Willibald Bebhardt (1861-1921): His life and His Achievements in Photomedicine."* Dermatologische Monatsschift, 1989, 175(11): 699-705.

Pancoast, Seth. *Blue and Red Light.* Philadelphia, PA: J. M. Stoddart & Co., 1877.

Pleasanton, Augustus J. *Blue and Sun-Lights.* Philadelphia, PA: Claxton, Remsen & Haffelfinger, 1876.

Sander, C.G. *Colors in Health and Disease.* London: C.W. Daniel Co., 1926.

Spitler, Harry Riley. *The Syntonic Principle.* The College of Syntonic Optometry, 1941. The thesis from which the practice of phototherapy by way of the eyes, known as Syntonics, was established.

Steiner, Rudolf. *Colour.* London: Rudolf Steiner Press, 1982.

Takeuchi, J., and W.J. Schwartz. *"Was Aesop A Chronobiologist?"* Lancet 1993: 341(8860): 1606.

"The Light Fantastic: Optoelectronics May Revolutionize Computers and a Lot More." Business Week, May 10, 1993: 44-50.

Vollmer, Herman. *"Studies in Biological Effect of Colored Light."* Archives of Physical Therapy, April, 1938.

Zajonc, Arthur. *Catching the Light: The Entwined History of Light and Mind,* New York, NY: Bantam, 1993.

2. LIGHT IN OPTOMETRY

The American College of Syntonic Optometry, *Journal of Optometric Phototherapy.* Contact Samuel Pesner, O.D., Editor. (See *Resource List* under *Light Years Ahead Authors*.)

Allen, Frank, and Manuel, Schwartz. *"The Effect of Stimulation of the Senses of Vision, Hearing, Taste and Smell Upon the Sensibility of the Organs of Vision."* Journal of General Physiology, September 20, 1940.

Berne, Samuel. *Creating a Personal Vision: A Mindbody Guide to Better Eyesight.* Santa Fe, N.M., Colorstone Press, 1994.

Birren, Faber. *"The Ophthalmic Aspects of Illumination, Brightness and Color."* Transactions of the American Academy of Ophthalmology and Otorlaryngology, May-June, 1948.

Ferree, C.E., and Gertrude Rand. *"Lighting and the Hygiene of the Eye."* Archives of Ophthalmology, July, 1929.

Gerard, Robert. *Differential Effects of Colored Lights on Psychophysiological Functions.* Doctoral Dissertation, Los Angeles: University of California, 1957.

Hitchcox, Lee. *Long Life Now: Strategies for Staying Alive.* Berkeley, CA: Celestial Arts Publishing, 1996.

Hollwich, Fritz. *The Influence of Ocular Light Perception on Metabolism in Man and in Animal.* New York, NY: Springer-Verlag, 1979.

Kaplan, Robert-Michael, *"Changes in Form Visual Fields in Reading Disabled Children Produced by Syntonic (Colored Light) Stimulation."* The International Journal of Biosocial Research 1983, 5(1): 20-33.

Kaplan, Robert-Michael, *Seeing Beyond 20/20.* Hillsboro, OR: Beyond Words Publishing, 1987.

Liberman, Jacob. *Light, Medicine of the Future.* Santa Fe, NM: Bear & Co. Publishing, 1991. This is the most current and far-ranging text on the subject of light as a therapeutic tool. It covers medical and psychological uses of light, contains an extensive bibliography, and is must reading for anyone interested in the subject.

Liberman, Jacob. *Take Off Your Glasses and See.* New York, N.Y.: Random House, 1995.

Reme, C.E, and M. Terman. *"Does Light Therapy Present An Ocular Hazard?"* American Journal of Psychiatry, 1992, 149(12): 1762-3.

Waxler, M.; R.H. James; G.C. Brainard; D.E. Moul; D.A. Oren; N.E. Rosenthal. *"Retinopathy and Bright Light Therapy."* American Journal of Psychiatry, 1992, 149(11): 1610-1.

3. LIGHT IN MEDICINE

Adler, J.S.; D.F. Kripke; R.T. Loving; S.T. Berga. *"Peripheral Vision Suppression of Melatonin."* Journal of Pineal Research, 1992, March 12(2): 49-52.

American Medical Association, The. *Encyclopedia of Medicine.* Clayman, Charles (editor) New York,: Random House 1989.

Anderson, J.L; R.G. Vasile; J.J. Mooney; K.L. Bloomingdale; J.A. Samson; J.J. Schildkraut. *"Changes in Norepinephrine Output Following Light Therapy for Fall/Winter Seasonal Depression."* Biological Psychiatry, 1992, 32(8): 700-4.

Arushanian, E.B., and K.B. Ovanesov. *"The Role of the Epiphysis in the Pathogenesis of Depressions."* Zhurnal Vysshei Nervnoi Deiatelnosti Imeni I. P. Pavlova, 1991, July-August.

Autier, P.; M. Joarlette; F. Lejeune; D. Lienard; J. Andre; G. Achten. *"Cutaneous Malignant Melanoma and Exposure to Sunlamps and Sunbeds: A Descriptive Study in Belgium."* Melanoma Research 1991, 1(1): 69-74.

Azuma, H.; A. Yamatodani, A. Yagi; T. Nishimura; H. Wada. *"Effect of Bright Light in the Morning on Diurnal Variations of Pineal Indoles in NZBWF1 Mice."* Neuroscience Letters 1991, 131(2): 210-2.

Ben-Hur, Ehud, and Ionel Rosenthal (Editors). *Photomedicine.* Boca Raton, FL: CRFC Press, 1987.

Burkhart, C.G.; J.P. Anders. *"Are City Sun Parlor Ordinances Necessary?"* Ohio *Medicine,* 1991, 87(9): 428-9.

Clayman, Charles (editor). American Medical Association, The. *Encyclopedia of Medicine.* New York, N.Y: Random House, 1989.

Cohen, R.M.; M. Gross; T.E. Nordahl; W.E. Semple; D.A. Oren; N.E. Rosenthal. *"Preliminary Data On The Metabolic Brain Pattern of Patients with Winter Seasonal Affective Disorder."* Archives of General Psychiatry, 1992, 49(7): 545-52.

Grob, J.J., and J.J. Bonerandi. *"New Sun, New Dermatology."* Anales et Dermatologie det de Venereologie, 1991, 118(12): 925-9.

Grob, J.J.; L. Buglieimina; J. Bouvernet; H. Zarour; L. Noe; J.J. Bonerandi. *"Study of Sunbathing Habits in Children and Adolescents: Application to the Prevention of Melanoma."* Dermatology, 1993, 186(2): 94-8.

Hawkins, L. *"Seasonal Affective Disorders: The Effects of Light on Human Behavior."* Endeavour, 1992, 16(3): 122-7.

Higgins, E.M.; R.W. Du Vivier. *"Possible Induction of Malignant Melanoma by Sunbed Use."* Clinical and Experimental Dermatology, 1992, 17(5): 357-9.

Joffe, R.T.; A.J. Levitt; S.H. Kennedy. *"Thyroid Function and Phototherapy in Seasonal Affective Disorder."* American Journal of Psychiatry, 1991, 148(3): 393.

Joseph-Vanderpool, M.; N.E. Rosenthal; G.P. Chrousos; T.A. Wehr; R. Skwerer; S. Kasper; P.W. Gold. *"Abnormal Pituitary-Adrenal Responses to Corticotropin-Releasing Hormone in Patients with Seasonal Affective Disorder: Clinical and Pathophysiological Implications."* Journal of Clinical Endocrinology and Metabolism, 1991, 72(6): 1382-7.

Kasper, S.; N.E. Rosenthal; S. Barberi; A. Williams; L. Tamarkin; S.L. Rogers; S.R. Pillemer. *"Immunological Correlates of Seasonal Fluctuations in Mood and Behavior."* Psychiatry Research, 1991, 36(3): 253-64.

Kupfer, David J.; T.H. Monk; J.D. Barchas (editors). *Biological Rhythms and Mental Disorders.* New York, N.Y.: Guilford Press, 1988.

Lam, R.W. *"Seasonal Affective Disorder Presenting As Chronic Fatigue Syndrome."* Canadian Journal of Psychiatry, 1991, 36(9): 680-2.

Levitt, A.J.; R.T. Joffe; S.H. Kennedy. *"Bright Light Augmentation in Antidepressant Nonresponders."* Journal of Clinical Psychiatry, 1991, 52(8): 336-7.

Lewy, A.; D. Sack; C. Singer; D. White. *"The Phase Shift Hypotheses for Bright Light's Therapeutic Mechanism of Action: Theoretical Considerations and Experimental Evidence."* Psychopharmacology Bulletin, 1987, Vol. 23, 349-353.

Lim, Henry W., and Nicholas A. Soter (editors). *Clinical Photomedicine.* New York, NY: M. Dekker, 1993.

Lindgren, C.E., and I. Jennings. *"Indoor Tanning — Physiological Abnormalities Induced by Ultraviolet."* A Journal of the Royal Society of Health, 1990, 110(2): 43-4.

Lowe, N.J. *"Home Ultraviolet Phototherapy."* Seminars in Dermatology, 1992, 11(4): 284-6.

McIntyre, I.M.; I.R. Norman; G.D. Burrows; S.M. Armstrong. *"Melatonin, Cortisol and Prolactin Response to Acute Nocturnal Light Exposure in Healthy Volunteers."* Psychoneuroendocrinology, 1992, 17(2-3): 243-8.

Meltzer, H.Y. *"Beyond Serotonin."* Journal of Clinical Psychiatry, 1991, 52: 58-62.

Petitto, J.M.; J.D. Folds; H. Ozer; D. Quade; D.L. Evans. *"Abnormal Diurnal Variation in Circulating Natural Killer Cell Phenotypes and Cytotoxic Activity in Major Depression."* American Journal of Psychiatry, 1992, 149(5): 694-6.

Rao, M.L.; B. Muller-Oerlinghausen; A. Mackert; B. Strebel; R.D. Stieglitz; H.P. Volz. *"Blood Serotonin, Serum Melatonin and Light Therapy in Healthy Subjects and in Patients with Nonseasonal Depression."* Acta Psychiatrica Scandinavica, 1992, 86(2): 127-32.

Reiter, R.J., and M. Karasek. *Advances in Pineal Research.* (Vol. 1.) London-Paris: John Libbey, 1986.

Rosenthal, N.; M. Jacobson; D. Sack; J. Arendt. *"Atenolol in Seasonal Affective Disorder: A Test of Melatonin Hypothesis."* American Journal of Psychiatry, 1988, 45:(1), 52-6.

Shafii, Mohammad, and Sharon Lee Shafii. *Biological Rhythms, Mood Disorders, Light Therapy, and the Pineal Gland.* Washington, DC: American Psychiatric Press, 1990.

Siegfried, E.C.; M.S. Stone; K.C. Madison. *"Ultraviolet Light Burn: A Cutaneous Complication of Visible Light Phototherapy of Neonatal Jaundice."* Pediatric Dermatology, 1992, 9(3): 278-82.

Snellman, E. *"Comparison of the Antipsoriatic Efficacy of Heliotherapy and Ultraviolet B: A Cross-over Study."* Photodermatology, Photoimmunology and Photomedicine, 1992, 90(2): 83-5.

Snellman, E.; J. Lauharanta; A. Reunanen; C.T. Jansen; T. Jyrkinen-Pakkasvirta; M. Kallio; J. Luoma; A. Aromaa; J. Waal. *"Effect of Heliotherapy on Skin and Joint Symptoms in Psoriasis, a Six-Month Follow-Up Study."* British Journal of Dermatology, 1993, 128(2): 172-7.

Snellman, E.; E.T. Jansen; J. Lauharanta; P. Kolari. *"Solar Ultraviolet (UV) Radiation and UV Doses Received by Patients During Four-Week Climate Therapy Periods in the Canary Islands."* Photodermatology, Photoimmunology and Photomedicine, 1992, 9(1): 40-3.

Society for Light Treatment and Biological Rhythms. (SLTBR) *Newsletter.* See *Resource List.*

Szadoczky, E.; A. Falus; A. Nemeth; G. Teszeri; E. Moussong-Kovacs. *"Effect of Phototherapy on ^{3}H-Imipramine Binding Sites in Patients with SAD, non-SAD and in Healthy Controls."* Journal of Affective Disorders, 1991, 22(4): 179-84.

Van Buskirk, C. *"The Effect of Different Modalities of Light on the Activation of the EEG."* EEG Clinic Neurophysiology, 1952, 4.

Weinstock, M.A. *"Assessment of Sun Sensitivity by Questionnaire: Validity of Items and Formulation of a Prediction Rule."* Journal of Clinical Epidemiology, 1992, 45(5): 547-52.

Wirz-Justice, Anna; P. van der Velde; A. Bucher; R. Nil. *"Comparison of Light Treatment with Citalopram in Winter Depression: A Longitudinal Single Case Study."* International Clinical Psychopharmacology, 1992, 7(2): 109-16.

Wurtman, Richard J.; Michael Baum; John Potts, Jr. *The Medical and Biological Effects of Light.* New York, NY: Academy of Sciences, Volume 453, 1979.

4. LIGHT IN PSYCHOLOGY AND EDUCATION

Avery, D.H.; M.A. Bolte; S.R. Dager; L.G. Wilson; M. Weyer; G.B. Cox; D.L. Dunner. *"Dawn Simulation Treatment of Winter Depression: A Controlled Study."* American Journal of Psychiatry, 1993, 150(1): 113-7.

Avery, D.H.; M.A. Bolte; M.S. Millet. *"Bright Dawn Simulation Compared with Bright Morning Light in the Treatment of Winter Depression."* Acta Psychiatrica Scandinavica, 1992, 85(6): 430-4.

Avery, D.H.; M.A. Bolte; S. Cohen; M.S. Millet. *"Gradual Versus Rapid Dawn Simulation Treatment of Winter Depression."* Journal of Clinical Psychiatry, 1992, 53(10): 359-63.

Boyce, P., and G. Parker. *"Seasonal Affective Disorder in the Southern Hemisphere."* American Journal of Psychiatry. 1988, 145(1): 96-9.

Budzynski, Thomas H. *The Clinical Guide to Light/Sound Instrumentation and Therapy.* Synectic Systems, 1992.

Dalton, Katherina. *Once A Month.* Alameda, CA: Hunter House, 1990.

Deltito, J.A.; M. Moline; C. Pollak; L.Y. Martin; I. Maremmani. *"Effects of Phototherapy on Non-Seasonal Unipolar and Bipolar Depressive Spectrum Disorders."* Journal of Affective Disorders, 1991, 23(4): 231-7.

Garvey, M.; R. Wesner; M. Godes. *"Comparison of Seasonal and Nonseasonal Affective Disorders."* American Journal of Psychiatry, 145(1): 100-2.

Glicksohn, J. *"Photic Driving and Altered States of Consciousness: An Exploratory Study."* Imagination, Cognition and Personality Journal, 1986, 6: 167-182.

Guilford, J.P. *"The Affective Value of Color as a Function of Hue, Tint, and Chroma."* Journal of Experimental Psychology, June, 1934.

Harmon, D.B. *"Lighting and Child Development."* Illuminating Engineering, April, 1945.

Hoflich, G.; S. Kasper; H.J. Moller. *"Successful Treatment of Seasonal Compulsive Syndrome with Phototherapy."* Nervenarzt, 1992, 63(11): 701-4.

Irlen, Helen. *Reading By The Colors: Overcoming Dyslexia and Other Reading Disabilities Through The Irlen Method.* Garden City Park, NY: Avery Publishing Group, 1991.

Kanofsky, J.D.; R. Sandy; S. Kaplan; J.A. Yaryura-Tobias. *"Seasonal Panic Disorder Responsive to Light Therapy."* Lancet, 1991, 337(8749): 1103-4.

Kantor, D.A.; M. Browne; A. Ravindran; E. Horn. *"Manic-like Response to Phototherapy."* Canadian Journal of Psychiatry, 1991, 36(9): 697-8.

Kids Discover Magazine, *"Light" Special Edition,* October, 1993. New York, NY: 170 Fifth Avenue. (212) 242-5133.

Kripke, D.F.; D.J. Mullaney; M.R. Clauber; S.C. Risch; J.C. Gillin. *"Controlled Trial of Bright Light for Nonseasonal Major Depressive Disorders."* Biological Psychiatry 1992, 31(2):119-34.

Kripke, D.F. *"Timing of Phototherapy and Occurrence of Mania."* Biological Psychiatry, 1991, 29(11): 156-7.

Lam, R.W.; A. Buchanan; J.A. Mador; M.R. Corral. *"Hypersomnia and Morning Light Therapy for Winter Depression."* Biological Psychiatry, 1992, 31(10): 1062-4.

Levitt, A.J.; R.T. Joffe; D.E. Moul; R.W. Lam; M.H. Teicher; B. Lebegue; M.G. Murray; D.A. Oren; P. Schwartz; A. Buchanan. *"Side Effects of Light Therapy in Seasonal Affective Disorder."* American Journal of Psychiatry, 1993, 150(4): 650-2.

Lewy, A.; H. Kern; N. Rosenthal; T. Wehr. *"Bright Artificial Light Treatment of a Manic-Depressive Patient with a Seasonal Mood Cycle."* American Journal of Psychiatry, 1992, 139: 1496-8.

Loving, R.T., and Daniel Kripke. *"Daily Light Exposure Among Psychiatric Inpatients."* Journal of Psychosocial Nursing and Mental Health Services, 1992, 30(11): 15-9.

Mackert, A.; H.P. Volz; R.D. Stieglitz; B. Muller-Oerlinghausen. *"Phototherapy in Nonseasonal Depression."* Biological Psychiatry, 1991, 30(3): 257-68.

Luscher, Max. *The Luscher Color Test.* New York, NY: Washington Square Press, 1969.

Parry, Barbara L. *"Morning Versus Evening Bright Light Treatment of Late Luteal Phase Dysphoric Disorder,"* American Journal of Psychiatry, 146:9.

Pressey, Sidney L. *"The Influence of Color Upon Mental and Motor Efficiency."* American Journal of Psychology, July, 1921.

Richardson, A., and F. McAndrew. *"The Effects of Photic Stimulation and Private Self-Consciousness on the Complexity of Visual Imagination Imagery."* British Journal of Psychology, 1990, 81: 381-94.

Roberts, Seth. *Artificial Morning Light Makes It Easier to Get Up.* Paper presented at the Twenty-Eighth Annual Meeting of the Psychonomic Society, Seattle, WA: November 6, 1987.

Rosenthal, Norman E. *Winter Blues: Seasonal Affect Disorder: What It Is and How To Overcome It.* New York, N.Y.: Guilford Press, 1993.

Rosenthal, Norman E. *"Diagnosis and Treatment of Seasonal Affective Disorder."* Journal of American Medical Association, 1993.

Rosenthal, Norman E.; D.E. Moul; C.J. Hellekson; D.A. Oren; Arlene Frank; G.C. Brainard; M.G. Murray; T.A. Wehr. *"A Multicenter Study of the Light Visor for Seasonal Affective Disorder: No Difference in Efficacy Found Between Two Different Intensities."* Neuropsychopharmacology, 1993, 8(2):151-60.

Rosenthal, Norman E., and Thomas A. Wehr. *"Seasonality and Affective Illness,"* American Journal of Psychiatry, 1989, 146(7).

Rosenthal, Norman E., and Mary Blehar (editors). **Seasonal Affective Disorders and Phototherapy.** New York, NY: Guilford Press, 1989.

Rosenthal, Norman E. **Seasons of the Mind.** New York, NY: Bantam, 1989.

Rosenthal, Norman E. *"Seasonal Affective Disorder: A Description of the Syndrome and Preliminary Findings with Light Therapy."* Archives of General Psychiatry, 1984, 41: 72-80.

Rubin, Herbert E., and Elias Katz. *"Auroratone Films for the Treatment of Psychotic Depressions in an Army General Hospital."* Journal of Clinical Psychology, October, 1946.

Thompson, C., and T. Silverstone (editors). **Seasonal Affective Disorders.** London: CNS Neuroscience Press, 1990.

Vazquez, Steven. **Brief Strobic Photostimulation.** Hurst, TX: Health Institute of North Texas, 1995.

Volz, H.P.; A. Mackert; R.D. Stieglitz. *"Side-Effects of Phototherapy in Nonseasonal Depressive Disorder."* Pharmacopsychiatry, 1991, 4:141-3.

Wetterberg, L. *"Light Therapy of Depression; Basal and Clinical Aspects."* Pharmacology and Toxicology, 1992, 71, Suppl. 1:96-106.

Yoney, T.H.; T.R. Pigott; I.R. L'Heureux; N.E. Rosenthal. *"Seasonal Variation in Obsessive-Compulsive Disorder: Preliminary Experience with Light Treatment."* American Journal of Psychiatry, 1991, 148(12):1727-9.

5. CHRONOBIOLOGY:
(Jet Lag, Sleep Disorders, Shift Work Problems and Circadian Rhythms)

Agishi, Y., and G. Hildebrandt. **Chronobiological Aspects of Physical Therapy and Cure Treatment.** Sapporo, Japan: Hokkaido University School of Medicine, 1989.

Arendt, J.; D.S. Minor; J.M. Waterhouse. **Biological Rhythms in Clinical Practice.** London and Boston: Wright, 1989.

Brock, M.A. *"Chronobiology and Aging."* Journal of the American Geriatrics Society. 1991, 39(1):74-91.

Bruguerolle, B.; and B. Lemmer. ***"Recent Advances in Chronopharmacokinetics: Methodological Problems."*** *Life Sciences,* 1993, 52(23):1809-24.

Carr, C.J. ***"Chronopharmacology and Therapeutic Drug Regulations."*** *Chronobiology International,* 1991, 8(6):539-40.

Daimon, K.; N. Yamada; T. Tsujimoto; T. Shioiri; K. Hanada; S. Tahahashi. ***"Effects of Phototherapy on Circadian Rhythms of Body Temperature in Affective Disorders."*** *Japanese Journal of Psychiatry and Neurology,* 1992, 46(1):240.

Del Rio, G.; C. Carani; A. Baldini; P. Marrama; L. Della Casa. ***"Chronobiology of Catecholamine Excretion in Normal and Diabetic Men."*** *Journal of Endrocrinological Investigation,* 1990, 13(7):575-80.

Dinges, R.J., and R. Broughton (editors). ***Sleep and Alertness: Chronobiological, Behavioral and Medical Aspects of Napping.*** New York, NY: Raven Press, 1989.

Ellis, C.R. ***"Chronobiological Aspects of Epileptic Phenomena: A Literature Review, Implications for Nursing and Suggestions for Research."*** *Journal of Neuroscience Nursing,* 1992, 24(6):335-9.

Gwinner, E. ***"Annual Rhythms: Perspective, and Circannual Systems."*** *Biological Rhythms Handbook of Behavioural Neurobiology,* (Vol. 4), New York, NY: Plenum Publishing, 1988.

Gwirtsman, H.; D. Wolf; M. Piletz. ***"Apparent Phase Advance in Diurnal MHPG Rhythm in Depression."*** *American Journal of Psychiatry,* 1989, 146: 1427-34.

Halaris, A. ***Chronobiology and Psychiatric Disorders.*** New York, NY: Elsevier, 1987.

Haye, D.K.; J.E. Pauly; R.J. Reiter (editors). ***Chronobiology: It's Role in Clinical Medicine, General Biology and Agriculture.*** Proceedings of the XIX International Conference of the International Society for Chonobiology, Bethesda, Maryland: June 20-24, 1989. New York, NY: Wiley-Liss, 1990.

Hekkens, J.M.; G. Kerkhof; W.L. Rietveld. ***Trends in Chronobiology.*** Proceedings of the XVIIIth Conference of the International Society for Chronobiology, held in conjunction with Third Annual Meeting of the European Society for Chronobiology, July 12-17, 1987, Leiden, The Netherlands. New York, NY: Pergamon, 1988.

Hermida, R.C.; D.E. Ayala; J.J. Lopez-Franco; R.J. Arroyave. ***"Circannual Variation in the Incidence of Uterine Cervix Cancer."*** *Chronobiology International,* 1993, 10(1): 54-62.

Klemfuss, H. ***"Rhythms and the Pharmacology of Lithium."*** *Pharmacology and Therapeutics,* 1992, 56(1):53-78.

Kristal-Boneh, E.; G. Harari; M.S. Green. *"Circannual Variations in Blood Cholesterol Levels."* Chronobiology International, 1993: 10(1):37-42.

Lahaie, U. *"Shift-Workers and Seasonal Affective Disorder."* Canadian Nurse, 1991, 87(5):33-4.

Lothman, E.W. *"Functional Anatomy: A Challenge for the Decade of the Brain."* Epilepsia, 1991, 32 Suppl. 5:3-13.

Martin, R.J. *"Nocturnal Asthma: Circadian Rhythms and Therapeutic Interventions."* American Review of Respiratory Disease. 1993, 147(6):825-8.

McGovern, J.P.; M.H. Smolensky; A. Reinberg (editors). *Chronobiology in Allergy and Immunology.* Springfield, IL: C.C. Thomas, 1977.

Mizuma, H.; T. Kotorii; Y. Nakazawa. *"Seasonal Affective Disorder (SAD) with Non-24-hour Sleep-Wake Rhythm During Depressive Phase."* Japanese Journal of Psychiatry and Neurology, 1992, 46(1):215-6.

Moore-Edge, M.C.; F.M. Sulzman; C.A. Fuller. *The Clocks That Time Us.* Cambridge, MA: A Commonwealth Fund Book (Harvard College), 1982.

Nappi, G., and O. Sjaastad. *Chronobiological Correlates of Headache.* Capri Symposium, May 27-28, 1983. Oslo, Norway: Universitetsforlaget, 1983.

Oren, Dan; Reich, Walter; Rosenthal, Norman; Wehr, Thomas. *"How to Beat Jet Lag: A Practical Guide for Air Travellers."* New York: Henry Holt & Co, 1993.

Pancheri, P., and L. Zichelle (editors). *Biorhythms and Stress in the Physiopathology of Reproduction.* New York, NY: Hemisphere Publishing, 1988.

Pauly, J.E., and L.E. Scheving (editors). *Advances in Chronobiology.* The XVIIth International Conference of the International Society for Chronobiology, held in Little Rock, Arkansas: November 3-6, 1987. New York, NY: Liss Publishing.

Rosenthal, N.E. *"Light Pulses Shift Astronaut's Rhythms."* N.Y. Times, Science Magazine, April 23, 1991.

Russa, B.K. (editor). *"The Society of Research on Biological Rhythms."* The Journal of Biological Rhythms, New York, NY: Guilford Press, 1991.

Satlin, A.; L. Volicer; V. Ross; L. Herz; S. Campbell. *"Bright Light Treatment of Behavioral and Sleep Disturbances In Patients with Alzheimer's Disease."* American Journal of Psychiatry, 1992, 149(8):1028-32.

Smolansky, M.H., and G.E. D'Alonzo. *"Medical Chronobiology: Concepts and Applications."* American Review of Respiratory Disease. 1993, 147(6):12-19.

Stampi, Caludio (editor). ***Why We Nap: Evolution, Chronobiology and Functions of Polyphasic and Ultrashort Sleep.*** Boston, MA: Birkhauser, 1992.

"The Right Time? Chronopharmacology — A New Science." *Nursing Research,* 1992, 7(10):23-26.

Van Cauter, E., and F. Turek. ***"Strategies for Resetting the Human Circadian Clock."*** *The New England Journal of Medicine,* 1990: 1306-08.

Van Sweden, B.; A. Wauquier; B. Kemp; H.A. Kamphuisen. ***"Variability of Normal Sleep Patterns in 40 Consecutive Ambulatory Sleep-Wakefulness Records."*** *Electroencephalograph and Clinical Neurophysiology,* 1991, 78(1):66-70.

Wehr, T., and F. Goodwin. ***Circadian Rhythms in Psychiatry.*** The Boxwood Press, 1983.

6. LIGHT IN HOMEOPATHY AND ACUPUNCTURE
(Colorpuncture and Kirlian Photography)

Aesklepeon of Light, ***Therapeutic Effects of Monochromatic Red Light.*** The Light Co., Seattle, WA: 1991.

Amaro, John A. ***"Lasers, Have We Been Duped?"*** *Dynamic Chiropractic,* 1991:26-7.

Belkin, Michael, and Michael Schwartz. ***"New Biological Phenomena Associated With Laser Radiation."*** *Health Physics,* 1989, 56(5):687-90.

Bergold, O. ***"The Effect of Light and Color on Human Physiology."*** *(For use in Acupuncture). Raum & Zeit,* 1989, 1:33-9.

Button, Graham. ***"Improvement on Copper Bracelets: The Use of Low-Powered Lasers in Pain Relief."*** *Forbes,* November 7, 1994.

Cousens, Gabriel. ***Spiritual Nutrition and The Rainbow Diet.*** Boulder, CO: Cassandra Press, 1986.

East Asian Medical Studies Society. ***Fundamentals of Chinese Medicine.*** Brookline, MA: Paradigm Productions, 1985.

Ericsson, Arthur D. ***"The Helium-Neon Laser: Pain Relief — A Clinical Study."*** *Raum & Zeit,* 1991, 3:11-4.

Ericsson, Arthur D., and W. LaValley. ***"Pain Management and Wound Healing."*** *Explore.* 1993, 4:12-3.

Ferguson, M. *"Soviets Hope to Account for Dramatic Laser Healing."* Brain/Mind Bulletin, May, 1989.

Fing, C.; J. Cleland; C. Knowles; J. Jackson. *"Effects of Healing: Neon Laser Experimental Auriculotherapy on Pain Threshold."* Physical Therapy, 1990, 70:24-30.

Gerber, Richard. *Vibrational Medicine: New Choices for Healing Ourselves.* Santa Fe, NM: Bear & Company, 1988.

Hammer, Leon. *Dragon Rises, Red Bird Flies: Psychology, Energy and Chinese Medicine.* New York, NY: Station Hill Press, 1990.

Karu, Tiina. *"Photobiology of Low-Power Laser Effects."* Health Physics, May, 1989, 56:691-702.

Kenyon, Julian N. *Modern Techniques of Acupuncture.* (3 volumes). Wellingborough, UK: Thorsons Publishers, 1985.

Kleinkort, J., and R. Foley. *"Laser Acupuncture: Its Use in Physical Therapy."* American Journal of Acupuncture. 1984, 12:51-56.

Light Energy Company. *Portable Phototherapy Unit Operating Guide.* Seattle, WA: Light Energy Company, 1995.

MacIvor, V. S., and L. LaForest. *Vibrations, Healing Through Color, Homeopathy and Radionics.* New York, NY: Samuel Weiser, Inc., 1979.

Mandel, Peter. *Esogetics: The Sense and Nonsense of Sickness and Pain.* Wassubrun, Germany: Energetik-Verlag, Gmbh, Sulzbach/Taunus, 1993.

Mandel, Peter. *Practical Compendium of Colorpuncture.* (German language edition). Bruschal, Germany: Edition Energetik Verlag, 1986.

Mandel, Peter. *The Practical Compendium of Colorpuncture.* (English translation). Bruschal, Germany: Energetik-Verlag, 1986.

Mandel, Peter. *The Pharmacy of Light.* Bruschal, Germany: Mandel-Institut für Esogetische Medizin, Bruschal, Germany: 1995.

McWilliams, Charles H. *Electro-Acupuncture Up-To-Date.* Health Sciences Research, 1981.

Shapiro, R.S., and H.E. Stockard. *"Electroencephalographic Evidence Demonstrates Altered Brainwave Patterns by Acupoint Stimulation."* American Journal of Acupuncture. 1989, 17(1).

Snyder-Mackler, L.; C. Bork; B. Bouron. *"Effects of Neon-Helium Laser on Musculo-skeletal Trigger Points."* Physical Therapy Journal. 1988, 66:1087-90.

Stelian, J.; I. Gil; B. Habot; M. Rosenthal; I. Abramovici; N. Kutok; A. Khahil. ***"Improvement of Pain and Disability in Elderly Patients with Degenerative Osteoarthritis of the Knee Treated with Narrow-Band Light Therapy."*** *Journal of the American Geriatrics Society*, 1992, 40:23-6.

White, James J., and Kendra Kaesberg-White. ***"Laser Therapy and Pain Relief."*** *Dynamic Chiropractic*, Oct. 7, 1994.

7. LIGHT IN HEALTH

Ceder, Ken, ***"Healthy Office Lighting: A Bright Idea."*** *The Healthy Office Report*, publication of National Safe Workplace Institute, May 15, 1992, 2(5).

Fairechild, Diana. ***Jet Lag, Jet Smart: How Flying Endangers Your Health.*** Hilo, HI: Flyana Rhyme, 1992.

Ferguson Marilyn. ***"Full-Spectrum Light Outshines Others In Classroom."*** *Brain/Mind Bulletin*, September, 1993, p. 6.

Gilbert, Susan. ***"Harnessing the Power of Light."*** *NY Times Magazine*, April 26, 1992.

Hutchison, Michael. ***Megabrain: New Tools and Techniques for Brain Growth and Mind Expansion,*** New York, NY: William Morrow, 1986.

Hyman, Jane Wegscheider. ***The Light Book: How Natural and Artificial Light Affect Our Health, Mood and Behavior.*** Los Angeles, CA: Tarcher, 1990.

Ott, John Nash. ***Health and Light.*** Old Greenwich, CT: The Devin-Adair Company, 1973. Republished by Ariel Press, Columbus, OH: 1978. John Nash Ott is probably one of our greatest living authorities on light and its healing properties. This is an excellent summary of his work, covering the effects of natural and artificial light on man and other living things. Any book by Ott is recommended.

Ott, John Nash. ***Light, Radiation and You.*** Old Greenwich, CT: The Devin-Adair Company, 1982.

Ott, John Nash. ***My Ivory Cellar.*** Chicago, IL: Twentieth Century Press, Inc., 1958.

Ott, John Nash. ***Exploring the Spectrum.*** Parts I and II. Film.

Ott, John Nash. ***Color and Light: Their Effects on Plants, Animals and People.*** Kensington Press, (Vol. 7) 1985. POB 1174, Tacoma, WA, 98401.

Rynk, Peggy. *"Fluorescent Lighting: How Does it Affect Health?"* *Let's Live,* May 1993.

Seem, Mark, and Joan Kaplan. *Bodymind Energetics: Towards a Dynamic Model of Health.* Rochester, NY: Thorsons Publishers, 1987.

Sobel, Michael. *Light.* Chicago and London: University of Chicago Press, 1987. An introduction to the science and technology of light. The author describes light's important role in the physics and biochemistry of everyday life. Very clear explanations of modern physics and a thorough exploration of light phenomena in the micro and macrocosmic dimensions.

Wurtman, Richard J. *"The Effects of Light on the Human Body."* *Scientific American,* July, 1975:69-77

Young, Patrick. *"Turning On Light Turns Off Disease."* *National Observer,* May 29, 1976.

8. COLOR THERAPY

Amber, R.B. *Color Therapy: Healing with Color.* Calcutta, India: Firma LKM Private Ltd., 1964; reprinted, 1976.

Anderson, Mary. *Colour Healing: Chromotherapy and How It Works.* New York, NY: Samuel Weiser, Inc., 1975.

Clark, Linda. *The Ancient Art of Color Therapy.* New York, NY: Pocket Books, 1975. A very extensive historical review. Out-of-print and worth looking for.

Birren, Faber. *Color Psychology and Color Healing.* Secaucus, NJ: Citadel Press, 1961.

Birren, Faber. *Color Psychology and Color Therapy.* Secaucus, NJ: Carol Publishing Group, 1989.

Cayce, Edgar. *The Power of Color and Stones: How to Understand the World Around You.* Virginia Beach, VA: The Edgar Cayce Foundation, 1985.

Color Healing: An Exhaustive Survey Compiled by Health Research from the 21 Works of the Leading Practitioners of Chromotherapy. Mokelumne Hill, CA: Health Research Press, 1956.

Howat, R. Douglas. *Elements of Chromotherapy.* London, UK: Actinic Press, 1938.

Hunt, Roland. *The Seven Keys to Colour Healing.* Ashingdon, England, UK: C.W. Daniel, 1940. Republished by Harper & Row, San Francisco, CA: 1971. Explains the basic principle of "color breathing," using color to enhance or restore physical, mental and spiritual well-being.

Hunt, Roland. *The Eighth Key to Colour.* England, UK: L.N. Fowler & Co., 1965. The operative principles of Hunt's work, describing how each color ray is related to our psychological make-up.

9. THE PHYSICS OF LIGHT

Becker, Robert O., and Gary Seldon. *The Body Electric.* New York, NY: William Morrow, 1985.

Capra, Fritjof. *The Turning Point.* New York, NY: Simon & Schuster, 1982.

Chiao, R.Y.; P.G. Kwiat; A.M. Steinberg. *"Faster than Light? Experiments in Quantum Optics Show that Two Distant Events can Influence Each Other Faster Than Any Signal Could Have Traveled Between Them".* Scientific American, August, 1993.

Feynman, Richard P. *The Strange Theory of Light and Matter.* Princeton, NJ: Princeton University Press, 1988.

Konikiewicz, Leonhard C., and Leonhard Griff. *Bioelectrography: A New Method for Detecting Cancer and Monitoring Body Physiology.* Harrisburg, PA: Leonhard Associates Press, 1984.

Mandel, Peter. *Energy Emission Analysis: A New Application of Kirlian Photography for Holistic Health.* Wessobrunn, West Germany: Sythesis Verlag, 1984.

Rubik, Beverly. *"Natural Light from Organisms."* Noetic Sciences Review, Summer, 1993: pp10-15.

Zajonc, Arthur. *Catching The Light, The Entwined History of Light and Mind.* New York, NY: Bantam, 1993.

10. THE METAPHYSICS OF LIGHT
(Chakras and Subtle Energies)

Bailey, Alice. *Esoteric Healing.* London, England: Lucis Press Ltd., 1972.

Besant, Annie. *A Study in Consciousness: A Contribution to the Science of Psychology.* Wheaton, London: The Theosophical Publishing House, 1972. lst published in 1938.

Besant, Annie, and C.W. Leadbeater. *Thought-Forms.* Wheaton, IL: Theosophical Publishing House, 1971.

Blavatsky, H.P. *The Secret Doctrine: The Synthesis of Science, Religion and Philosophy.* 3 volumes. Wheaton, IL: Theosophical Publishing House, 1888.

Bragdon, Emma. *The Call of Spiritual Emergency, From Personal Crisis to Personal Transformation: How to Deal with the Disorientation that Can Accompany Death, Illness, Injury, Childbirth, Drug Experiences, Sex, Meditation, and all Life-Transforming Experiences.* San Francisco, CA: Harper & Row, 1990.

Brennan, Barbara. *Light Emerging.* New York, NY: Bantam Books, 1993.

Brennan, Barbara. *Hands of Light: A Guide to Healing Through the Human Energy Field.* The best source for pictures of the chakras and the subtle energy bodies. An outstanding integration of classical body-oriented psychotherapy and subtle energy healing. New York, NY: Bantam Books, 1988.

Brennan, Barbara. *Function of the Human Energy Field in the Dynamic Process of Health, Health and Disease.* New York, NY: Institute for New Age, 1980.

Bruyere, Rosalyn. *Wheels of Light.* Glendale, CA: Healing Light Center, 1987.

Complementary Medicine Magazine. Volume 2(4), March-April 1987. Entire issue is devoted to *"Subtle Energies in Medicine."*

Fadiman, Dorothy. *Radiance, The Experience of Light and Celebration.* Video. San Francisco: Art Group, New Era Media 1985. A sumptuous feast of visuals and music reveals the multiple facets of light which the sensitive narration weaves into a universal totality.

Grey, Alex. *Sacred Mirrors: The Sacred Art of Alex Grey,* Rochester, VT: Inner Traditions International, 1990.

Haas, Elson M. *Staying Healthy with Nutrition: The Complete Guide to Diet and Nutritional Medicine.* Berkeley, CA: Celestial Arts, 1992.

Haas, Elson M. *Staying Healthy with the Seasons.* Berkeley, CA: Celestial Arts, 1981.

Haas, Elson M. *Diet for the Seasons.* Berkeley, CA: Celestial Arts, 1995.

Heline, Corinne. *Healing and Regeneration Through Color/Music.* A spiritual, metaphysical look at color and music in the processes of healing and regeneration. Marina del Rey, CA: De Vorss & Co., 1983.

Hunt, Valerie; W. Massey; R. Weinberg; R. Bruyere; P. Hahn. *A Study of Structural Integration from Neuromuscular, Energy Field, and Emotional Approaches.* Los Angeles, CA: U.C.L.A. Press, 1977.

Johari, Harish. *Chakras: Energy Centers of Transformation.* Rochester, VT: Destiny Books, 1987.

Judith, Anodea, and Selene Vega. *The Sevenfold Journey: Reclaiming Mind, Body and Spirit Through the Chakras.* Freedom, CA: The Crossing Press, 1993.

Judith, Anodea. *Wheels of Life.* A user's guide to the chakra system. Extensive, comprehensive, and well-written. St. Paul, MN: 1990.

Kilner, W.J. *The Human Aura* new edition retitled: *The Human Atmosphere.* New Hyde Park, NY: University Books, 1965.

Krieger, D. *The Therapeutic Touch.* Englewood Cliffs, NJ: Prentice-Hall, 1979.

Kunz, Dora, and Erik Peper. *Fields and Their Clinical Implications.* *The American Theosophist*, December, 1982.

Leadbeater, Charles W. *The Chakras.* London, England: Theosophical Publishing House, 1974.

Leadbeater, Charles W. *Man Visible and Invisible.* London, England: Theosophical Publishing Society, 1920.

Le Shan, Lawrence. *The Medium, the Mystic, and the Physicist.* New York, NY: Ballantine Books, 1966.

Lowen, Alexander. *The Spirituality of the Body, Bioenergetics for Grace and Harmony.* New York, NY: MacMillan, 1990.

Lowen, Alexander. *Physical Dynamics of Character Structure.* New York, NY: Grune & Stratton, 1958.

Mann, John, and L.T. Short. *The Body of Light, History and Practical Techniques for Awakening Your Subtle Body.* New York, NY: Globe Press Books. 1990.

Motoyama, Hiroshi. ***Theories of the Chakras: Bridge to Higher Consciousness.*** Wheaton, IL: The Theosophical Publishing House, 1988.

Peat, F. David, *"**Subtle Energies: Towards a Process Theory of Healing: Energy, Activity and Global Form.**"* Volume 3,(2): 1-40.

Pierrakos, John C. ***Core Energetics: Developing the Capacity to Love and Heal.*** Mendocino, CA: Life Rhythm Publications, 1989.

Pierrakos, Eva. ***The Pathwork of Self-Transformation.*** New York, NY: Bantam Books, 1990.

Russell, Walter. ***The Secret of Light.*** Waynesboro, VA: University of Science and Philosophy, 1974.

Sannella, Lee. ***The Kundalini Experience.*** Lower Lake, CA: Integral Publishing, 1992.

Schwarz, Jack. ***Human Energy Systems.*** New York, NY: E.P. Dutton, 1980.

Schwarz, Jack. ***Voluntary Controls.*** New York, NY: E.P. Dutton, 1978.

Shapiro, Debbie. ***The Body/mind Workbook: Exploring How the Mind and The Body Work Together.*** UK: Element Books, Ltd., 1990.

Sharamon, Shalila, and Bodo J. Baginski. ***The Chakra Handbook: From Basic Understanding to Practical Application.*** Wilmot, WI: Lotus Light Publications, 1991.

Sui, Choa Kok. ***Pranic Healing.*** York Beach, ME: Samuel Weiser, 1990.

Tansley, David. ***Radionics and the Subtle Anatomy of Man.*** Rustington, Sussex, England: Health Science Press, 1972.

Unity School of Christianity. ***The Light that Shines for You.*** Unity Village, MO: Unity Publishing: 1994.

White, George Starr. ***The Story of the Human Aura.*** Los Angeles, CA: published by author, 1928.

Wood, Betty. ***The Healing Power of Color, How to Use Color to Improve Your Mental, Physical and Spiritual Well-Being.*** Rochester, VT: Destiny Books, 1985.

Yogananda, Paramahansa. ***Let There Be Light.*** Self Realization Fellowship, Los Angeles, CA: Self Realization Fellowship, 1992.

Yogananda, Paramahansa. ***The Great Light of God.*** Audiotape. Los Angeles, CA: Self Realization Fellowship, 1993.

11. THE BUSINESS OF LIGHT
(Professional Legal Considerations)

Jerry A. Green, J.D,. is the author of the following professional articles:

"Medicine and the Scope of Practice Boundaries." *Townsend Letter For Doctors,* February/March 1995 pp. 79-82.

"Compliers, Consenters, Collaborators, and Deciders: Know Your Patient's Decision-Making Preferences." *Medical Malpractice Prevention,* September 1991, pp. 17-19.

"Shared Planning: A New Foundation For Quality Criteria." *Physician Executive,* Volume 15 (3) May/June 1989, pp. 15-19.

"Minimizing Malpractice Risks by Role Clarification: The Confusing Transition from Tort to Contract." *Annals of Internal Medicine,* 109, August 1988, pp. 234-241.

"The Health Care Contract: A Model For Sharing Responsibility." *Somatics,* 3 (4) 1982 pp. 364-374.

"The Health Care Contract: Key to Minimizing Malpractice Risks." *Professional Liability Newsletter,* 3/1982, Insurance Corporation of America.

SECTION X
Index

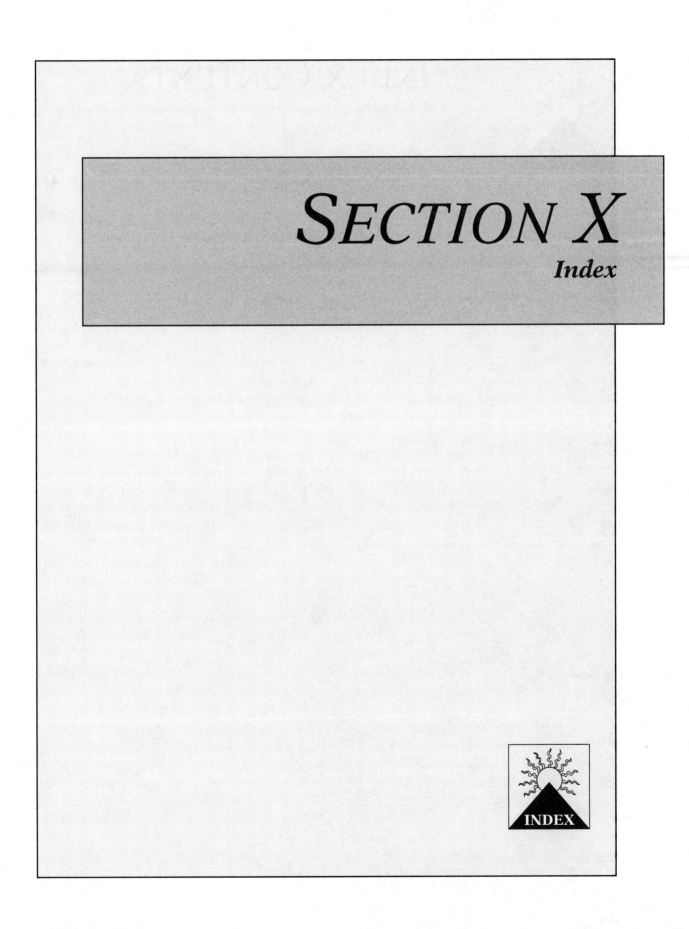

INDEX

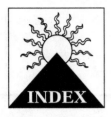

INDEX CONTENTS

LIGHT YEARS AHEAD
INDEX

LIGHT YEARS AHEAD

LIGHT YEARS AHEAD
INDEX OF CHARTS